Updates on Imaging of Common Urogenital Neoplasms

Updates on Imaging of Common Urogenital Neoplasms

Guest Editor
Athina C Tsili

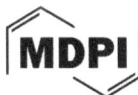

Basel • Beijing • Wuhan • Barcelona • Belgrade • Novi Sad • Cluj • Manchester

Guest Editor
Athina C Tsili
Department of Clinical Radiology
University of Ioannina
Ioannina
Greece

Editorial Office
MDPI AG
Grosspeteranlage 5
4052 Basel, Switzerland

This is a reprint of the Special Issue, published open access by the journal *Cancers* (ISSN 2072-6694), freely accessible at: www.mdpi.com/journal/cancers/special_issues/4VQN8NWIOU.

For citation purposes, cite each article independently as indicated on the article page online and using the guide below:

Lastname, A.A.; Lastname, B.B. Article Title. *Journal Name* **Year**, *Volume Number*, Page Range.

ISBN 978-3-7258-3166-1 (Hbk)
ISBN 978-3-7258-3165-4 (PDF)
https://doi.org/10.3390/books978-3-7258-3165-4

Cover image courtesy of Athina C. Tsili

© 2025 by the authors. Articles in this book are Open Access and distributed under the Creative Commons Attribution (CC BY) license. The book as a whole is distributed by MDPI under the terms and conditions of the Creative Commons Attribution-NonCommercial-NoDerivs (CC BY-NC-ND) license (https://creativecommons.org/licenses/by-nc-nd/4.0/).

Contents

Athina C. Tsili
Updates on Imaging of Common Urogenital Neoplasms
Reprinted from: *Cancers* 2024, *17*, 84, https://doi.org/10.3390/cancers17010084 1

Charis Bourgioti, Marianna Konidari and Lia Angela Moulopoulos
Manifestations of Ovarian Cancer in Relation to Other Pelvic Diseases by MRI
Reprinted from: *Cancers* 2023, *15*, 2106, https://doi.org/10.3390/cancers15072106 9

Antonella Borrelli, Martina Pecoraro, Francesco Del Giudice, Leonardo Cristofani, Emanuele Messina and Ailin Dehghanpour et al.
Standardization of Body Composition Status in Patients with Advanced Urothelial Tumors: The Role of a CT-Based AI-Powered Software for the Assessment of Sarcopenia and Patient Outcome Correlation
Reprinted from: *Cancers* 2023, *15*, 2968, https://doi.org/10.3390/cancers15112968 37

Amreen Shakur, Janice Yu Ji Lee and Sue Freeman
An Update on the Role of MRI in Treatment Stratification of Patients with Cervical Cancer
Reprinted from: *Cancers* 2023, *15*, 5105, https://doi.org/10.3390/cancers15205105 52

Camilla Panico, Silvia Bottazzi, Luca Russo, Giacomo Avesani, Veronica Celli and Luca D'Erme et al.
Prediction of the Risk of Malignancy of Adnexal Masses during Pregnancy Comparing Subjective Assessment and Non-Contrast MRI Score (NCMS) in Radiologists with Different Expertise
Reprinted from: *Cancers* 2023, *15*, 5138, https://doi.org/10.3390/cancers15215138 72

Carlotta Pozza, Marta Tenuta, Franz Sesti, Michele Bertolotto, Dean Y. Huang and Paul S. Sidhu et al.
Multiparametric Ultrasound for Diagnosing Testicular Lesions: Everything You Need to Know in Daily Clinical Practice
Reprinted from: *Cancers* 2023, *15*, 5332, https://doi.org/10.3390/cancers15225332 85

Valentina Miceli, Marco Gennarini, Federica Tomao, Angelica Cupertino, Dario Lombardo and Innocenza Palaia et al.
Imaging of Peritoneal Carcinomatosis in Advanced Ovarian Cancer: CT, MRI, Radiomic Features and Resectability Criteria
Reprinted from: *Cancers* 2023, *15*, 5827, https://doi.org/10.3390/cancers15245827 124

Leonie Van Vynckt, Philippe Tummers, Hannelore Denys, Menekse Göker, Sigi Hendrickx and Eline Naert et al.
Performance of MRI for Detection of ≥pT1b Disease in Local Staging of Endometrial Cancer
Reprinted from: *Cancers* 2024, *16*, 1142, https://doi.org/10.3390/cancers16061142 145

Athina C. Tsili, George Alexiou, Martha Tzoumpa, Timoleon Siempis and Maria I. Argyropoulou
Imaging of Peritoneal Metastases in Ovarian Cancer Using MDCT, MRI, and FDG PET/CT: A Systematic Review and Meta-Analysis
Reprinted from: *Cancers* 2024, *16*, 1467, https://doi.org/10.3390/cancers16081467 158

Marie-France Bellin, Catarina Valente, Omar Bekdache, Florian Maxwell, Cristina Balasa and Alexia Savignac et al.
Update on Renal Cell Carcinoma Diagnosis with Novel Imaging Approaches
Reprinted from: *Cancers* 2024, *16*, 1926, https://doi.org/10.3390/cancers16101926 193

Dean Y. Huang, Majed Alsadiq, Gibran T. Yusuf, Annamaria Deganello, Maria E. Sellars and Paul S. Sidhu
Multiparametric Ultrasound for Focal Testicular Pathology: A Ten-Year Retrospective Review
Reprinted from: *Cancers* **2024**, *16*, 2309, https://doi.org/10.3390/cancers16132309 . . . . **226**

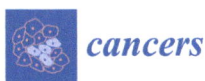

Editorial

Updates on Imaging of Common Urogenital Neoplasms

Athina C. Tsili

Department of Clinical Radiology, Faculty of Medicine, School of Health Sciences, University of Ioannina, 45110 Ioannina, Greece; atsili@uoi.gr

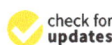

Received: 15 December 2024
Accepted: 24 December 2024
Published: 30 December 2024

Citation: Tsili, A.C. Updates on Imaging of Common Urogenital Neoplasms. *Cancers* **2025**, *17*, 84. https://doi.org/10.3390/cancers17010084

Copyright: © 2024 by the author. Licensee MDPI, Basel, Switzerland. This article is an open access article distributed under the terms and conditions of the Creative Commons Attribution (CC BY) license (https://creativecommons.org/licenses/by/4.0/).

Urogenital neoplasms represent some of the most common malignancies. Advances in imaging have given radiologists an increasingly significant role in the diagnosis, staging, treatment planning, and follow-up of patients with urogenital tumors.

In this Special Issue, the value of current imaging techniques is emphasized, including ultrasonography (US), computed tomography (CT), magnetic resonance imaging (MRI), and fluorodeoxyglucose (FDG)–positron emission tomography (PET)–CT, and the potential applications of novel imaging tools in the work-up of patients with urogenital neoplasms are discussed. This Special Issue contains four original studies and six reviews, which I briefly present in the following paragraphs.

Endometrial cancer is the most common gynecologic neoplasm in the United States and Europe, with incidence rates increasing by about 1–3% per year [1,2]. The updated 2023 FIGO staging system incorporates histological and molecular classifications to better reflect the complex nature and biological behavior of the different types of endometrial cancer, providing a more evidence-based context for treatment planning [3]. Although endometrial cancer is a surgically staged disease, preoperative MRI is recommended as it provides critical diagnostic information on tumor size and depth, the extent of myometrial and cervical invasion, extrauterine extent, and lymph node status, all of which are important in the planning of an appropriate treatment [1,2,4,5].

The important role of preoperative MRI in the local staging of endometrial cancer is validated in the original study of Van Vynckt et al. (contribution 2). The authors found that MRI has a good diagnostic performance for the detection of $\geq$pT1b endometrial cancer (i.e., tumor with an invasion of half or more of the myometrium, invasion of the cervical stroma, or extrauterine spread). The $\geq$pT1b threshold is one of the most important clinical factors in the T-staging of endometrial carcinoma, as it has significant prognostic value and direct implications for planning lymphadenectomy in addition to hysterectomy. In the same study, tumor size was proven to be a predictive factor of $\geq$pT1b disease, irrespective of MRI signs of invasion. Specifically, a tumor diameter measured via an MRI of $\geq$40 mm and a tumor volume of $\geq$20 mL proved highly predictive for the presence of $\geq$pT1b disease. More importantly, an endometrial carcinoma size of at least 5 mm was associated with $\geq$pT1b disease in more than 50% of cases, confirming the value of the size criterion as an independent prognostic factor of endometrial carcinoma and as a guide to determine the most appropriate surgical strategy.

Cervical cancer is the fourth most common carcinoma in women worldwide [6–8]. Despite advances in prevention and treatment, morbidity, and mortality in women with cervical cancer remain high. MRI is the preferred imaging modality in staging cervical cancer and is included into the 2018 FIGO staging system. The primary aim of the FIGO system is to risk stratify patients who are eligible for primary surgery and those who will benefit from chemoradiation. MRI allows for the accurate assessment of tumor size, parametrial and vaginal invasion, lymph node involvement, and urinary bladder and bowel invasion [6–8].

Shakur et al. (contribution 8) highlight MRI findings and pitfalls corresponding to the 2018 FIGO classification of cervical cancer and discuss their implications on treatment selection. This review also comments on the efficacy of MRI in assessing which patients are eligible for fertility-sparing surgery. For women with cervical cancer treated with chemoradiation, the authors present the role of MRI in radiotherapy planning alongside image-guided adaptive brachytherapy, the assessment of treatment response, the detection of tumor recurrence, and treatment complications.

Characterization of an ovarian mass is an important part of pretreatment evaluation. The referral of women with ovarian cancer to a gynecologic oncologist significantly improves survival rate. However, in cases of benign ovarian masses, alternative treatments, such as laparoscopic surgery or surveillance, may be recommended [9–11]. MRI is a highly accurate technique in the detection, localization, and characterization of ovarian masses, mainly used in cases of sonographically indeterminate adnexal mass lesions, allowing for appropriate subspecialty referral and optimal preoperative planning [9–13]. The introduction of the Ovarian-Adnexal Reporting and Data System (O-RADS) for MRI was a significant advancement in the work-up of patients with ovarian masses, standardizing the reporting of ovarian lesions, increasing diagnostic accuracy, and helping in the stratification of malignancy risk [12,13]. In the narrative review by Bourgioti et al. (contribution 9), discriminative MRI features of common and uncommon ovarian and non-ovarian pelvic masses are presented, providing helpful tips for lesion characterization. The authors also describe a stepwise approach to lesion localization, as the first question faced by radiologists when evaluating a suspicious pelvic mass is to suggest its origin, whether ovarian or extraovarian. In the same review, a special emphasis is placed on MRI features of ovarian masses detected in the pediatric population and during pregnancy [14–19].

Panico et al. (contribution 3), in their retrospective study, assessed the diagnostic accuracy of unenhanced MRI in the characterization of ovarian masses with inconclusive US findings in pregnant women. The study used both subjective assessment and a Non-Contrast MRI Score (NCMS) assessed by two radiologists with different expertise in gynecologic imaging. The NCMS is a quantitative tool, introduced in the literature by the same authors for the characterization of adnexal masses detected during pregnancy [20]. Although most adnexal masses seen in pregnancy are benign, malignant tumors are detected in approximately 1–8% of cases [17–19]. MRI represents the preferred imaging modality for the characterization of adnexal tumors in pregnant women, when sonographic findings are indeterminate [17–19]. The use of intravenous gadolinium-based contrast agents in pregnancy should be restricted to cases in which the potential benefits of MRI significantly outweigh the potential risks to the fetus [21,22]. This renders unenhanced MRI an important tool for the characterization of ovarian masses in this population. In the study, NCMS was proven to be a reliable tool in predicting the risk of malignancy in adnexal masses during pregnancy. More importantly, this score was extremely helpful for inexperienced radiologists, and therefore, could be used in centers not specialized in gynecologic imaging.

Peritoneal metastases represent the most common pathway for the spread of primary or recurrent ovarian cancer. Diagnostic work-up with CT, MRI, and/or FDG PET/CT plays a vital role in the accurate evaluation of the extent of peritoneal carcinomatosis in women with ovarian cancer. The accurate mapping of peritoneal metastases is pivotal in planning the appropriate therapeutic strategy, predicting the likelihood of optimal cytoreduction, and identifying potentially unresectable or difficult disease sites that may require surgical technique modifications [23,24].

Based on recently published joint recommendations by the European Society of Gastrointestinal and Abdominal Radiology, the European Society of Urogenital Radiology, the Peritoneal Surface Oncology Group International, and the European Association of Nuclear Medicine, MRI is considered the most accurate imaging technique to assess the extent of peritoneal metastases in ovarian cancer [23]. MRI allows for a better detection of subcentimeter peritoneal metastases and peritoneal carcinomatosis, involving certain anatomic areas, such as the bowel serosal surface, pelvis, right hypochondrium, and mesentery [24–27]. CT has limitations in the assessment of peritoneal carcinomatosis, including poor soft tissue contrast and diminished sensitivity in the detection of small peritoneal metastases and those in certain anatomic locations, including the mesentery and bowel serosa, especially in the absence of ascites [24,25,27]. However, CT is often used for the initial staging of ovarian cancer, treatment response monitoring, and evaluation of the extent of the disease in suspected recurrence, mainly due to its widespread availability [23]. The disadvantages of FDG PET/CT in the evaluation of peritoneal metastases include limited spatial resolution in the detection of small implants; difficulty in the evaluation of diffuse peritoneal disease; the presence of neoplasms with low FDG avidity, such as mucinous tumors; false positives due to inflammation, infection, and/or the normal physiologic activity in the bowel, gallbladder, vessels, ureters, and urinary bladder; limited availability; and high cost [25,27,28]. Therefore, FDG PET/CT is often used as a problem-solving technique in women with ovarian cancer suspected of recurrence, as it can help to detect extraperitoneal metastases that were potentially missed on prior imaging [23].

The superiority of MRI in the detection of peritoneal metastases in ovarian cancer is reported in an up-to-date systematic review and meta-analysis (contribution 10), comparing the diagnostic performance of multidetector CT, MRI (including diffusion-weighted imaging), and FDG PET/CT. Based on the results of this meta-analysis, MRI and FDG PET/CT had higher diagnostic performances in the detection of peritoneal metastases compared to CT on a per patient analysis. On a per lesion basis, sensitivity estimates were similar for all imaging modalities.

Based on a thorough literature search, Miceli et al. (contribution 6) review the diagnostic performance of traditional imaging modalities, including CT, MRI, and PET/CT in the detection of peritoneal carcinomatosis in patients with advanced ovarian cancer. The authors also present classification systems useful in diagnostic evaluation—including the Peritoneal Cancer Index and the Bowel, Upper Abdomen, Mesentery in Peritoneal Metastasis score—and describe diffusion pathways, the most frequent patterns of disease, and anatomic sites that are difficult to evaluate on imaging [24,29]. Comments on evolving imaging tools in the assessment of peritoneal metastases in ovarian cancer are included, such as PET/MRI and radiomics.

Although most intratesticular masses should be considered malignant, a possible diagnosis of benign testicular lesions substantially improves patient care and may decrease the number of unnecessary radical surgical explorations. Conventional US, including grayscale and color Doppler US, represents the imaging modality of choice for the assessment of testicular masses, with high diagnostic accuracy in lesion detection and characterization. However, US does not always allow for a confident characterization of the nature of an intratesticular mass [30,31].

Multiparametric US, including conventional grayscale and color Doppler US, contrast-enhanced US, and elastography, introduced into clinical practice in the last two decades, has greatly improved the diagnostic efficacy of US in the assessment of testicular diseases [32–34]. Pozza et al. (contribution 7) present a detailed roadmap of the multiparametric US features of several common and uncommon benign and malignant testicular lesions that is useful in daily clinical practice. This pictorial review, based on an extensive

Medline search, describes the clinical features, conventional US, contrast-enhanced US, and elastography findings of intratesticular masses that are helpful for lesion characterization.

Huang et al. (contribution 1) confirmed the adjunct role of multiparametric US in the increase in the diagnostic confidence in the characterization of focal intratesticular lesions by incorporating the 10-year experience of a tertiary center. The study includes the largest cohort published up to date.

The absence of contrast enhancement is considered as one of the most sensitive signs for predicting the benign nature of intratesticular masses. Color Doppler US may not depict blood flow in a testicular tumor, especially those with a diameter less than 1.5 cm [32]. Contrast-enhanced US can more reliably distinguish between vascularized and avascular focal testicular lesions, and therefore helping to exclude malignancy [32]. Dean Huang's study reported the presence of vascularity in all malignant testicular tumors on contrast-enhanced US, including cases of malignancies that were detected as "avascular" on color Doppler US. In addition, by using time-intensity curves, the authors showed the efficacy of contrast-enhanced US in the characterization of intratesticular tumors, and particularly in the differentiation between seminomas and benign Leydig cell tumors.

The widespread use of scrotal sonography in recent years has resulted in a rise in the detection of small, impalpable, incidentally found testicular tumors [33,35]. These lesions are often benign, and Leydig cell tumors with low malignant potential represent the most common histologic type. The preoperative characterization of Leydig cell tumors based on imaging findings is important, as conservative treatment may be strongly recommended. The authors found a distinct vascular pattern of prolonged enhancement on contrast-enhanced US, which is highly suggestive of the diagnosis of Leydig cell tumors.

Elastography is recognized as an essential part of the multiparametric US of the scrotum, providing additional information on tissue stiffness, aiming to further improve diagnostic efficacy in the characterization of testicular lesions [34]. Although a significant overlap exists between the elastographic characteristics of testicular mass lesions, Huang showed that the combined use of contrast-enhanced US and elastography had a higher specificity in the differentiation between malignant and benign testicular abnormalities compared to conventional US.

The increased use of cross-sectional imaging over the last few decades has resulted in a rise in the number of incidentally detected renal tumors and an increase in the incidence of renal cell carcinoma. Imaging has a pivotal role in the detection and characterization of renal tumors, as well as in the staging, prognosis, therapeutic management, and follow-up of patients with renal cell carcinoma [36,37].

Innovative imaging techniques have been introduced into clinical practice, aiming to improve the efficacy of conventional imaging in the work-up of renal masses [36–38]. The review by Bellin MF et al. (contribution 5) discusses the most promising, novel imaging approaches in renal cell carcinoma diagnosis, including Dual-Energy CT; Photon-Counting Detector CT; multiparametric MRI; contrast-enhanced US; innovative nuclear medicine techniques, such as sestamibi SPECT/CT and PMSA PET/CT; radiomics; and Artificial Intelligence. The authors also comment on recently proposed or updated imaging algorithms and guidelines used for the diagnosis of renal cell carcinoma, including the Bosniak Classification of Cystic Masses, Version 2019; Clear Cell Likehood Score for the characterization of solid renal tumors, based on multiparametric MRI findings; and the 2017 American Urological Association recommendations, focused on the evaluation and management of clinically localized sporadic renal masses suspicious for renal cell carcinoma in adults and renal mass biopsy.

Sarcopenia, the progressive, generalized skeletal muscle disorder characterized by a reduction in muscle mass and strength, develops as a consequence of the progression of cancer cachexia in oncologic patients. Sarcopenia may be used as an important biomarker in the work-up of patients with urogenital tumors [39–41]. The study by Borrelli et al. (contribution 4) describes an easy-to-use CT-based Artificial Intelligence-powered software assessing sarcopenia in patients with advanced urothelial neoplasms that may be used as a reliable predictor of clinical benefits in terms of tumor response to systemic chemotherapy and oncologic outcomes.

Sarcopenia is often measured by a cross-sectional skeletal muscle area in a single CT slice, more often at the level of the third lumbar vertebra. However, this technique is time-consuming and the measured single-slice area provides only an estimation of the total muscle mass [42]. CT-based Artificial Intelligence models can automate body composition and sarcopenia measurement, helping clinicians to offer a more tailored treatment to patients [43–45].

Artificial Intelligence and radiomics is an emerging field of research that aims to offer significant advancements in the diagnosis, prognosis, and management of urogenital malignancies [46–53]. Radiomics allows for a high throughput extraction of quantitative data from images, capturing the complex tissue microstructure; improving detection and characterization of malignancies, the determination of tumor grades, and metastatic potential; and predicting survival rates and risks of recurrence. Radiomics analysis and its integration with clinical data and other quantitative biologic information, such as genomics and proteomics, are expected to enhance both precision and personalization in medical treatments [46–53].

Funding: This research received no external funding.

Conflicts of Interest: The author declare no conflict of interest.

List of Contributions:

1. Huang, D.Y.; Alsadiq, M.; Yusuf, G.T.; Deganello, A.; Sellars, M.E.; Sidhu P.S. Multiparametric Ultrasound for Focal Testicular Pathology: A Ten-Year Retrospective Review. *Cancers* **2024**, *16*, 2309. https://doi.org/10.3390/cancers16132309.
2. Van Vynckt, L.; Tummers, P.; Denys, H.; Göker, M.; Hendrickx, S.; Naert, E.; Salihi, R.; Van de Vijver, K.; van Ramshorst, G.H.; Van Weehaeghe, D.; et al. Performance of MRI for Detection of ≥pT1b Disease in Local Staging of Endometrial Cancer. *Cancers* **2024**, *16*, 1142. https://doi.org/10.3390/cancers16061142.
3. Panico, C.; Bottazzi, S.; Russo, L.; Avesani, G.; Celli, V.; D'Erme, L.; Cipriani, A.; Mascilini, F.; Fagotti, A.; Scambia, G.; et al. Prediction of the risk of malignancy of adnexal masses during pregnancy comparing subjective assessment and non-contrast MRI score (NCMS) in radiologists with different expertise. *Cancers* **2023**, *15*, 5138. https://doi.org/10.3390/cancers15215138.
4. Borrelli, A.; Pecoraro, M.; Del Giudice, F.; Cristofani, L.; Messina, E.; Dehghanpour, A.; Landini, N.; Roberto, M.; Perotti, S.; Muscaritoli, M.; et al. Standardization of Body Composition Status in Patients with Advanced Urothelial Tumors: The Role of a CT-Based AI-Powered Software for the Assessment of Sarcopenia and Patient Outcome Correlation. *Cancers* **2023**, *15*, 2968. https://doi.org/10.3390/cancers15112968.
5. Bellin, M.F.; Valente, C.; Bekdache, O.; Maxwell, F.; Balasa, C.; Savignac, A.; Meyrignac, O. Update on Renal Cell Carcinoma Diagnosis with Novel Imaging Approaches. *Cancers* **2024**, *16*, 1926. https://doi.org/10.3390/cancers16101926.
6. Miceli, V.; Gennarini, M.; Tomao, F.; Cupertino, A.; Lombardo, D.; Palaia, I.; Curti, F.; Riccardi, S.; Ninkova, R.; Maccioni, F.; et al. Imaging of Peritoneal Carcinomatosis in Advanced Ovarian Cancer: CT, MRI, Radiomic Features and Resectability Criteria. *Cancers* **2023**, *15*, 5827. https://doi.org/10.3390/cancers15245827.
7. Pozza, C.; Tenuta, M.; Sesti, F.; Bertoletto, M.; Huang, D.Y.; Sidhu, P.S.; Maggi, M.; Isidori, A.M.; Lotti, F. Multiparametric Ultrasound for Diagnosing Testicular Lesions: Everything You Need

to Know in Daily Clinical Practice. *Cancers* **2023**, *15*, 5332. https://doi.org/10.3390/cancers15225332.
8. Shakur, A.; Lee, J.Y.J.; Freeman, S. An update on the role of MRI in treatment stratification of patients with cervical cancer. *Cancers* **2023**, *15*, 5105. https://doi.org/10.3390/cancers15205105.
9. Bourgioti, C.; Konidari, M.; Moulopoulos, L.A. Manifestations of Ovarian Cancer in Relation to Other Pelvic Diseases by MRI. *Cancers* **2023**, *15*, 2106. https://doi.org/10.3390/cancers15072106.
10. Tsili, A.C.; Alexiou, G.; Tzoumpa, M.; Siempis, T.; Argyropoulou, M.I. Imaging of Peritoneal Metastases in Ovarian Cancer Using MDCT, MRI, and FDG PET/CT: A Systematic Review and Meta-Analysis. *Cancers* **2024**, *16*, 1467. https://doi.org/10.3390/cancers16081467.

References

1. Sbarra, M.; Lupinelli, M.; Brook, O.R.; Venkatesan, A.M.; Nougaret, S. Imaging of Endometrial Cancer. *Radiol. Clin. N. Am.* **2023**, *61*, 609–625. [CrossRef] [PubMed]
2. Maheshwari, E.; Nougaret, S.; Stein, E.B.; Rauch, G.M.; Hwang, K.P.; Stafford, R.J.; Klopp, A.H.; Soliman, P.T.; Maturen, K.E.; Rockall, A.G.; et al. Update on MRI in Evaluation and Treatment of Endometrial Cancer. *Radiographics* **2022**, *42*, 2112–2130. [CrossRef]
3. Berek, J.S.; Matias-Guiu, X.; Creutzberg, C.; Fotopoulou, C.; Gaffney, D.; Kehoe, S.; Lindemann, K.; Mutch, D.; Concin, N.; Endometrial Cancer Staging Subcommittee; et al. FIGO staging of endometrial cancer: 2023. *Int. J. Gynaecol. Obstet.* **2023**, *162*, 383–394. [CrossRef] [PubMed]
4. Nougaret, S.; Horta, M.; Sala, E.; Lakhman, Y.; Thomassin-Naggara, I.; Kido, A.; Masselli, G.; Bharwani, N.; Sadowski, E.; Ertmer, A.; et al. Endometrial Cancer MRI staging: Updated Guidelines of the European Society of Urogenital Radiology. *Eur. Radiol.* **2019**, *29*, 792–805. [CrossRef] [PubMed]
5. Kido, A.; Himoto, Y.; Kurata, Y.; Minamiguchi, S.; Nakamoto, Y. Preoperative Imaging Evaluation of Endometrial Cancer in FIGO 2023. *J. Magn. Reson. Imaging* **2024**, *60*, 1225–1242. [CrossRef] [PubMed]
6. Chen, J.; Kitzing, Y.X.; Lo, G. Systematic Review-Role of MRI in Cervical Cancer Staging. *Cancers* **2024**, *16*, 1983. [CrossRef] [PubMed]
7. Pak, T.; Sadowski, E.A.; Patel-Lippmann, K. MR Imaging in Cervical Cancer: Initial Staging and Treatment. *Radiol. Clin. N. Am.* **2023**, *61*, 639–649. [CrossRef]
8. Manganaro, L.; Lakhman, Y.; Bharwani, N.; Gui, B.; Gigli, S.; Vinci, V.; Rizzo, S.; Kido, A.; Cunha, T.M.; Sala, E.; et al. Staging, recurrence and follow-up of uterine cervical cancer using MRI: Updated Guidelines of the European Society of Urogenital Radiology after revised FIGO staging 2018. *Eur. Radiol.* **2021**, *31*, 7802–7816. [CrossRef]
9. Fournier, L. The role of MR imaging in ovarian tumor risk stratification. *Diagn. Interv. Imaging* **2024**, *105*, 353–354. [CrossRef] [PubMed]
10. Avesani, G.; Panico, C.; Nougaret, S.; Woitek, R.; Gui, B.; Sala, E. ESR Essentials: Characterization and staging of adnexal masses with MRI and CT-practice recommendations by ESUR. *Eur. Radiol.* **2024**, *34*, 7673–7689. [CrossRef]
11. Jeong, Y.Y.; Outwater, E.K.; Kang, H.K. Imaging evaluation of ovarian masses. *Radiographics* **2000**, *20*, 1445–1470. [CrossRef]
12. Reinhold, C.; Rockall, A.; Sadowski, E.A.; Siegelman, E.S.; Maturen, K.E.; Vargas, H.A.; Forstner, R.; Glanc, P.; Andreotti, R.F.; Thomassin-Naggara, I. Ovarian-Adnexal Reporting Lexicon for MRI: A White Paper of the ACR Ovarian-Adnexal Reporting and Data Systems MRI Committee. *J. Am. Coll. Radiol.* **2021**, *18*, 713–729. [CrossRef]
13. Vara, J.; Manzour, N.; Chacón, E.; López-Picazo, A.; Linares, M.; Pascual, M.A.; Guerriero, S.; Alcázar, J.L. Ovarian Adnexal Reporting Data System (O-RADS) for Classifying Adnexal Masses: A Systematic Review and Meta-Analysis. *Cancers* **2022**, *14*, 3151. [CrossRef] [PubMed]
14. Birbas, E.; Kanavos, T.; Gkrozou, F.; Skentou, C.; Daniilidis, A.; Vatopoulou, A. Ovarian Masses in Children and Adolescents: A Review of the Literature with Emphasis on the Diagnostic Approach. *Children* **2023**, *10*, 1114. [CrossRef]
15. Heo, S.H.; Kim, J.W.; Shin, S.S.; Jeong, S.I.; Lim, H.S.; Choi, Y.D.; Lee, K.H.; Kang, W.D.; Jeong, Y.Y.; Kang, H.K. Review of ovarian tumors in children and adolescents: Radiologic-pathologic correlation. *Radiographics* **2014**, *34*, 2039–2055. [CrossRef]
16. Janssen, C.L.; Littooij, A.S.; Fiocco, M.; Huige, J.C.B.; de Krijger, R.R.; Hulsker, C.C.C.; Goverde, A.J.; Zsiros, J.; Mavinkurve-Groothuis, A.M.C. The diagnostic value of magnetic resonance imaging in differentiating benign and malignant pediatric ovarian tumors. *Pediatr. Radiol.* **2021**, *51*, 427–434. [CrossRef] [PubMed]
17. Kim, J.; Lim, J.; Sohn, J.W.; Lee, S.M.; Lee, M. Diagnostic imaging of adnexal masses in pregnancy. *Obstet. Gynecol. Sci.* **2023**, *66*, 133–148. [CrossRef] [PubMed]
18. Thomassin-Naggara, I.; Fedida, B.; Sadowski, E.; Chevrier, M.C.; Chabbert-Buffet, N.; Ballester, M.; Tavolaro, S.; Darai, E. Complex US adnexal masses during pregnancy: Is pelvic MR imaging accurate for characterization? *Eur. J. Radiol.* **2017**, *93*, 200–208. [CrossRef]

19. Causa Andrieu, P.I.; Wahab, S.A.; Nougaret, S.; Petkovska, I. Ovarian cancer during pregnancy. *Abdom. Radiol.* **2023**, *48*, 1694–1708. [CrossRef] [PubMed]
20. Sahin, H.; Panico, C.; Ursprung, S.; Simeon, V.; Chiodini, P.; Frary, A.; Carmo, B.; Smith, S.; Freeman, S.; Jimenez-Linan, M.; et al. Non-contrast MRI can accurately characterize adnexal masses: A retrospective study. *Eur. Radiol.* **2021**, *31*, 6962–6973. [CrossRef]
21. Webb, J.A.W.; Thomsen, H.S.; Morcos, S.K. Members of Contrast Media Safety Committee of European Society of Urogenital Radiology (ESUR). The use of iodinated and gadolinium contrast media during pregnancy and lactation. *Eur. Radiol.* **2005**, *15*, 1234–1240. [CrossRef]
22. Puac, P.; Rodríguez, A.; Vallejo, C.; Zamora, C.A.; Castillo, M. Safety of Contrast Material Use During Pregnancy and Lactation. *Magn. Reson. Imaging Clin. N. Am.* **2017**, *25*, 787–797. [CrossRef] [PubMed]
23. Vandecaveye, V.; Rousset, P.; Nougaret, S.; Stepanyan, A.; Otero-Garcia, M.; Nikolić, O.; Hameed, M.; Goffin, K.; de Hingh, I.H.J.; Lahaye, M.J.; et al. Imaging of peritoneal metastases of ovarian and colorectal cancer: Joint recommendations of ESGAR, ESUR, PSOGI, and EANM. *Eur. Radiol.* **2024**, *online ahead of print*. [CrossRef] [PubMed]
24. Nougaret, S.; Addley, H.C.; Colombo, P.E.; Fujii, S.; Al Sharif, S.S.; Tirumani, S.H.; Jardon, K.; Sala, E.; Reinhold, C. Ovarian carcinomatosis: How the radiologist can help plan the surgical approach. *Radiographics* **2012**, *32*, 1775–1800. [CrossRef]
25. An, H.; Lee, E.Y.P.; Chiu, K.; Chang, C. The emerging roles of functional imaging in ovarian cancer with peritoneal carcinomatosis. *Clin. Radiol.* **2018**, *73*, 597–609. [CrossRef] [PubMed]
26. Gagliardi, T.; Adejolu, M.; DeSouza, N.M. Diffusion-Weighted Magnetic Resonance Imaging in Ovarian Cancer: Exploiting Strengths and Understanding Limitations. *J. Clin. Med.* **2022**, *11*, 1524. [CrossRef]
27. Expert Panel on Women's Imaging; Kang, S.K.; Reinhold, C.; Atri, M.; Benson, C.B.; Bhosale, P.R.; Jhingran, A.; Lakhman, Y.; Maturen, K.E.; Nicola, R.; et al. ACR Appropriateness Criteria® Staging and Follow-Up of Ovarian Cancer. *J. Am. Coll. Radiol.* **2018**, *15*, S198–S207.
28. Lee, E.Y.P.; An, H.; Tse, K.Y.; Khong, P.L. Molecular Imaging of Peritoneal Carcinomatosis in Ovarian Carcinoma. *AJR Am. J. Roentgenol.* **2020**, *215*, 305–312. [CrossRef]
29. Nougaret, S.; Sadowski, E.; Lakhman, Y.; Rousset, P.; Lahaye, M.; Worley, M.; Sgarbura, O.; Shinagare, A.B. The BUMPy road of peritoneal metastases in ovarian cancer. *Diagn. Interv. Imaging* **2022**, *103*, 448–459. [CrossRef]
30. Dogra, V.S.; Gottlieb, R.H.; Oka, M.; Rubens, D.J. Sonography of the scrotum. *Radiology* **2003**, *227*, 18–36. [CrossRef]
31. Belfield, J.; Findlay-Line, C. Testicular Germ Cell Tumours-The Role of Conventional Ultrasound. *Cancers* **2022**, *14*, 3882. [CrossRef] [PubMed]
32. Sidhu, P.S.; Cantisani, V.; Dietrich, C.F.; Gilja, O.H.; Saftoiu, A.; Bartels, E.; Bertolotto, M.; Calliada, F.; Clevert, D.A.; Cosgrove, D.; et al. The EFSUMB Guidelines and Recommendations for the Clinical Practice of Contrast-Enhanced Ultrasound (CEUS) in Non-Hepatic Applications: Update 2017 (Long Version). *Ultraschall Med.* **2018**, *39*, e2–e44.
33. Maxwell, F.; Savignac, A.; Bekdache, O.; Calvez, S.; Lebacle, C.; Arama, E.; Garrouche, N.; Rocher, L. Leydig Cell Tumors of the Testis: An Update of the Imaging Characteristics of a Not So Rare Lesion. *Cancers* **2022**, *14*, 3652. [CrossRef] [PubMed]
34. Cantisani, V.; Di Leo, N.; Bertolotto, M.; Fresilli, D.; Granata, A.; Polti, G.; Polito, E.; Pacini, P.; Guiban, O.; Del Gaudio, G.; et al. Role of multiparametric ultrasound in testicular focal lesions and diffuse pathology evaluation, with particular regard to elastography: Review of literature. *Andrology* **2021**, *9*, 1356–1368. [CrossRef] [PubMed]
35. Rocher, L.; Ramchandani, P.; Belfield, J.; Bertolotto, M.; Derchi, L.E.; Correas, J.M.; Oyen, R.; Tsili, A.C.; Turgut, A.T.; Dogra, V.; et al. Incidentally detected non-palpable testicular tumours in adults at scrotal ultrasound: Impact of radiological findings on management Radiologic review and recommendations of the ESUR scrotal imaging subcommittee. *Eur. Radiol.* **2016**, *26*, 2268–2278. [CrossRef] [PubMed]
36. Abou Elkassem, A.M.; Lo, S.S.; Gunn, A.J.; Shuch, B.M.; Dewitt-Foy, M.E.; Abouassaly, R.; Vaidya, S.S.; Clark, J.I.; Louie, A.V.; Siva, S.; et al. Role of Imaging in Renal Cell Carcinoma: A Multidisciplinary Perspective. *Radiographics* **2021**, *41*, 1387–1407. [CrossRef]
37. Chung, A.; Raman, S.S. Radiologist's Disease: Imaging for Renal Cancer. *Urol. Clin. N. Am.* **2023**, *50*, 161–180. [CrossRef] [PubMed]
38. Schawkat, K.; Krajewski, K.M. Insights into renal cell carcinoma with novel imaging approaches. *Hematol. Oncol. Clin. N. Am.* **2023**, *37*, 863–875. [CrossRef] [PubMed]
39. Fukushima, H.; Koga, F. Impact of sarcopenia in the management of urological cancer patients. *Expert Rev. Anticancer Ther.* **2017**, *17*, 455–466. [CrossRef] [PubMed]
40. Fukushima, H.; Yokoyama, M.; Nakanishi, Y.; Tobisu, K.; Koga, F. Sarcopenia as a prognostic biomarker of advanced urothelial carcinoma. *PLoS ONE* **2015**, *10*, e0115895. [CrossRef] [PubMed]
41. Pickl, C.; Engelmann, S.; Girtner, F.; Gužvić, M.; van Rhijn, B.W.G.; Hartmann, V.; Holbach, S.; Kälble, S.; Haas, M.; Rosenhammer, B.; et al. Body Composition as a Comorbidity-Independent Predictor of Survival following Nephroureterectomy for Urothelial Cancer of the Upper Urinary Tract. *Cancers* **2023**, *15*, 450. [CrossRef] [PubMed]

42. Mourtzakis, M.; Prado, C.M.; Lieffers, J.R.; Reiman, T.; McCargar, L.J.; Baracos, V.E. A practical and precise approach to quantification of body composition in cancer patients using computed tomography images acquired during routine care. *Appl. Physiol. Nutr. Metab.* **2008**, *33*, 997–1006. [CrossRef] [PubMed]
43. Bedrikovetski, S.; Seow, W.; Kroon, H.M.; Traeger, L.; Moore, J.W.; Sammour, T.; Seow, W.; Kroon, H.M.; Traeger, L.; Moore, J.W.; et al. Artificial intelligence for body composition and sarcopenia evaluation on computed tomography: A systematic review and meta-analysis. *Eur. J. Radiol.* **2022**, *149*, 110218. [CrossRef]
44. Roblot, V.; Giret, Y.; Mezghani, S.; Auclin, E.; Arnoux, A.; Oudard, S.; Duron, L.; Fournier, L. Validation of a deep learning segmentation algorithm to quantify the skeletal muscle index and sarcopenia in metastatic renal carcinoma. *Eur. Radiol.* **2022**, *32*, 4728–4737. [CrossRef]
45. Ying, T.; Borrelli, P.; Edenbrandt, L.; Enqvist, O.; Kaboteh, R.; Trägårdh, E.; Ulén, J.; Kjölhede, H. Automated artificial intelligence-based analysis of skeletal muscle volume predicts overall survival after cystectomy for urinary bladder cancer. *Eur. Radiol. Exp.* **2021**, *5*, 50. [CrossRef] [PubMed]
46. Gelikman, D.G.; Rais-Bahrami, S.; Pinto, P.A.; Turkbey, B. AI-powered radiomics: Revolutionizing detection of urologic malignancies. *Curr. Opin. Urol.* **2024**, *34*, 1–7. [CrossRef]
47. Thomas, R.; Qin, L.; Alessandrino, F.; Sahu, S.P.; Guerra, P.J.; Krajewski, K.M.; Shinagare, A.M. A review of the principles of texture analysis and its role in imaging of genitourinary neoplasms. *Abdom. Radiol.* **2019**, *44*, 2501–2510. [CrossRef] [PubMed]
48. Manganaro, L.; Nicolino, G.M.; Dolciami, M.; Martorana, F.; Stathis, A.; Colombo, I.; Rizzo, S. Radiomics in cervical and endometrial cancer. *Br. J. Radiol.* **2021**, *94*, 20201314. [CrossRef]
49. Lefebvre, T.L.; Ueno, Y.; Dohan, A.; Chatterjee, A.; Vallières, M.; Winter-Reinhold, E.; Saif, S.; Levesque, I.R.; Zeng, X.Z.; Forghani, R.; et al. Development and Validation of Multiparametric MRI-based Radiomics Models for Preoperative Risk Stratification of Endometrial Cancer. *Radiology* **2022**, *305*, 375–386. [CrossRef]
50. Nougaret, S.; Tardieu, M.; Vargas, H.A.; Reinhold, C.; Vande Perre, S.; Bonanno, N.; Sala, E.; Thomassin-Naggara, I. Ovarian cancer: An update on imaging in the era of radiomics. *Diagn. Interv. Imaging* **2019**, *100*, 647–655. [CrossRef]
51. Panico, C.; Avesani, G.; Zormpas-Petridis, K.; Rundo, L.; Nero, C.; Sala, E. Radiomics and Radiogenomics of Ovarian Cancer: Implications for Treatment Monitoring and Clinical Management. *Radiol. Clin. N. Am.* **2023**, *61*, 749–760. [CrossRef] [PubMed]
52. Raman, A.G.; Fisher, D.; Yap, F.; Oberai, A.; Duddalwar, V.A. Radiomics and Artificial Intelligence: Renal Cell Carcinoma. *Urol. Clin. N. Am.* **2024**, *51*, 35–45. [CrossRef] [PubMed]
53. Lubner, M.G. Radiomics and Artificial Intelligence for Renal Mass Characterization. *Radiol. Clin. N. Am.* **2020**, *58*, 995–1008. [CrossRef] [PubMed]

Disclaimer/Publisher's Note: The statements, opinions and data contained in all publications are solely those of the individual author(s) and contributor(s) and not of MDPI and/or the editor(s). MDPI and/or the editor(s) disclaim responsibility for any injury to people or property resulting from any ideas, methods, instructions or products referred to in the content.

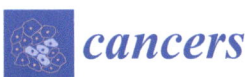

Review

Manifestations of Ovarian Cancer in Relation to Other Pelvic Diseases by MRI

Charis Bourgioti *, Marianna Konidari and Lia Angela Moulopoulos

Department of Radiology, School of Medicine, National and Kapodistrian University of Athens, Aretaieion Hospital, 76 Vas. Sofias Ave., 11528 Athens, Greece
* Correspondence: chbourg@med.uoa.gr

Simple Summary: Characterization of an adnexal mass may be challenging since there are several benign and malignant pelvic conditions with similar appearances on imaging. The aim of this study is to comprehensively review discriminative MRI features of common and uncommon adnexal masses in order to help radiologists more accurately diagnose ovarian cancer. Imaging findings of ovarian tumors in specific settings, including adolescence and pregnancy, are also discussed.

Abstract: Imaging plays a pivotal role in the diagnostic approach of women with suspected ovarian cancer. MRI is widely used for preoperative characterization and risk stratification of adnexal masses. While epithelial ovarian cancer (EOC) has typical findings on MRI; there are several benign and malignant pelvic conditions that may mimic its appearance on imaging. Knowledge of the origin and imaging characteristics of a pelvic mass will help radiologists diagnose ovarian cancer promptly and accurately. Finally, in special subgroups, including adolescents and gravid population, the prevalence of various ovarian tumors differs from that of the general population and there are conditions which uniquely manifest during these periods of life.

Keywords: ovarian cancer; malignancy; benign tumors; mimickers; MR

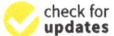

Citation: Bourgioti, C.; Konidari, M.; Moulopoulos, L.A. Manifestations of Ovarian Cancer in Relation to Other Pelvic Diseases by MRI. *Cancers* **2023**, *15*, 2106. https://doi.org/10.3390/cancers15072106

Academic Editor: Edward J. Pavlik

Received: 12 February 2023
Revised: 29 March 2023
Accepted: 30 March 2023
Published: 31 March 2023

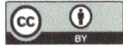

Copyright: © 2023 by the authors. Licensee MDPI, Basel, Switzerland. This article is an open access article distributed under the terms and conditions of the Creative Commons Attribution (CC BY) license (https:// creativecommons.org/licenses/by/ 4.0/).

1. Introduction

1.1. Data Search

Literature search for this narrative review was conducted using MEDLINE (PubMed) Library. Applied key words included the following terms: ovarian neoplasms; ovarian masses; ovarian malignancy; probability of malignancy; ovarian benign tumors; ovarian tumor mimickers; MRI. The search period extended from July 1997 to November 2022. Studies with prospectively and retrospectively collected data and review articles including systematic meta-analyses were considered. All authors agreed on the following inclusion criteria: acceptable methodology, adequate data collection, use of clear diagnostic evidence, sufficient statistical analysis, and reproducibility of results. A total of 122 studies was considered eligible and included in this review.

1.2. Epidemiology

The ovary is made of a variety of different cell types and is, therefore, the site of diverse tumors. Ovarian neoplasms are divided into four main categories depending on the cell of origin: epithelial, germ cell, sex cord–stromal tumors, and metastases. Epithelial neoplasms account for the majority of primary ovarian tumors, followed by germ cell tumors [1]. Most of these tumors are benign or borderline, however, malignant epithelial neoplasms are a serious public health issue since they often manifest as advanced stage disease. Ovarian cancer is the second most frequent gynecologic malignancy. With a total of 313,959 new cases recorded globally in 2020, an age-standardized incidence rate of 6.6/100,000 and an age-standardized mortality rate of 4.2/100,000 women/year, ovarian cancer is the fifth leading cause of cancer death in women [2]. Most ovarian cancer deaths are caused by epithelial cell carcinomas, specifically high-grade serous cystadenocarcinoma, which is the most common subtype and accounts for approximately 64% of all epithelial ovarian cancers.

Pitfalls and Diagnostic Challenges

Imaging plays a significant role in the diagnostic approach of women with suspected ovarian cancer. The two main challenges faced by radiologists when assessing a suspicious pelvic mass include (a) confirming its origin (ovarian or extraovarian) and (b) characterizing its nature (benign or malignant and, if possible, the most likely diagnosis). Both these are important for narrowing the differential diagnosis and helping decision making (Figure 1). All imaging modalities including Ultrasound (US), Magnetic Resonance Imaging (MRI), and Computed Tomography (CT) can be used to assess pelvic masses, each having different advantages and offering complementary information.

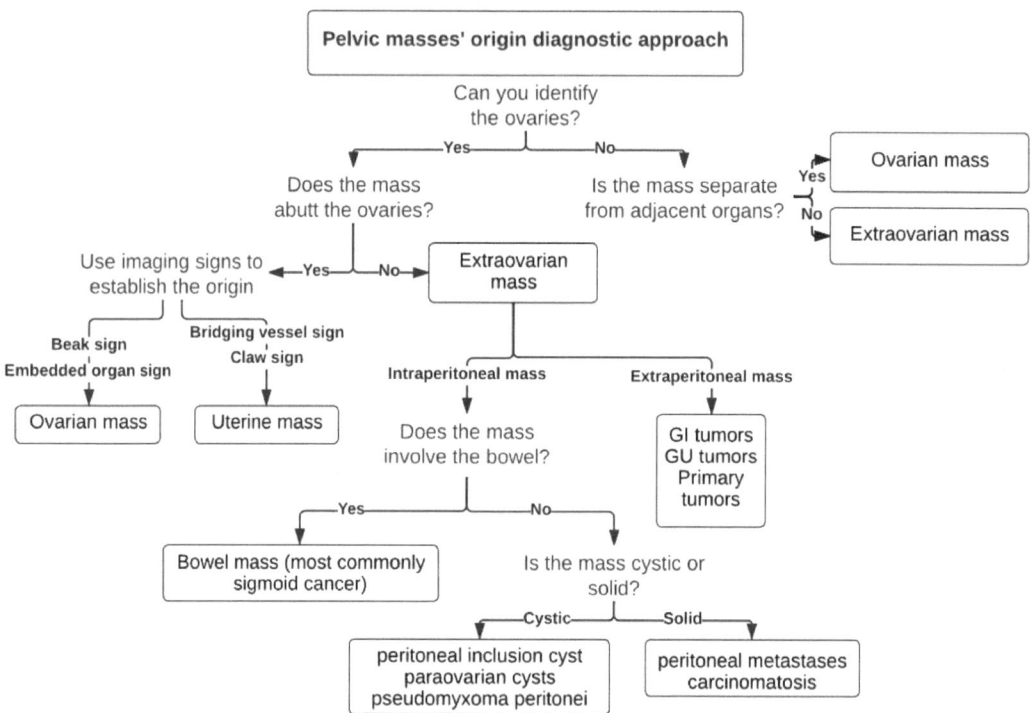

Figure 1. Imaging approach of pelvic masses' origin.

Pelvic US is the modality of choice for the initial evaluation of an adnexal mass and, in most cases, can accurately characterize the ovarian lesion as benign or malignant. However, a varying range of ovarian lesions (5–40%), depending on the experience of the sonographer, may remain indeterminate after initial evaluation [3–7].

1.3. Origin and Characterization of a Pelvic Mass

To establish an ovarian origin of a pelvic mass, the following stepwise approach may be used:

- Identify the ovaries.

An oblique coronal T2-weighted sequence parallel to the endometrium, is particularly useful in determining ovarian versus extraovarian origin of a pelvic mass. If a normal ipsilateral ovary is identified, the mass cannot be of ovarian origin. Note that when finding the ovary on MR images is difficult, e.g., in postmenopausal women, you may follow the gonadal vessels anterior to the psoas muscle and all the way to the ovary [8]. This is facilitated on contrast-enhanced images of the pelvis. When a normal ovary cannot be identified (e.g., in large pelvic masses), but the mass appears separate from other pelvic organs (bladder, bowel, or uterus) and the gonadal vessels run into it, then an ovarian origin is highly likely [9]. However, advanced ovarian cancer is often seen to invade adjacent pelvic structures, in which case establishing the primary site can still be difficult.

- Describe relationship to the ovary.

Mass abutting the ovary: If a mass abuts the ovary, this does not necessarily indicate an ovarian origin, since it can as well originate from adjacent pelvic structures. Several previously described imaging signs are useful for determining the ovarian origin of a pelvic mass, such as the presence of the beak sign, created by the ovarian tissue partly enveloping the mass and forming sharp angles with it and the embedded sign, when the ovary appears to be engulfed by the tumor [10]. However, the bridging vessel sign as well as the claw sign are indicative of uterine origin. The bridging vessel sign is present when vessels extend between the uterus and the mass, while the claw sign is present when uterine tissue is draped around the mass; both signs are commonly seen in cases of uterine leiomyomas [11].

Ovary not involved: If the ovary is not involved but the mass is intraperitoneal, one should consider the bowel as the site of origin, particularly the sigmoid colon. If the mass is intraperitoneal but separate from the ovary or bowel, it is important to determine its nature. Cystic masses may be of benign nature, such as peritoneal inclusion and para-ovarian cysts or they may be malignant, such as pseudomyxoma peritonei. Solid masses more commonly include peritoneal metastases or carcinomatosis. Extraperitoneal masses most often result from direct extension of gastrointestinal (rectal) or genitourinary (bladder, uterine, cervical) tumors. However, primary tumors, mainly of mesenchymal or neurogenic origin, can also occur in the extraperitoneal spaces.

Characterization of an ovarian mass is based on a combination of clinical information (i.e., age, elevated levels of tumor markers etc.) and imaging findings.

MRI is a problem-solving tool for preoperative characterization and subsequent risk stratification of indeterminate adnexal masses [12–15]. MRI provides better contrast resolution between different soft-tissue components (e.g., fat, hemorrhage, fibrous tissue) without the use of ionizing radiation [16]. The Ovarian-Adnexal Reporting and Data System (O-RADS) MRI is a recently developed and validated scoring system which is now proposed for risk assignment of sonographically indeterminate adnexal masses. This MRI scoring system includes six categories with different risks of malignancy and it is based on MRI features with high positive and high negative predictive values in distinguishing benign from malignant masses [17] (Figure 2).

Computed Tomography (CT) is recommended for ovarian cancer staging as it provides excellent spatial resolution and very short examination times [18]; however, it does not assist the characterization of an adnexal mass apart from identifying fat and calcifications (mostly in cases of teratomas).

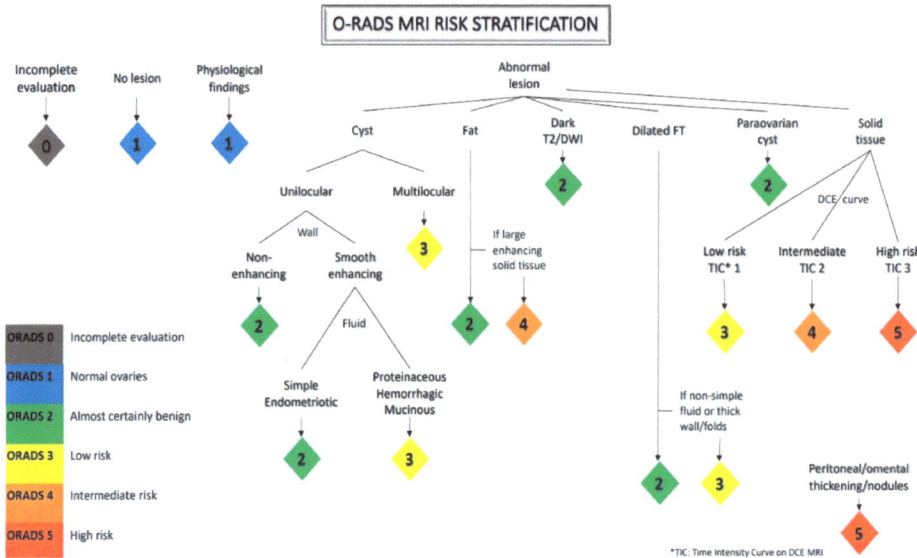

Figure 2. Ovarian-adnexal reporting and data MRI risk stratification system.

1.4. Importance of Accurate Diagnosis in Treatment Decisions

Accurate differential diagnosis of pelvic masses based on imaging is crucial since it largely affects the clinical management and treatment decisions.

Establishing the site of origin and providing the most likely diagnosis of a pelvic mass can help determine whether the patient should be referred to a gynecologist (benign lesions), gynecologic oncologist (malignancy), or other specialist (suspected metastases to the ovary or non-gynecologic tumor), and which is the best treatment option.

Regarding management of ovarian neoplasms, benign ovarian tumors may be followed-up or treated with conservative surgery. Malignant epithelial ovarian neoplasms are most often present at an advanced stage with peritoneal dissemination. Cytoreductive surgery followed by adjuvant chemotherapy is the treatment of choice. Primary neoadjuvant chemotherapy may be applied in cases of extensive peritoneal disease, followed by interval debulking surgery [19]. Fertility-sparing surgery (i.e., unilateral salpingo-oophorectomy (USO) with preservation of the uterus and contralateral ovary), may be an option in cases of malignant germ cell tumors of any stage, sex-cord stromal and borderline histology, or even early-stage epithelial carcinomas [20,21].

In general, the clinical management is mainly influenced by the tumor's nature (benign or malignant), histologic subtype and stage, since these are the main prognostic factors [22]. Imaging can provide useful information for all the above. The established US and MRI scoring systems are helpful tools in stratifying the risk of malignancy and discriminating between benign and malignant tumors. Several US-based models have been employed to differentiate benign from malignant adnexal masses, such as the IOTA group Simple Rules or ADNEX model, the Gynecologic Imaging Reporting and Data System (GI-RADS) and more recently the O-RADS US risk stratification and management system by the ACR Ovarian-Adnexal Reporting and Data System Committee [23–26]. Regarding different histologic subtypes, although some of them have distinguishing imaging features, findings are often overlapping and nonspecific. Even though final diagnosis requires histopathologic analysis, specific features and typical imaging findings of ovarian neoplasms may limit the differential diagnosis. Finally, accurate staging of ovarian cancer is vital, given the fact that the extent of disease as well as residual disease after surgery affect prognosis and survival. CT and DWI MRI both have high sensitivity in depicting peritoneal disease and can provide valuable information to clinicians for selecting the best treatment option [27].

1.5. Special Subgroups

1.5.1. Adolescence

Ovarian tumors in children and adolescents differ from those in adults, regarding incidence, histology, and presentation. In general, ovarian neoplasms in childhood are uncommon and usually benign, with germ cell tumors (GCTs) being the most common type, followed by epithelial and stromal cell tumors [28]. In many cases, they present with abnormal hormonal secretion, unusual sexual development, and increased serum tumor markers (i.e., AFP in immature teratoma and yolk sac tumor, β-hCG in dysgerminoma, CA-125 in epithelial neoplasms). Imaging can help discriminate between benign and malignant ovarian neoplasms since malignant masses usually appear predominantly solid, more heterogeneous, and larger than benign tumors. In a recent study MRI showed 100% specificity and sensitivity in differentiating benign and malignant pediatric ovarian tumors [29].

1.5.2. Pregnancy

Adnexal masses are common during pregnancy, discovered in 0.1 to 2.4% of pregnant women. Most adnexal lesions in the gravid population are benign, mostly functional, with only 1–5% being malignant [30,31]. Germ cell tumors, sex cord (stromal) tumors, and borderline tumors are the most common malignant ovarian neoplasms in the gravid population [32], whereas epithelial ovarian cancer accounts for only 35% of ovarian cancers in pregnancy [33].

Evaluation of adnexal masses in the gravid population is challenging because they may undergo morphologic changes due to the altered hormonal status and may demonstrate features that can mimic malignancy on imaging. The most common pregnancy-related adnexal masses are the corpus luteum of pregnancy and the theca lutein cyst; both are expected to resolve after gestational week 18, although a few may persist until after delivery [34]. Other conditions that can mimic malignancy at imaging are decidualized endometriomas and leiomyomas with red degeneration. Decidualized endometriomas are the result of progesterone action and increased glandular endometrial secretion and are characterized by increased blood flow and intraluminal papillary projections [35]. Red degeneration is a subtype of hemorrhagic infarction of leiomyomas that often occurs during pregnancy due to venous thrombosis within the periphery of the mass or rupture of intra-tumoral arteries [36].

2. Typical and Atypical Findings of Ovarian Cancer and Mimickers on MRI

2.1. Borderline and Malignant Neoplasms

Imaging findings indicative of borderline or malignant tumors include mural nodules, papillary projections, enhancing solid tissue (except those of fatty or fibrous nature), thickened, irregular walls or septa (i.e., diameter > 3 mm and highly vascular), and necrosis. Large size and the involvement of lymph nodes or peritoneal dissemination may suggest a borderline or malignant tumor [37].

The epithelial subtype accounts for most borderline and malignant ovarian neoplasms. According to the 2014 WHO classification, epithelial ovarian neoplasms include serous, mucinous, endometrioid, clear cell, seromucinous, Brenner, and undifferentiated tumors [1]. Serous malignant tumors can be further classified into low- and high-grade tumors.

2.1.1. High-Grade Serous Cystadenocarcinoma (HGSC)

HGSC is the most common histological type of ovarian malignancy accounting for almost half of ovarian cancer cases [2]. It usually affects postmenopausal women (mean age: 60 years), and most often presents at an advanced stage. Serum CA-125 levels are elevated in up to 90% of patients with HGSC [38].

HGSC usually manifests as bilateral (58% of cases), predominantly cystic masses with differing amounts of solid tissue. A few of such tumors are entirely solid. The solid component often demonstrates restricted diffusion and intense enhancement on dynamic contrast enhanced images with type 3 Time Intensity Curve (TIC) (i.e., initial slope greater than myometrium and marked increase in signal intensity with a plateau or washout) [17,39]. It usually presents with extraovarian disease at diagnosis, including peritoneal dissemination, pelvic organ invasion, ascites, and lymphadenopathy [40] (Figure 3).

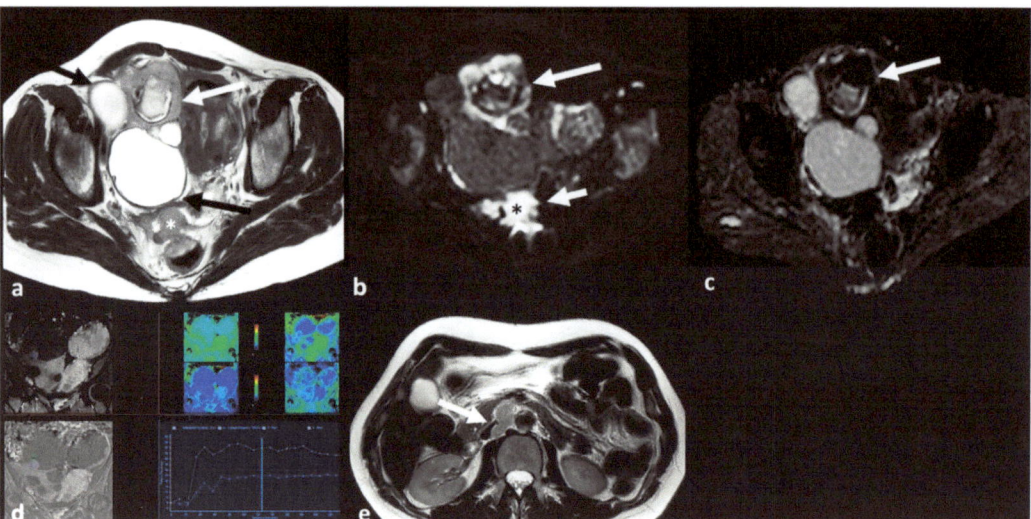

Figure 3. High grade serous cystadenocarcinoma with peritoneal and lymph node metastases. Axial T2 weighted image (**a**) shows a multiloculated right ovarian cystic mass (black arrows) with a large solid component (white arrow). The solid portion (white arrow) demonstrates high signal on axial 1200 b value DWI (**b**) and low signal on ADC map (**c**). DCE image analysis (**d**) demonstrates an intermediate-risk time intensity curve of the solid tissue (TIC type 2, orange line: myometrium, blue line: solid tissue). Axial T2 weighted image of the upper abdomen of the same patient (**e**) shows right paraaortic lymphadenopathy (white arrow). Shown also is a large peritoneal implant in the pelvis (asterisk in (**a**); asterisk and short arrow in (**b**)).

2.1.2. Serous Borderline Neoplasms and Low-Grade Serous Cystadenocarcinoma

The most often diagnosed borderline tumor is a serous borderline neoplasm (65–70%). It is most common in young women (mean age: 42 years) compared to their high-grade counterparts and has excellent overall prognosis [41].

Low-grade serous cystadenocarcinoma (LGSC) is uncommon, accounting for only 2.5% of ovarian malignancies. Interestingly, it can arise from and co-exist with a non-invasive serous borderline component. Compared to borderline neoplasms, women with LGSC often present at a later stage and have a poorer prognosis since LGSC is platinum-resistant [42] (Figure 4).

Tumors of borderline and low-grade serous histology, manifest as multilocular cystic masses, with solid tissue in the form of papillary projections or mural nodules and rarely, surface nodules. The solid elements enhance after intravenous contrast administration, usually with type 2 TIC on DCE images (i.e., initial slope less than myometrium, moderate increase in signal intensity with a plateau or washout). Compared to their mucinous counterparts, borderline and low-grade serous neoplasms are more often bilateral (around one-third of serous borderline tumors and the majority of LGSC) with an increased number of papillary projections [43] (Figure 5).

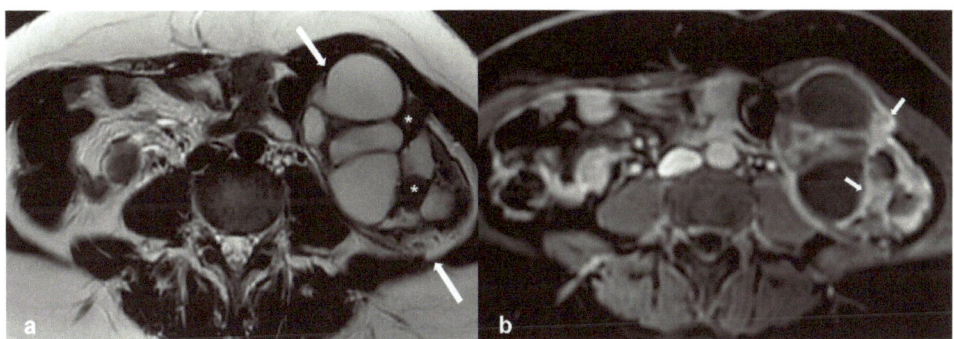

Figure 4. Low grade serous cystadenocarcinoma. Axial T2 weighted image (**a**) shows a multiloculated, predominantly cystic mass at the left ovary (white arrows) with solid tissue (asterisks) showing avid enhancement on the T1 weighted FS CE image ((**b**), white arrows).

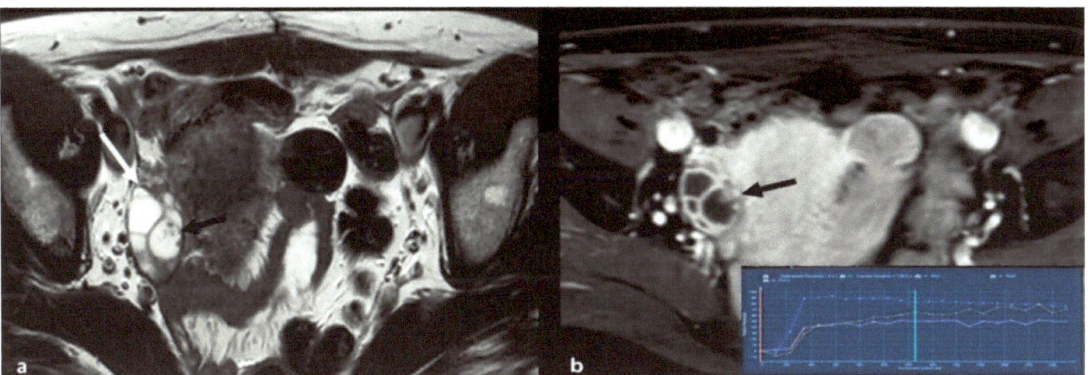

Figure 5. Serous epithelial borderline ovarian tumor. Axial T2 weighted image (**a**) shows a multiloculated cystic lesion at the right ovary (white arrow). A small, papillary projection (black arrow) is present, with avid enhancement on the T1 weighted FS CE image ((**b**), black arrow). An intermediate-risk time intensity curve (TIC type 2) was detected on DCE image analysis (inset in b, blue line: myometrium, orange/pink lines: papillary projection).

Tip: Epithelial tumors of low malignant potential exhibit an increased number of papillary projections. Although these can also be found in invasive carcinomas, the latter usually have a dominant solid component. According to a previously published study with CT and MRI, papillary projections were detected more frequently in ovarian tumors of low malignant potential (67%) followed by malignant (38%) and benign (13%) neoplasms [44].

2.1.3. Mucinous Borderline Neoplasms and Mucinous Cystadenocarcinoma

Tumors of mucinous histology account for 10–15% of all ovarian neoplasms; malignant mucinous tumors are quite rare [45]. In general, mucinous borderline neoplasms involve younger women than their serous counterparts and they are associated with an excellent outcome [41]. Conversely, mucinous adenocarcinoma, which accounts for 9.4% of all invasive epithelial tumors, has the poorest prognosis of all ovarian malignancies, with low survival rates [46].

Mucinous neoplasms are usually unilateral, confined to the ovary, and larger when diagnosed compared with serous tumors. At imaging, they appear as multilocular, predominantly cystic masses. The signal intensity of the locules may vary on MRI, because of different mucin content, the so-called stained-glass appearance [45] (Figure 6).

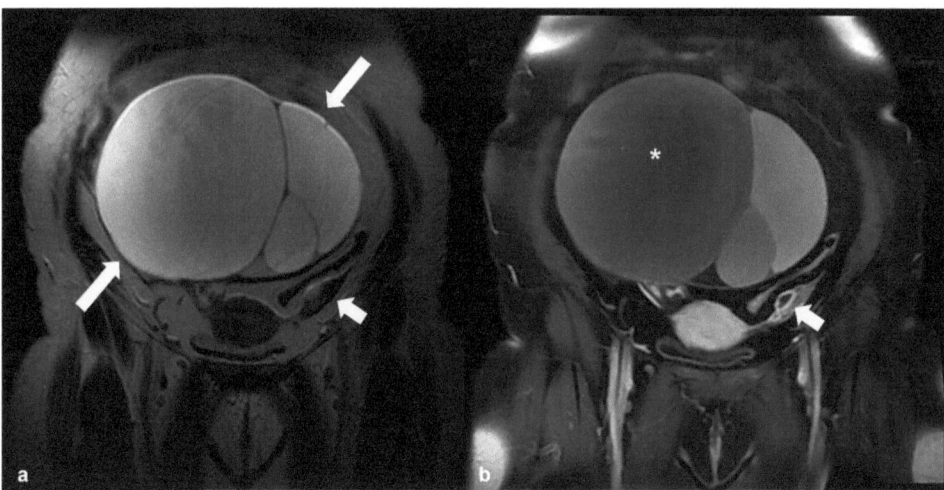

Figure 6. Mucinous cystadenoma. T2 weighted image (**a**) in the coronal plane, shows a large multilocular cystic mass originating from the right ovary (arrows). Corresponding T1 CE FS image (**b**) shows different signal intensity of various compartments (asterisk), the so-called 'stained-glass' appearance. Shown also is the normal left ovary (short arrow in (**a**,**b**)).

Papillary solid elements, described in serous neoplasms, are not a common finding [44]. Intramural (often linear) calcifications are present in about one-third of cases [47]. Discrimination between benign and borderline mucinous neoplasms can be challenging. Features indicative of a borderline histology, include increasing size and number of locules, fluid content with high T1 or low T2 signal intensity, and mural nodules or septa > 5 mm thick [48]. Typical features of mucinous cystadenocarcinomas include large solid component and size > 10 cm, with internal smaller loculi (i.e., a honeycomb appearance) [49]. Rupture of a mucinous cystadenocarcinoma into the peritoneal cavity results in pseudomyxoma peritonei (PMP); however, in most cases, PMP is caused by rupture of a mucinous neoplasm of the appendix and, less frequently, rupture of a primary ovarian mucinous tumor [50].

2.1.4. Endometrioid Carcinoma and Clear Cell Carcinoma

Endometrioid and clear cell ovarian carcinomas are typically invasive and aggressive, although typically they are low grade neoplasm [51]. Both commonly affect women in their fifties in the 5th decade and present at an early stage, leading to better clinical outcomes [46]. There is an increased incidence of these tumors with Lynch syndrome [52], endometrial carcinoma, and endometriosis (39% and 41%, respectively) [53].

Imaging findings of endometrioid and clear cell carcinomas are nonspecific. High-grade endometrioid carcinoma can be indistinguishable from HGSC. Both are typically present as a mass with varying solid and cystic parts, usually more solid than serous and mucinous neoplasms, often with evidence of hemorrhage. When they develop in an endometrioma, diagnosis may be suggested by the presence of an enhancing mural nodule within an otherwise typical endometrioma (particularly with large endometriomas in women > 45 years) [54,55] (Figure 7). Loss of T2 shading on MRI may be another sign of malignancy due to dilution of hemorrhagic contents by non-hemorrhagic fluid produced by the malignant tissue [55].

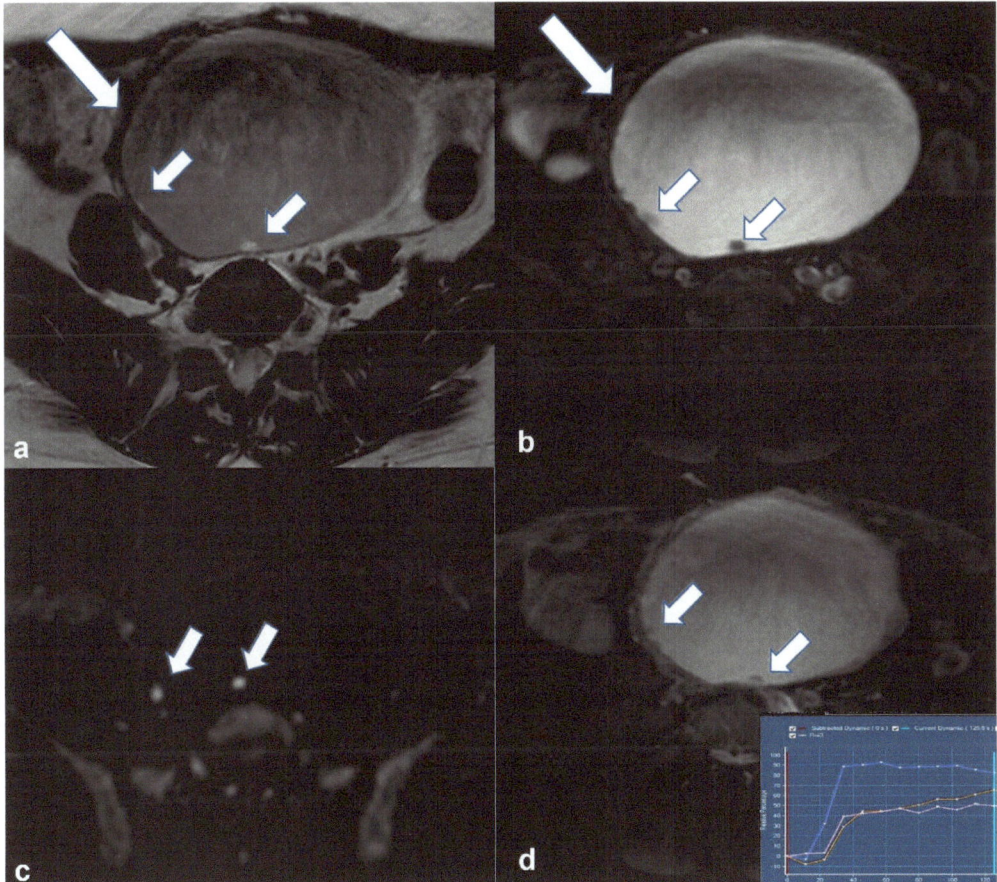

Figure 7. Endometrioid borderline ovarian tumor Axial T2 weighted image (**a**) shows a cystic mass (large arrow) originating from the right ovary with hemorrhagic content on corresponding axial T1 weighted FS image (**b**). There are small mural nodules in the right posterolateral aspect of the lesion (small arrows in a and (**b**)) with restricted diffusivity on corresponding axial high b value DWI image (small arrows in (**c**)). Note the enhancement of the nodules on the corresponding axial T1 weighted FS CE image (small arrows in (**d**)). DCE analysis showed a type 2 time–intensity curve (inset in (**d**), blue line: uterus; yellow/pink line: nodules).

Tip: Concurrent with ovarian tumor endometrial thickening or mass may suggest endometrioid carcinoma [56] (Figure 8). Thromboembolic episodes (which may occur as a complication in 1/3 of clear cell tumors), hypercalcemia and a mostly solid ovarian mass should suggest a diagnosis of clear cell carcinoma [57,58].

Tip: Although rare, endometrioid carcinoma is the most common malignancy arising within an endometriotic cyst, followed by clear cell carcinoma.

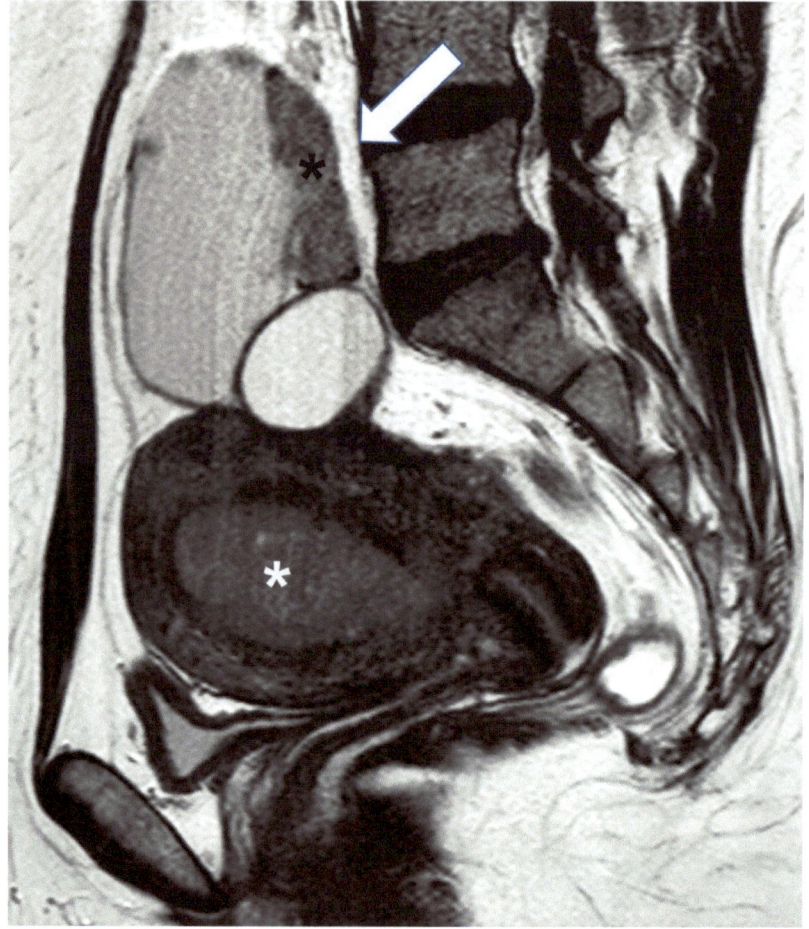

Figure 8. Synchronous ovarian and endometrial endometrioid adenocarcinoma. Sagittal T2 weighted image shows a soft-tissue mass occupying the endometrial cavity (white asterisk). Note a solid and cystic mass of the right ovary (arrow) with the solid component (black asterisk) exhibiting similar signal intensity to that of the endometrial mass.

2.2. Benign Tumors That Can Mimic EOC

2.2.1. Cystadenofibroma

Adenofibromas and cystadenofibromas are rare epithelial–stromal neoplasms most often of the serous subtype that are almost always benign. They are usually discovered incidentally but sometimes they may cause symptoms related to hormone production; most commonly vaginal bleeding due to excessive estrogen secretion. They rarely have borderline or malignant features, but even the benign subtypes can mimic malignant neoplasms at imaging [59].

Typically, they appear as mixed solid and cystic masses, often with papillary projections. At MRI, the solid components which correspond to the fibrous stroma are characteristically quite hypointense on T2 weighted images, of lower signal intensity compared to muscle, often with internal cysts and minimal enhancement [60]. The low T2 signal of the septa, together with the high T2 signal of the cystic spaces give the tumor a characteristic 'black sponge' appearance (Figure 9). If the fibrous component displays higher T2 signal intensity or stronger enhancement, based on occasional case reports, the extremely rare malignant cystadenocarcinofibroma may be considered [61].

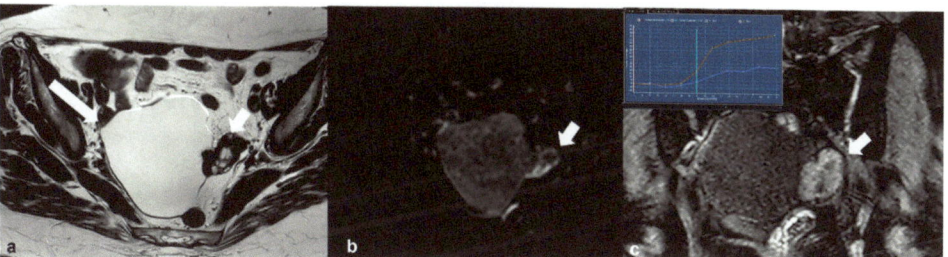

Figure 9. Cystadenofibroma. Axial T2 weighted image (**a**) shows a right-sided ovarian cystic mass (long arrow) with a peripheral solid component of very low signal intensity (short arrow). Corresponding axial high b value (1200) diffusion weighted image (**b**) shows no restricted diffusion of the solid tissue (arrow). Dynamic contrast-enhanced image (**c**) demonstrates avid enhancement of the solid part of the lesion (arrow) and a type 2 time–intensity curve (yellow line: uterus; blue line: lesion in inset).

2.2.2. Fibrothecoma

Fibromas, thecomas, and fibrothecomas are benign stromal ovarian tumors. Usually, they are incidentally found and are asymptomatic, however, occasionally, they may manifest with abdominal pain, in the event of torsion, or with abnormal vaginal bleeding due to estrogen secretion from the thecoma component [62,63].

Typically, on MRI, they present as solid ovarian masses with low T2 signal intensity relative to muscle. However, T2 signal intensity may be higher when oedema or cystic degeneration co-exist (most often in thecomas) [64]. In most cases, they demonstrate low signal intensity both on DWI and ADC maps (known as the T2 blackout effect) due to the presence of fibrous tissue [65,66]. On DCE, they demonstrate minimal enhancement initially, which increases on delayed images; this perfusion pattern corresponds to TIC type 1 (i.e., mild and gradual increase in signal over time with no well-defined shoulder and no plateau) [66] (Figure 10).

Tip: Functioning thecomas and cellular fibromas may show restricted diffusivity due to higher cellularity [67].

Tip: The degree of contrast enhancement differs with the amount of fibrous tissue. While the fibrous tissue demonstrates delayed weak enhancement on DCE, the theca cells are highly vascularized. That explains why thecomas may demonstrate a TIC type 2 or 3 compared to the typical TIC type 1 of fibrothecomas on DCE [17,68].

Fibrothecomas are often indistinguishable from other fibrous tumors such as Brenner tumors which are also hypointense on T2 weighted images. Fibrothecomas are usually of larger size than Brenner tumors and calcifications are not so common, although dense calcifications may sometimes be present [64,69].

In some cases, they may be misinterpreted for a pedunculated leiomyoma, but this usually displays more intense homogeneous enhancement similar to that of the myometrium and possibly, the bridging vessel sign [11] (Figure 11).

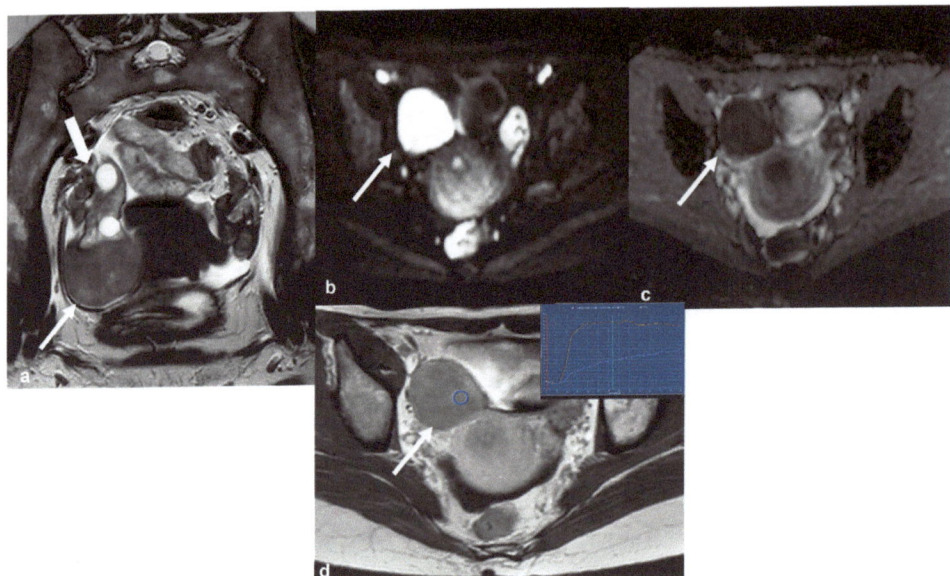

Figure 10. Cellular fibrothecoma. T2 weighted image in the axial oblique plane (**a**) demonstrates a rather low signal intensity lesion (long white arrow) attached to the lower pole of the right ovary (short white arrow). Corresponding axial high b value (1200) diffusion weighted image (**b**) and ADC map (**c**) show restricted diffusion of the lesion (arrow in (**b**,**c**)). The lesion shows avid contrast uptake on axial CE T1 weighted image ((**d**), arrow). DCE analysis of the lesion shows a type 1 time–intensity curve (inset in (**d**), blue line: lesion; orange line: uterus; blue circle: region of interest (ROI) within the lesion).

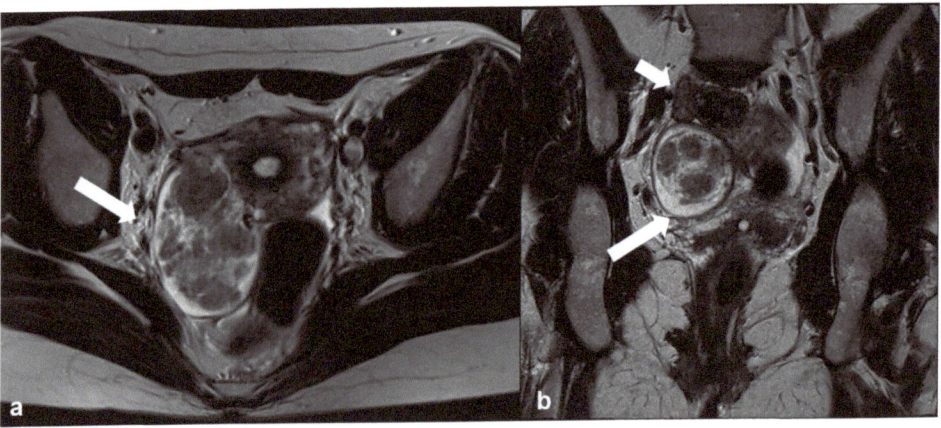

Figure 11. Degenerative pedunculated leiomyoma mimicking ovarian lesion. Axial T2 weighted image (**a**) shows a large inhomogeneous mass within the right broad ligament (arrow). Coronal oblique T2 weighted image (**b**) of the same patient shows the right ovary (short arrow) separate from the mass (long arrow).

2.2.3. Pelvic Inflammatory Disease—Tubo-Ovarian Abscess (TOA)

Patients with PID and tubo-ovarian abscesses, usually present with typical clinical symptoms such as fever and abdominal pain, and the diagnosis is made with transvaginal

US. However, in some cases, especially in older patients, unusual causes, or chronic stage, the imaging findings may be indeterminate and mimic malignancy.

MRI usually demonstrates a low T1 signal-intensity cystic mass with heterogeneous high signal intensity on T2-weighted images depending on the content and protein concentration [70]. T2-shading at the periphery of the cyst and a hyperintense halo on T1-weighted images have also been described and may help the differential diagnosis [71]. Typical MRI features of pyosalpinx include fluid-filled tubular structures with enhancing, thick walls usually adjacent to and inseparable from a TOA (Figure 12).

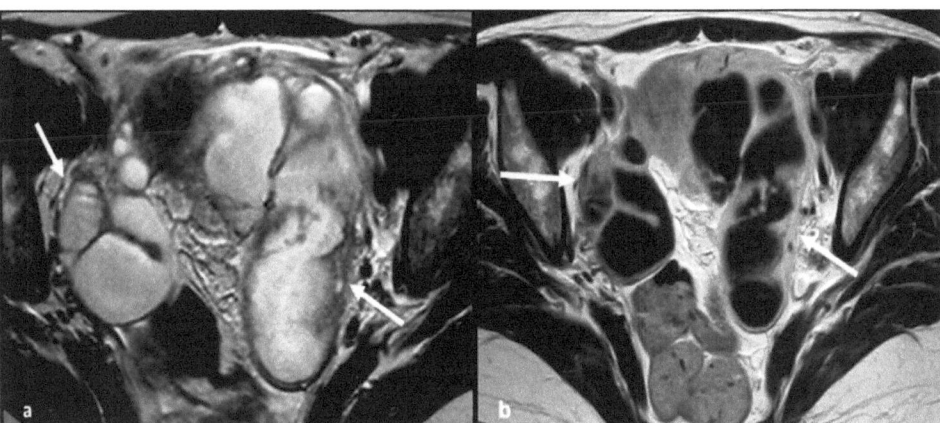

Figure 12. Acute pelvic inflammatory disease. Axial T2 weighted image (**a**) shows large tubular pelvic structures bilaterally (arrows) with thick, smooth walls and incomplete folds, containing non-simple fluid, consistent with dilated tubes. Corresponding T1 weighted contrast-enhanced image (**b**) demonstrates enhancement of the tubal wall but no internal enhancing solid tissue.

The presence of gas is pathognomonic of a tubo-ovarian abscess although only seen in 22–38% of cases [72]. There is infiltration of the perilesional fat and in chronic cases, adhesions. In acute PID, diffusion restriction is commonly seen due to highly viscous internal proteinaceous material. However, diffusion restriction may be absent in chronic abscesses or TOA after antibiotic treatment [73].

2.3. Rare Ovarian Neoplasms That Can Mimic EOC

2.3.1. Brenner Tumor

Brenner tumors are uncommon neoplasms of epithelial-stromal origin, almost always benign with only a few reports of borderline and malignant histology [74].

At imaging, their size varies from microscopic to huge; in a series by Moon et al. including eight tumors, the mean size was reported to be 11 cm [75]. In addition, about half of the cases demonstrated extensive amorphous punctuate calcifications [75]. Characteristically, the solid component exhibits markedly low T2 signal intensity on MRI because of dense fibrous stroma [37,75]. Brenner tumors can coexist with mucinous tumors in the same ovary. Findings suggestive of malignancy in a Brenner tumor, include large cystic parts and an inhomogeneous solid component (i.e., with mild enhancement, due to coexistence of fibrous and malignant components [74,75] (Figure 13).

Tip: Predominantly solid ovarian masses with very low (lower than muscle) signal intensity on T2-weighted MR images are indicative of fibroma, Brenner tumor, and, occasionally, fibrothecoma.

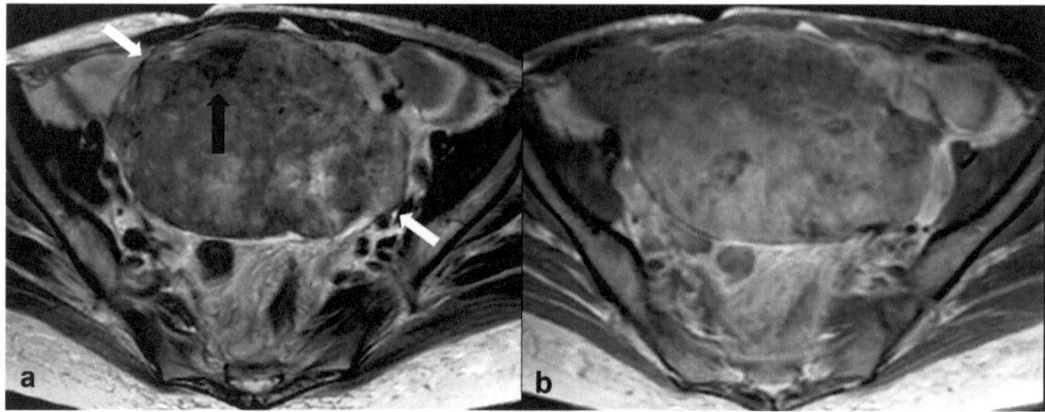

Figure 13. Malignant Brenner tumor. Axial T2 weighted image (**a**) shows a large, predominantly solid mass of moderately high signal intensity (white arrows) with areas of lower T2 signal (black arrow), occupying the pelvis. Axial T1 weighted CE image (**b**) shows mild, heterogeneous enhancement of the mass.

2.3.2. Monodermal Teratoma (Struma Ovarii)

Monodermal (specialized) teratomas are rare. They consist mainly of mature cells, most commonly of thyroid origin (struma ovarii) [76]. Struma ovarii tumors may manifest with hyperthyroidism. Malignant transformation, most often to papillary carcinoma, may occur [77].

At imaging, they present with a variable mixed solid and cystic component or appear entirely solid (Figure 14). They often coexist with a mature teratoma in which cases the solid component demonstrates avid enhancement. When struma ovarii is suspected, CT may be helpful in narrowing the differential diagnosis, since the solid component is often hyperattenuating on unenhanced images because of the iodine content in the thyroid tissue [78].

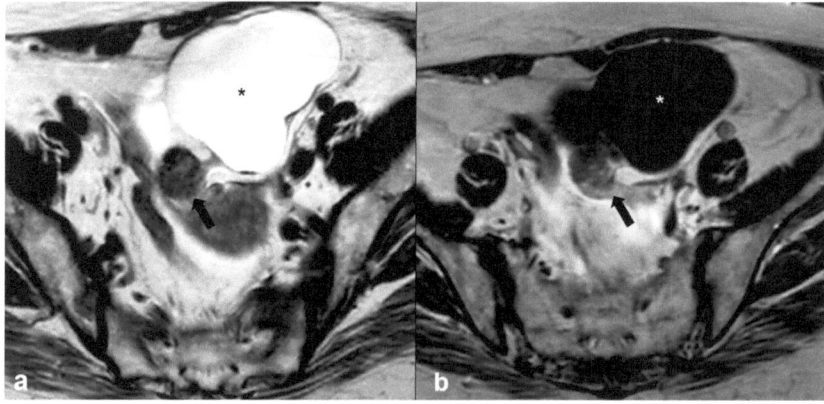

Figure 14. Struma ovarii tumor. Axial T2 weighted image (**a**) shows a predominantly cystic mass (asterisk) with a posteriorly located solid nodule (arrow) in the left ovary showing mild enhancement on the T1 weighted contrast-enhanced image (arrows in (**b**)) and corresponding to ectopic thyroid tissue.

2.3.3. Granulosa Cell Tumor

Granulosa cell tumors (GCT) belonging to the sex-cord stromal tumors, are low grade malignant tumors and most are estrogen producing.

Imaging characteristics of GCT vary and may overlap with those of malignant epithelial cell tumors [79]. GCTs are usually present as large (mean size: 10–12 cm), multilocular masses with both solid and cystic components and areas of hemorrhage; they can also be purely solid or cystic. Their most characteristic appearance is that of a solid mass with a spongelike ("Swiss cheese") appearance; the tumor's cystic compartments may be hemorrhagic fluid with high T1 signal and fluid-fluid levels [80].

Discriminative features of GCTs from malignant epithelial cell neoplasms include absence of intracystic papillary projections, unilateral location, and confinement to the ovary. Additionally, there is a low incidence of peritoneal disease at diagnosis [79]. Endometrial thickening or endometrioid carcinoma may co-exist due to the estrogenic effect [81].

Tip: Ovarian tumors with estrogen secretion such as, endometrioid carcinoma, granulosa cell tumor, and, occasionally, thecoma or fibrothecoma, can be associated with endometrial hyperplasia or carcinoma.

2.3.4. Lymphoma

Lymphoma of the ovary is usually secondary, occurring as part of systemic disseminated disease; primary lymphoma of the ovary is rare [82].

MRI features of lymphoma of the ovary include the presence of bilateral homogeneous solid masses with mild, homogenous enhancement [83] and rather low T2 signals, due to the presence of myeloperoxidase [84].

Helpful signs for diagnosing ovarian lymphoma are bilaterality, bulky abdominal or pelvic nodal conglomerates, and no ascites. Other characteristic imaging signs include the presence of small peripheral cysts, which correspond to preserved ovarian follicles, and encasement of vessels and bowel by the mass without obstruction [84] (Figure 15).

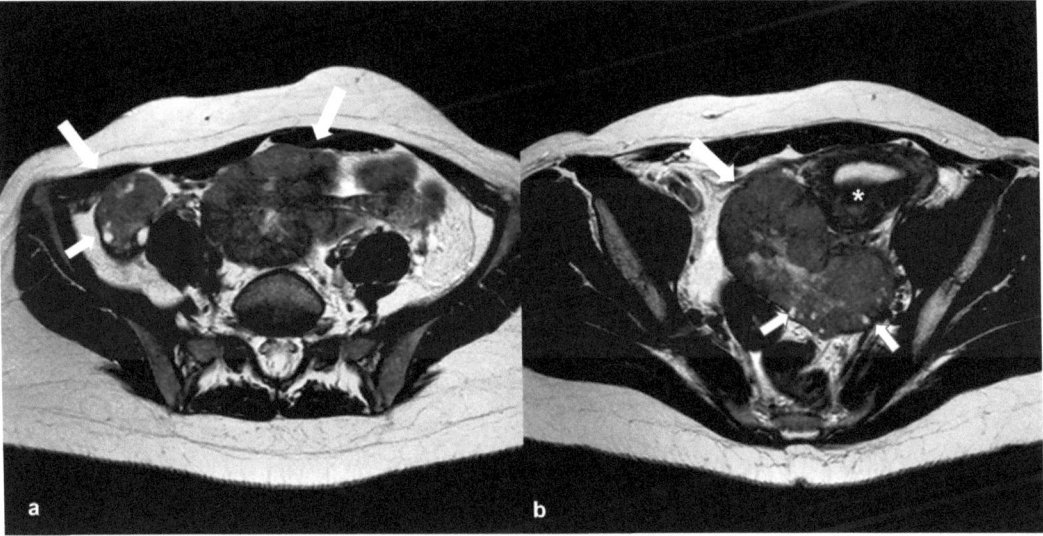

Figure 15. Primary ovarian lymphoma. Axial T2 weighted images (**a**,**b**) show bilateral ovarian enlargement (long arrows) with abnormal stromal signal intensity and peripheral displacement of the ovarian follicles (short arrows). The uterus is displaced to the left side of the pelvis by the enlarged left ovary (asterisk in (**b**)).

2.3.5. Metastases

Metastases to the ovary notably occur from tumors of the gastrointestinal tract (colon, appendix, stomach, pancreas), as well as from breast or lung primaries [85].

They are bilateral in most cases [86]. Imaging manifestations of metastases depend on their site of origin. Predominantly solid metastases usually originate from gastric or breast primaries, while other GI tract metastases (i.e., appendiceal, colorectal, and pancreaticobiliary) often have larger cystic components [87] (Figure 16). At imaging, if bilateral highly vascular ovarian masses measuring less than 10 cm (or for some authors less than 15 cm) are present, metastases should be considered, especially in cases of known history of malignancy or when an extraovarian primary neoplasm with peritoneal carcinomatosis is depicted [88,89]. They are usually associated with heterogeneous hyperintense signal on T2-weighted images because of the variable degree of cystic degeneration; T2-hypointense components may be seen within the metastatic tumor, yet not of lower signal compared to muscle [87].

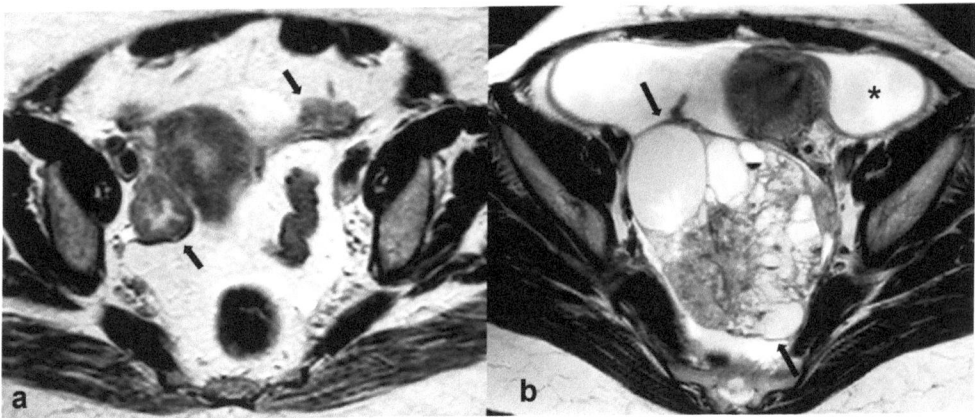

Figure 16. Metastatic ovarian cancer. Axial T2 weighted image (**a**) of a postmenopausal woman with primary gastric cancer. Note the presence of small predominantly solid masses in both ovaries (black arrows). Axial T2 weighted image (**b**) of a premenopausal woman shows a large, mixed cystic, and solid mass in the right adnexa (black arrows) originating from a colon primary. Shown also is a large amount of ascites (asterisk).

Radiologists are often challenged to differentiate a primary ovarian mucinous neoplasm from metastasis by an extraovarian mucinous carcinoma, especially when involvement of the ovary is the initial finding, and the primary neoplasm remains unknown. Accurate differential diagnosis is crucial since it highly impacts the right specialty referral and subsequently, treatment.

Imaging signs supporting the diagnosis of mucinous ovarian metastasis over primary borderline or malignant mucinous tumor include (a) size < 10 cm (or for some authors <15 cm), (b) bilateral involvement, and (c) peritoneal dissemination [88,89].

A helpful sign in distinguishing primary borderline and malignant serous tumors from metastases (since they may both present as bilateral tumors with peritoneal spread), is the presence of papillary projections in the former. An imaging feature indicative of ovarian metastases from colorectal tumors is the 'mille-feuille sign' which consists of fine, alternating layers of tumor cells and necrosis with a width/length of $\geq 10/20$ mm within the metastatic tumor [90]. Tumor markers may be used as an additional tool by the radiologist to try and reach a diagnosis and help further work-up since high levels of CA-125 are more often observed in primary serous neoplasms, while CEA is often increased in gastrointestinal cancers. It should be noted though that normal assays of tumor markers do not exclude malignancy, because they may not be elevated in small masses or early clinical stages of ovarian cancers.

2.4. Adolescence-Germ Cell Tumors

Germ cell tumors represent the second largest category of ovarian neoplasms in the general population; however, they are the most frequently occurring subtype in adolescents and young adults [91]. Histological types include teratoma (mature, immature, and monodermal), dysgerminoma, yolk sac tumor (also known as endodermal sinus tumor), embryonal carcinoma, polyembryoma, and choriocarcinoma. The vast majority of these tumors (95%) are benign; in a number of cases germ cell tumors may be associated with elevated tumor markers including human chorionic gonadotropin (HCG), alfa-fetoprotein (AFP), and the recently introduced embryonic serum microRNAs (MiRNA), which helps in the diagnosis and monitoring of such tumors [92].

2.4.1. Mature Cystic Teratoma (Dermoid)

Mature cystic teratoma is the most common benign ovarian neoplasm in children and adolescents, constituting almost half of all neoplasms in this age population. Bilaterality occurs in 10–25% of cases [93]. Typically, it is asymptomatic; however, complications include torsion (3–16%), rupture (1–4%) and less likely infection (1%), and malignant transformation (1–2%) [94].

Imaging characteristics of a mature teratoma include presence of a cystic, fat-containing mass usually with solid components (i.e., dermoid plug or Rokitansky nodule) [95].

At MRI, detection of fatty elements (i.e., high T1 and T2 signal and suppression of signal on fat-suppressed images) is virtually pathognomonic for teratoma. T1-weighted images with saturation of fat is the key sequence for discriminating between fat and hemorrhage (which remains T1 hyperintense). The fat-containing mass shows chemical shift artifact in a significant number of cases (62–87%) [96]. In 25–33% of cases, fat may not be detected within the mass and mature cystic teratomas may, thus, resemble cystic epithelial tumors. In such cases, the wall of the cyst should be carefully inspected for the identification of small T1 and T2 hyperintense foci. Loss of signal intensity on opposed-phase MRI, may assist the diagnosis of intralesional fat [96] (Figure 17). Moreover, DWI may be useful since almost all mature cystic teratomas, even the lipid poor, are known to have a keratinoid component which shows restricted diffusion [97].

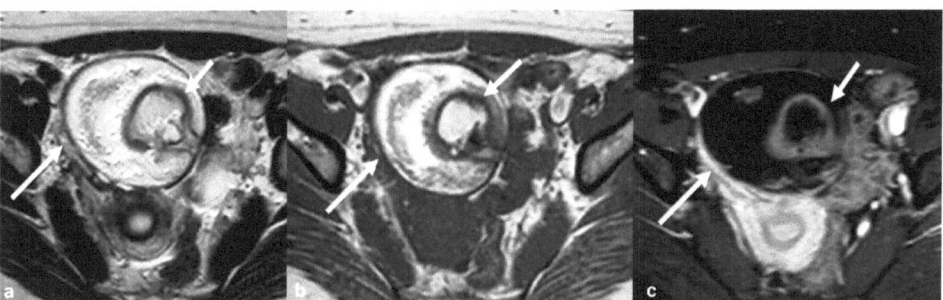

Figure 17. Mature teratoma. Axial T2 weighted image (**a**) shows a large, high signal intensity mass (long white arrow) in the right side of the pelvis. The mass demonstrates high signal intensity on corresponding axial T1 weighted image (**b**) and significant signal drop on T1 weighted FS CE image (**c**), typical of fatty content (long white arrow). Shown also is the typical fat-containing intra-tumoral Rokitansky nodule (short arrow in (**a**) and (**b**)) with peripheral contrast enhancement (short arrow in (**c**)).

Other imaging characteristics of mature teratoma depend on its histologic composition and the presence of sebum, hair, teeth/calcification (in 31% of cases, presenting with low signal intensity at both T1 and T2 weighted images), bone, or cartilage [96].

The solid component of a benign dermoid cyst may show a TIC type 1, 2, or even 3 on DCE which is related to the specific content of the solid tissue of the lesion, without necessarily indicating malignancy (e.g., thyroidal tissue) [98]. Typically, a Rokitansky nodule shows peripheral enhancement, and the lesion is classified as O-RADS MRI 2; however, the presence of large enhancing components within the dermoid, with irregular margins particularly when there is invasion of the cystic wall may indicate malignancy and the lesion is then classified as O-RADS 4 [17]. Most malignant transformations of teratomas (>80%) are of squamous cell histology (SCCs) arising from the ectoderm; less frequently, malignant transformation to carcinoid tumors or adenocarcinomas may occur [99]. Apart from arising in a cystic teratoma, ovarian SCC has been associated with prolonged exposure to various carcinogens and high-risk human papillomavirus (HPV) infection [100].

2.4.2. Immature Teratoma

Immature teratoma is the second most common malignant germ cell tumor in children and adolescents, accounting for 10–20% of all ovarian malignancies in girls younger than 20 years [28]. It is often associated with elevated serum AFP levels (33–65%) [93].

At MRI, in contrast to benign mature teratomas, it tends to be unilateral and larger, more heterogeneous, with more solid elements which enhance, only small, scattered foci of fat and cystic components with usually simple fluid content. In addition, the calcification pattern seems to differ, since calcifications in immature teratoma are irregular and multiple while in mature tumors they are coarsened or toothlike [96,101] (Figure 18).

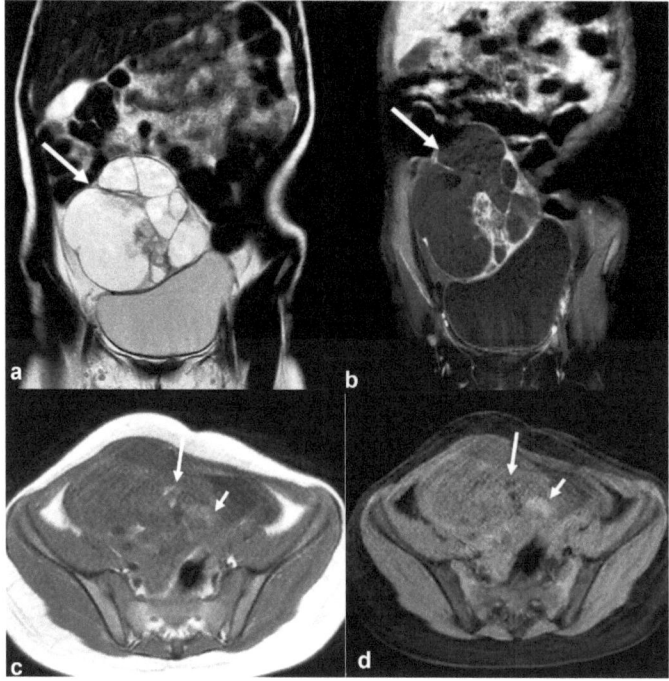

Figure 18. Immature teratoma in a 7-year-old girl. Coronal T2 weighted image (**a**) shows a large cystic right-sided pelvic mass (white arrow) with internal septations and smaller solid components which are enhanced on the T1 weighted FS CE image ((**b**), white arrow). Axial T1 weighted image (**c**) shows tiny foci of high signal intensity (long arrow) with signal loss on the T1 weighted FS image ((**d**), long arrow). Note also a few hemorrhagic foci with high T1 signal intensity on both T1 weighted images (short arrows in (**c**,**d**)).

Tip: Calcifications may be seen in mature or immature teratoma, Brenner tumor, and less commonly, fibrothecoma of the ovary.

Tip: The presence of fat in an ovarian lesion is virtually pathognomonic of a teratoma. Mature cystic teratomas have an increased number of cystic elements and coarse calcifications, and the solid component presents as a Rokitansky nodule. Immature teratomas contain larger amounts of solid tissue, small foci of fat, and scattered calcifications. Although histological diagnosis cannot be reached with imaging, the suspicion of an immature teratoma can certainly be raised.

2.4.3. Dysgerminoma

Dysgerminoma is the most common malignant germ cell tumor in children and adolescents. Predisposing factors include gonadal dysgenesis, abnormal gonads (gonadoblastoma), and chromosomal syndromes (e.g., Turner syndrome) [102]. Tumor markers, such as LDH and ALP or, rarely β-hCG, are elevated.

Unlike immature teratoma, dysgerminoma may involve both ovaries in a small number of cases (10–15%) and may occasionally spread to the retroperitoneal lymph nodes [102].

Dysgerminoma is typically seen as a large, lobulated predominantly solid mass with internal fibrovascular septa. Because of their fibrous nature, the septa demonstrate low T2 signal intensity and intense, homogenous enhancement [103]. Necrosis, hemorrhage, or speckled calcifications are less frequently seen within the tumor (Figure 19).

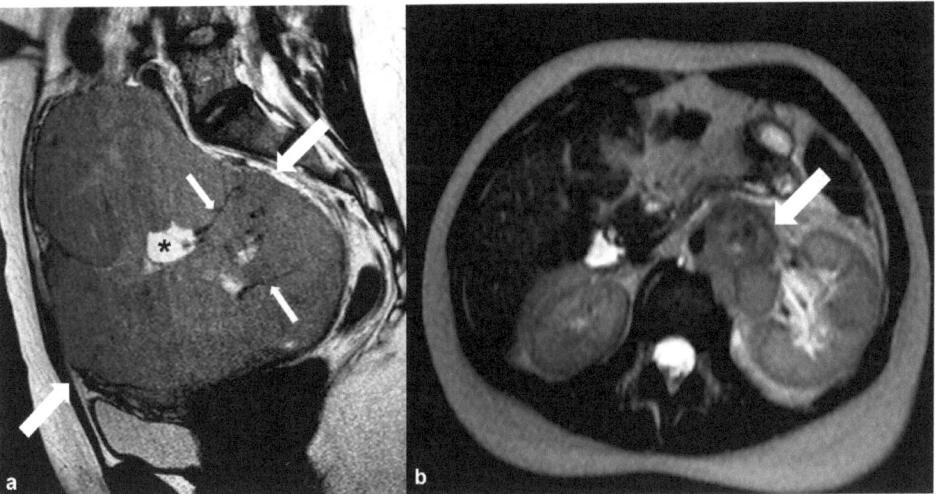

Figure 19. Dygerminoma. Axial T2 weighted image (**a**) shows a predominantly solid ovarian mass (large arrows) with thin low signal intensity internal septa (thin arrows) and cystic/necrotic area (asterisk). T2 weighted image (**b**) of the same patient at the level of the renal hilum shows multiple enlarged left paraaortic lymph nodes (arrow).

Note that, in contrast to other fibrous ovarian tumors (i.e., Brenner tumor and fibroma/fibrothecoma), the T2 signal intensity of fibrous tissue in dysgerminomas is not lower but slightly hyperintense to muscle [104].

2.5. Pregnancy

2.5.1. Corpus Luteum Cysts/Theca Lutein Cysts

Corpus luteum cysts, accounting for 13–17% of cystic, pregnancy-related adnexal masses, result from failure of involution of the corpus luteum. The corpus luteum normally forms after ovulation and produces progesterone during the first 8–9 weeks until the placenta takes over [105]. At MRI, corpus luteum cysts appear with variable signal intensity, ragged internal walls, and avid peripheral enhancement [33].

Hyperreactio luteinalis (theca lutein cysts) is a rare condition caused by increased levels of β-hCG and manifests as bilateral, multicystic ovarian masses (spoke-wheel appearance), which can mimic ovarian hyperstimulation syndrome or mucinous borderline tumors (Figure 20). It is highly associated with gestational trophoblastic disease and only rarely seen in normal uncomplicated pregnancies [106].

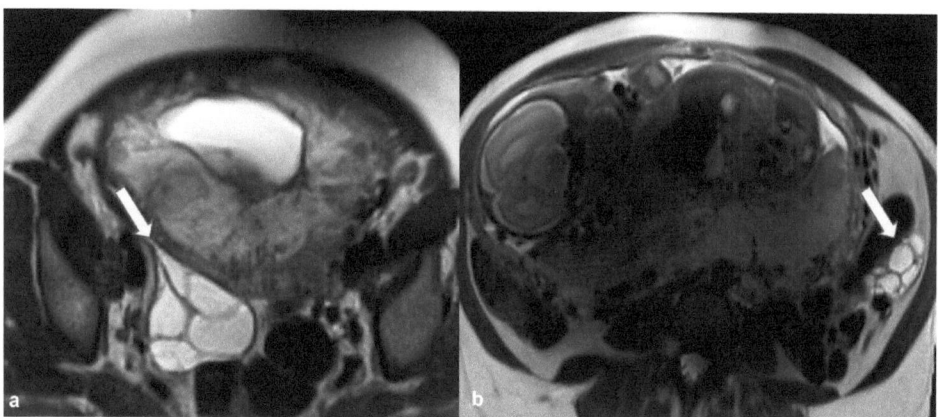

Figure 20. Hyperreactio luteinalis (theca lutein cysts) in third-trimester pregnancy. Axial T2 weighted images shows bilateral, multicystic ovarian masses with a spoke-wheel appearance (arrows in (**a**,**b**)). No solid tissue is present.

Luteoma of pregnancy is a rare, non-neoplastic ovarian lesion consisting of proliferating luteinized stromal cells, which under the influence of β-hCG, replace normal ovarian parenchyma. As it is a purely solid mass, its discrimination from solid ovarian neoplasms of stromal origin based on imaging is virtually impossible; however, these tumors are usually associated with androgen secretion which may induce maternal and female fetus virilization. If there is suspicion of ovarian luteoma, intervention is not recommended since these lesions spontaneously regress during the early postpartum period [107].

2.5.2. Decidualized Endometrioma

During pregnancy, the ectopic endometrium is characterized by increasing glandular epithelial secretion, stromal vascularity, and oedema due to increased progesterone levels, a change defined as decidualization [108]. At imaging, decidualized endometrioma often appears as a cystic mass with hemorrhagic fluid and a variable amount of enhancing solid component, which can mimic mucinous borderline neoplasms [35,109]. However, decidualized nodules are usually smaller, with signal intensity similar to that of normal placenta, demonstrating higher signal intensity on T2-weighted images and no restricted diffusion on DWI compared to ovarian cancers [110].

2.5.3. Epithelial Ovarian Cancer

Imaging appearances of ovarian cancer in pregnant women do not differ from those in the general population. Evaluation of size and morphologic features can help in distinguishing benign from malignant lesions and the established US and MRI scoring systems can be applied. However, an important limitation of the O-RADS MRI classification system in the gravid population is that gadolinium administration is strongly discouraged for the characterization of a lesion's solid component since there are still safety issues regarding the effect of paramagnetic contrast media on the fetus [111,112] (Figure 21).

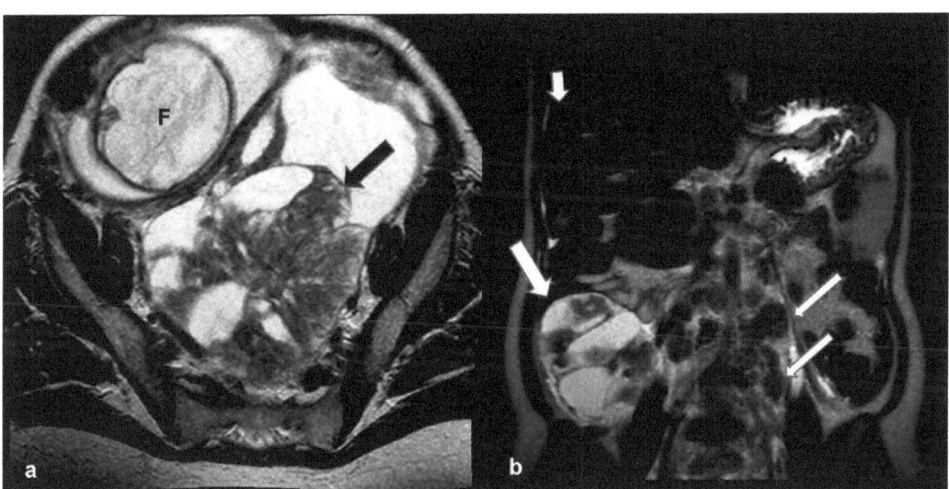

Figure 21. Bilateral high grade epithelial ovarian cancer in a 26 gestational week pregnant woman with twins. Axial T2 weighted image (**a**) shows a mixed cystic-solid left ovarian mass (black arrow). Coronal T2 weighted image (**b**) of the same patient shows a mixed cystic-solid mass in the contralateral ovary (thick white arrow). Shown also are enlarged left paraaortic lymph nodes (thin arrows) and hepatic metastases (short arrows). F: fetus.

2.6. Non-Ovarian Masses

2.6.1. Mucinous Rectosigmoid Cancer

Sigmoid colon adenocarcinoma typically invades the bowel circumferentially narrowing its lumen. At MRI, tumor enhancement and restricted diffusion are common findings. Occasionally, a primary colonic cancer can directly invade or metastasize to the ovaries, making it challenging to accurately identify its origin (Figure 22). Another ambitious task is differentiating between the mucinous subtype of rectal cancer and primary mucinous ovarian neoplasms, since in the case of a large mucin-containing mass, it can be difficult to establish the primary site [113].

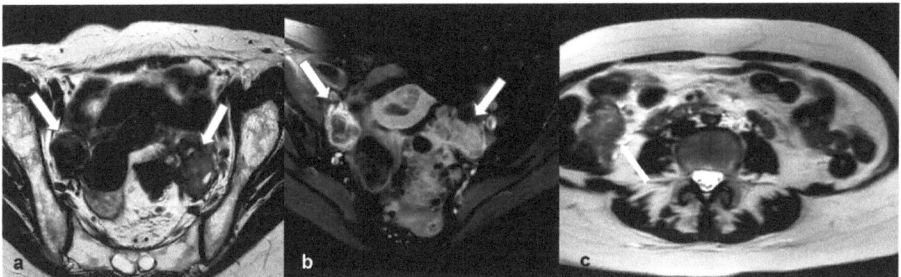

Figure 22. Bilateral ovarian metastases (Krukenberg tumors) from colon cancer. T2 weighted axial image (**a**) shows bilateral ovarian soft-tissue masses ((**a**),arrows) exhibiting inhomogeneous enhancement on corresponding T1 weighted FS CE image ((**b**), arrows). Axial T2 weighted image (**c**) of the upper abdomen of the same patient shows extensive circumferential wall thickening of the ascending colon (arrows).

2.6.2. Appendiceal Mucocele—PMP

Mucocele of the appendix presents as a distended appendix with mucinous content. It is more commonly seen in middle-aged women and in most cases, it is incidentally found [114]. Underlying histology of an appendiceal mucocele may be that of a simple retention cyst, mucosal hyperplasia, cystadenoma, and cystadenocarcinoma. On MRI, a tubular structure communicating with the base of the caecum with high T2 signal fluid content will be seen [115]. If there is irregular thickening of the wall of the dilated appendix or enhancing nodules cystadenocarcinoma should be suspected.

Accurate preoperative diagnosis and differentiation from mucinous ovarian neoplasms is important in order to avoid rupture during surgery and subsequent pseudomyxoma peritonei formation (i.e., mucinous implants throughout the peritoneal cavity) [116]. On MRI, pseudomyxoma peritonei deposits manifest as low T1 and high T2 foci displacing bowel loops centrally and encasing the bowel lumen, causing bowel obstruction. Frequently, large, complex cystic metastases can also be identified in the ovaries. Characteristically, PMP results in scalloped appearance of the liver and spleen, a useful sign to distinguish mucinous implants from loculated ascites [117].

Tip: PMP is more often the result of a ruptured mucinous adenocarcinoma of the appendix—rupture of mucinous ovarian neoplasms rarely occurs.

2.6.3. Liposarcoma/Schwannoma

Sometimes, distinguishing a large ovarian mass that extends in the upper abdominal spaces from a primary retroperitoneal tumor can be challenging. These tumors are usually of mesenchymal (leiomyoma, sarcoma, solitary fibrous tumor) or neurogenic origin (schwannomas, neurofibromas).

To narrow the differential diagnosis, the first step is to assess the presence of intralesional macroscopic fat. Increased signal intensity on T1-weighted images and signal loss after fat saturation is indicative of a fat-containing lesion. If a fatty mass presents with irregular and ill-defined borders, then the diagnosis of liposarcoma should be considered. Liposarcomas are the most common type of retroperitoneal sarcomas [118]. They typically occur in the 5th and 6th decades of life, mostly in females. At imaging, three distinctive patterns are recognized: mixed, solid, and pseudocystic. The most frequent is the mixed pattern, consisting of a fatty mass with soft-tissue component(s) that usually displaces adjacent organs. Well-differentiated liposarcomas contain an increased amount of fat, whereas high-grade liposarcomas are associated with large soft-tissue components, with appearances similar to those of other sarcomas [119].

If the mass appears predominantly solid or has a myxoid component, one should consider a tumor of neurogenic origin. Schwannoma is a benign, encapsulated tumor of neurogenic origin, commonly seen in young to middle-aged women [120]. On MRI, a low T1 and high T2 signal lesion is seen eccentrically located to a nerve. Areas of cystic degeneration, a pseudocapsule, calcifications, or hemorrhagic foci may also be seen.

Several imaging signs have been described and are associated with benign neurogenic tumors [120]. These include: (a) the fat split sign (a thin rim of high T1 signal corresponding to fat around the lesion), (b) the target sign (peripheral high T2 signal myxoid material and central low T2 signal fibrous component), and (c) the fascicular sign (multiple T2 hypointense ring-like structures surrounded by high T2 signal, representing the fascicular bundles within the nerves).

Ancient schwannoma is a rare benign variant characterized by degenerative changes. On imaging, these tumors appear more heterogeneous compared to a typical schwannoma and due to their cystic component, are often misdiagnosed as malignant tumors. Helpful imaging signs in the differential diagnosis include a smooth enhancing fibrous capsule and degenerative areas with enhancing circumference [121].

Their malignant counterpart, MPNST (Malignant Peripheral Nerve Sheath Tumor), is extremely uncommon and rarely occurs in the retroperitoneum. Peripheral enhancement with non-cystic appearance and heterogeneous enhancement may suggest the diagnosis. Other helpful imaging features to differentiate MPNST from BPNST include: (1) size > 5 cm with ill-defined margins, (2) peritumoral edema, (3) intra-tumoral lobulation, (4) absence of target sign, and (5) bone destruction [122] (Figure 23).

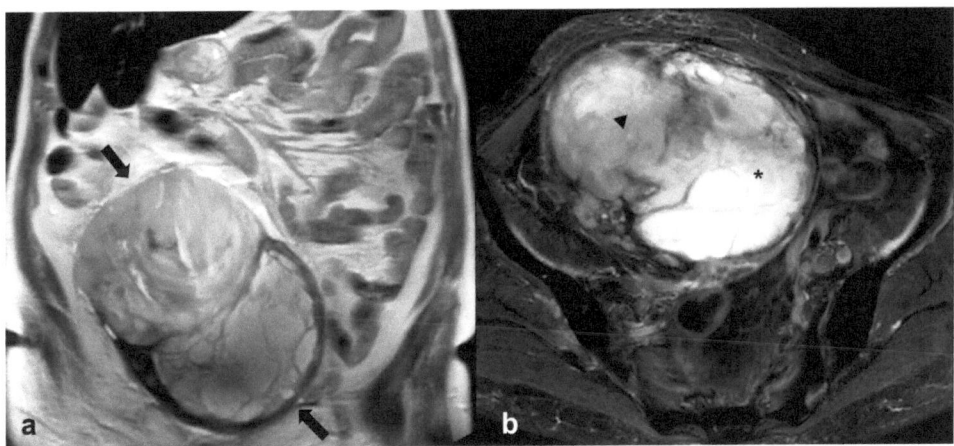

Figure 23. Malignant peripheral nerve sheath tumor (MPNST). Coronal T2 weighted image (**a**) shows a large, encapsulated pelvic mass extending in the upper abdomen (arrows). On the axial T2 weighted FS image (**b**), the mass consists of a high signal intensity, lobulated component on the left (asterisk) and a lower signal intensity component on the right (arrowhead).

3. Conclusions

Accurate differential diagnosis of suspicious pelvic masses based on imaging is crucial since it largely affects clinical management. MRI, with its superior contrast resolution and tissue characterization, can be a useful tool for radiologists. Introduction of 3T magnets in daily clinical routine and application of the O-RADS diagnostic criteria may further familiarize radiologists with the appearances of ovarian cancer and other pelvic diseases that may act as mimickers, increasing their confidence in establishing the site of origin and providing the most likely diagnosis.

Author Contributions: Conceptualization, C.B. and L.A.M.; methodology, C.B.; validation, C.B. and M.K.; formal analysis, M.K.; investigation, M.K.; resources, M.K.; data curation, M.K.; writing—original draft preparation, C.B. and M.K.; writing—review and editing, C.B. and L.A.M.; visualization, C.B. and L.A.M.; supervision, L.A.M.; project administration, C.B.; All authors have read and agreed to the published version of the manuscript.

Funding: This research received no external funding.

Institutional Review Board Statement: Ethical review and approval were waived for this review study.

Informed Consent Statement: Patient consent was waived for this review study.

Data Availability Statement: All imaging data were provided by the Department of Radiology, School of Medicine, National and Kapodistrian University of Athens, Aretaieion Hospital, Athens, Greece. These data can be available upon request, while they are not fully uploaded to publicly accessible links due to the General Data Protection Regulation (GDPR) policy of the Hospital.

Conflicts of Interest: The authors declare no conflict of interest.

References

1. Kurman, R.; Carcanjiu, M.; Herrington, S.; Young, R. Tumours of the Ovary. In *World Health Organization Classification of Tumours of the Female Reproductive Organs*; IARC: Lyon, France, 2014; pp. 11–86.
2. Huang, J.; Chan, W.C.; Ngai, C.H.; Lok, V.; Zhang, L.; Lucero-Prisno, D.E.; Xu, W.; Zheng, Z.-J.; Elcarte, E.; Withers, M.; et al. Worldwide Burden, Risk Factors, and Temporal Trends of Ovarian Cancer: A Global Study. *Cancers* **2022**, *14*, 2230. [CrossRef] [PubMed]

3. Timmerman, D.; Van Calster, B.; Testa, A.C.; Guerriero, S.; Fischerova, D.; Lissoni, A.A.; Van Holsbeke, C.; Fruscio, R.; Czekierdowski, A.; Jurkovic, D.; et al. Ovarian Cancer Prediction in Adnexal Masses Using Ultrasound-Based Logistic Regression Models: A Temporal and External Validation Study by the IOTA Group. *Ultrasound Obstet. Gynecol.* **2010**, *36*, 226–234. [CrossRef] [PubMed]
4. Van Holsbeke, C.; Daemen, A.; Yazbek, J.; Holland, T.K.; Bourne, T.; Mesens, T.; Lannoo, L.; Boes, A.-S.; Joos, A.; Van De Vijver, A.; et al. Ultrasound Experience Substantially Impacts on Diagnostic Performance and Confidence When Adnexal Masses Are Classified Using Pattern Recognition. *Gynecol. Obstet. Investig.* **2010**, *69*, 160–168. [CrossRef]
5. Adusumilli, S.; Hussain, H.K.; Caoili, E.M.; Weadock, W.J.; Murray, J.P.; Johnson, T.D.; Chen, Q.; Desjardins, B. MRI of Sonographically Indeterminate Adnexal Masses. *Am. J. Roentgenol.* **2006**, *187*, 732–740. [CrossRef]
6. Sadowski, E.A.; Paroder, V.; Patel-Lippmann, K.; Robbins, J.B.; Barroilhet, L.; Maddox, E.; McMahon, T.; Sampene, E.; Wasnik, A.P.; Blaty, A.D.; et al. Indeterminate Adnexal Cysts at US: Prevalence and Characteristics of Ovarian Cancer. *Radiology* **2018**, *287*, 1041–1049. [CrossRef] [PubMed]
7. Zhang, X.; Mao, Y.; Zheng, R.; Zheng, Z.; Huang, Z.; Huang, D.; Zhang, J.; Dai, Q.; Zhou, X.; Wen, Y. The Contribution of Qualitative CEUS to the Determination of Malignancy in Adnexal Masses, Indeterminate on Conventional US—A Multicenter Study. *PLoS ONE* **2014**, *9*, e93843. [CrossRef]
8. Karaosmanoglu, D.; Karcaaltincaba, M.; Karcaaltincaba, D.; Akata, D.; Ozmen, M. MDCT of the Ovarian Vein: Normal Anatomy and Pathology. *Am. J. Roentgenol.* **2009**, *192*, 295–299. [CrossRef]
9. Lee, J.H.; Jeong, Y.K.; Park, J.K.; Hwang, J.C. "Ovarian Vascular Pedicle" Sign Revealing Organ of Origin of a Pelvic Mass Lesion on Helical CT. *Am. J. Roentgenol.* **2003**, *181*, 131–137. [CrossRef]
10. Arikawa, S.; Uchida, M.; Shinagawa, M.; Tohnan, T.; Hayabuchi, N. Significance of the "Beak Sign" in the Differential Diagnosis of Uterine Lipoleiomyoma from Ovarian Dermoid Cyst. *Kurume Med. J.* **2006**, *53*, 37–40. [CrossRef]
11. Kim, J.C.; Kim, S.S.; Park, J.Y. "Bridging Vascular Sign" in the MR Diagnosis of Exophytic Uterine Leiomyoma. *J. Comput. Assist. Tomogr.* **2000**, *24*, 57–60. [CrossRef]
12. Sahin, H.; Panico, C.; Ursprung, S.; Simeon, V.; Chiodini, P.; Frary, A.; Carmo, B.; Smith, J.; Freeman, S.; Jimenez-Linan, M.; et al. Non-contrast MRI can accurately characterize adnexal masses: A retrospective study. *Eur. Radiol.* **2021**, *31*, 6962–6973. [CrossRef] [PubMed]
13. Lee, S.I.; Kang, S.K. MRI Improves the Characterization of Incidental Adnexal Masses Detected at Sonography. *Radiology* **2023**, *307*, e222866. [CrossRef] [PubMed]
14. Liu, B.; Liao, J.; Gu, W.; Wang, J.; Li, G.; Wang, L. ADNEX Model-Based Diagnosis of Ovarian Cancer Using MRI Images. *Contrast Media Mol. Imaging* **2021**, *2021*, 2146578. [CrossRef] [PubMed]
15. Forstner, R.; Thomassin-Naggara, I.; Cunha, T.M.; Kinkel, K.; Masselli, G.; Kubik-Huch, R.; Spencer, J.A.; Rockall, A. ESUR Recommendations for MR Imaging of the Sonographically Indeterminate Adnexal Mass: An Update. *Eur. Radiol.* **2017**, *27*, 2248–2257. [CrossRef]
16. Jeong, Y.-Y.; Outwater, E.K.; Kang, H.K. Imaging Evaluation of Ovarian Masses. *RadioGraphics* **2000**, *20*, 1445–1470. [CrossRef]
17. Thomassin-Naggara, I.; Poncelet, E.; Jalaguier-Coudray, A.; Guerra, A.; Fournier, L.S.; Stojanovic, S.; Millet, I.; Bharwani, N.; Juhan, V.; Cunha, T.M.; et al. Ovarian-Adnexal Reporting Data System Magnetic Resonance Imaging (O-RADS MRI) Score for Risk Stratification of Sonographically Indeterminate Adnexal Masses. *JAMA Netw. Open* **2020**, *3*, e1919896. [CrossRef]
18. Kang, S.K.; Reinhold, C.; Atri, M.; Benson, C.B.; Bhosale, P.R.; Jhingran, A.; Lakhman, Y.; Maturen, K.E.; Nicola, R.; Pandharipande, P.V.; et al. ACR Appropriateness Criteria for Staging And Follow-Up of Ovarian Cancer. *J. Am. Coll. Radiol.* **2018**, *15*, S198–S207. [CrossRef]
19. Kobal, B.; Noventa, M.; Cvjeticanin, B.; Barbic, M.; Meglic, L.; Herzog, M.; Bordi, G.; Vitagliano, A.; Saccardi, C.; Skof, E. Primary Debulking Surgery versus Primary Neoadjuvant Chemotherapy for High Grade Advanced Stage Ovarian Cancer: Comparison of Survivals. *Radiol. Oncol.* **2018**, *52*, 307–319. [CrossRef]
20. McEvoy, S.H.; Nougaret, S.; Abu-Rustum, N.R.; Vargas, H.A.; Sadowski, E.A.; Menias, C.O.; Shitano, F.; Fujii, S.; Sosa, R.E.; Escalon, J.G.; et al. Fertility-Sparing for Young Patients with Gynecologic Cancer: How MRI Can Guide Patient Selection Prior to Conservative Management. In *Abdominal Radiology*; Springer: New York, NY, USA, 2017; pp. 2488–2512. [CrossRef]
21. Colombo, N.; Ledermann, J.A. Updated Treatment Recommendations for Newly Diagnosed Epithelial Ovarian Carcinoma from the ESMO Clinical Practice Guidelines. *Ann. Oncol.* **2021**, *32*, 1300–1303. [CrossRef]
22. Mutch, D.G.; Prat, J. 2014 FIGO Staging for Ovarian, Fallopian Tube and Peritoneal Cancer. *Gynecol. Oncol.* **2014**, *133*, 401–404. [CrossRef]
23. Timmerman, D.; Testa, A.C.; Bourne, T.; Ameye, L.; Jurkovic, D.; Van Holsbeke, C.; Paladini, D.; Van Calster, B.; Vergote, I.; Van Huffel, S.; et al. Simple Ultrasound-Based Rules for the Diagnosis of Ovarian Cancer. *Ultrasound Obstet. Gynecol.* **2008**, *31*, 681–690. [CrossRef] [PubMed]
24. Viora, E.; Piovano, E.; Baima Poma, C.; Cotrino, I.; Castiglione, A.; Cavallero, C.; Sciarrone, A.; Bastonero, S.; Iskra, L.; Zola, P. The ADNEX Model to Triage Adnexal Masses: An External Validation Study and Comparison with the IOTA Two-Step Strategy and Subjective Assessment by an Experienced Ultrasound Operator. *Eur. J. Obstet. Gynecol. Reprod. Biol.* **2020**, *247*, 207–211. [CrossRef] [PubMed]
25. Amor, F.; Vaccaro, H.; Alcázar, J.L.; León, M.; Craig, J.M.; Martinez, J. Gynecologic Imaging Reporting and Data System. *J. Ultrasound Med.* **2009**, *28*, 285–291. [CrossRef] [PubMed]

26. Andreotti, R.F.; Timmerman, D.; Strachowski, L.M.; Froyman, W.; Benacerraf, B.R.; Bennett, G.L.; Bourne, T.; Brown, D.L.; Coleman, B.G.; Frates, M.C.; et al. O-RADS US Risk Stratification and Management System: A Consensus Guideline from the ACR Ovarian-Adnexal Reporting and Data System Committee. *Radiology* **2020**, *294*, 168–185. [CrossRef]
27. Low, R.N.; Barone, R.M.; Lucero, J. Comparison of MRI and CT for Predicting the Peritoneal Cancer Index (PCI) Preoperatively in Patients Being Considered for Cytoreductive Surgical Procedures. *Ann. Surg. Oncol.* **2015**, *22*, 1708–1715. [CrossRef]
28. Northridge, J.L. Adnexal Masses in Adolescents. *Pediatr. Ann.* **2020**, *49*, e183–e187. [CrossRef]
29. Janssen, C.L.; Littooij, A.S.; Fiocco, M.; Huige, J.C.B.; de Krijger, R.R.; Hulsker, C.C.C.; Goverde, A.J.; Zsiros, J.; Mavinkurve-Groothuis, A.M.C. The Diagnostic Value of Magnetic Resonance Imaging in Differentiating Benign and Malignant Pediatric Ovarian Tumors. *Pediatr. Radiol.* **2021**, *51*, 427–434. [CrossRef]
30. Webb, K.E.; Sakhel, K.; Chauhan, S.P.; Abuhamad, A.Z. Adnexal Mass during Pregnancy: A Review. *Am. J. Perinatol.* **2015**, *32*, 1010–1016. [CrossRef]
31. Telischak, N.A.; Yeh, B.M.; Joe, B.N.; Westphalen, A.C.; Poder, L.; Coakley, F.V. MRI of Adnexal Masses in Pregnancy. *Am. J. Roentgenol.* **2008**, *191*, 364–370. [CrossRef]
32. Botha, M.H.; Rajaram, S.; Karunaratne, K. Cancer in Pregnancy. *Int. J. Gynecol. Obstet.* **2018**, *143*, 137–142. [CrossRef]
33. Yacobozzi, M.; Nguyen, D.; Rakita, D. Adnexal Masses in Pregnancy. *Semin. Ultrasound CT MRI* **2012**, *33*, 55–64. [CrossRef] [PubMed]
34. Bourgioti, C.; Konidari, M.; Gourtsoyianni, S.; Moulopoulos, L.A. Imaging during Pregnancy: What the Radiologist Needs to Know. *Diagn. Interv. Imaging* **2021**, *102*, 593–603. [CrossRef] [PubMed]
35. Yin, M.; Wang, T.; Li, S.; Zhang, X.; Yang, J. Decidualized Ovarian Endometrioma Mimicking Malignancy in Pregnancy: A Case Report and Literature Review. *J. Ovarian Res.* **2022**, *15*, 33. [CrossRef]
36. Murase, E.; Siegelman, E.S.; Outwater, E.K.; Perez-Jaffe, L.A.; Tureck, R.W. Uterine Leiomyomas: Histopathologic Features, MR Imaging Findings, Differential Diagnosis, and Treatment. *RadioGraphics* **1999**, *19*, 1179–1197. [CrossRef]
37. Jung, S.E.; Lee, J.M.; Rha, S.E.; Byun, J.Y.; Jung, J.I.; Hahn, S.T. CT and MR Imaging of Ovarian Tumors with Emphasis on Differential Diagnosis. *RadioGraphics* **2002**, *22*, 1305–1325. [CrossRef] [PubMed]
38. Seidman, J.; Russell, P.; Kurman, R. Surface Epithelial Tumors of the Ovary. In *Blaustein's Pathology of the Female Genital Tract*; Springer: New York, NY, USA, 2002; pp. 791–904.
39. Thomassin-Naggara, I.; Aubert, E.; Rockall, A.; Jalaguier-Coudray, A.; Rouzier, R.; Daraï, E.; Bazot, M. Adnexal Masses: Development and Preliminary Validation of an MR Imaging Scoring System. *Radiology* **2013**, *267*, 432–443. [CrossRef] [PubMed]
40. Boger-Megiddo, I.; Weiss, N.S. Histologic Subtypes and Laterality of Primary Epithelial Ovarian Tumors. *Gynecol. Oncol.* **2005**, *97*, 80–83. [CrossRef]
41. Hart, W.R. Borderline Epithelial Tumors of the Ovary. *Mod. Pathol.* **2005**, *18*, S33–S50. [CrossRef]
42. Folkins, A.K.; Longacre, T.A. Low-Grade Serous Neoplasia of the Female Genital Tract. *Surg. Pathol. Clin.* **2019**, *12*, 481–513. [CrossRef]
43. Bazot, M.; Haouy, D.; Daraï, E.; Cortez, A.; Dechoux-Vodovar, S.; Thomassin-Naggara, I. Is MRI a Useful Tool to Distinguish between Serous and Mucinous Borderline Ovarian Tumours? *Clin. Radiol.* **2013**, *68*, e1–e8. [CrossRef]
44. Outwater, E.K.; Huang, A.B.; Dunton, C.J.; Talerman, A.; Capuzzi, D.M. Papillary Projections in Ovarian Neoplasms: Appearance on MRI. *J. Magn. Reson. Imaging* **1997**, *7*, 689–695. [CrossRef] [PubMed]
45. Marko, J.; Marko, K.I.; Pachigolla, S.L.; Crothers, B.A.; Mattu, R.; Wolfman, D.J. Mucinous Neoplasms of the Ovary: Radiologic-Pathologic Correlation. *RadioGraphics* **2019**, *39*, 982–997. [CrossRef] [PubMed]
46. Peres, L.C.; Cushing-Haugen, K.L.; Köbel, M.; Harris, H.R.; Berchuck, A.; Rossing, M.A.; Schildkraut, J.M.; Doherty, J.A. Invasive Epithelial Ovarian Cancer Survival by Histotype and Disease Stage. *JNCI J. Natl. Cancer Inst.* **2019**, *111*, 60–68. [CrossRef]
47. Okada, S.; Ohaki, Y.; Inoue, K.; Kawamura, T.; Hayashi, T.; Kato, T.; Kumazaki, T. Calcifications in Mucinous and Serous Cystic Ovarian Tumors. *J. Nippon. Med. Sch.* **2005**, *72*, 29–33. [CrossRef] [PubMed]
48. Zhao, S.H.; Qiang, J.W.; Zhang, G.F.; Wang, S.J.; Qiu, H.Y.; Wang, L. MRI in Differentiating Ovarian Borderline from Benign Mucinous Cystadenoma: Pathological Correlation. *J. Magn. Reson. Imaging* **2014**, *39*, 162–166. [CrossRef]
49. Okamoto, Y.; Tanaka, Y.O.; Tsunoda, H.; Yoshikawa, H.; Minami, M. Malignant or Borderline Mucinous Cystic Neoplasms Have a Larger Number of Loculi than Mucinous Cystadenoma: A Retrospective Study with MR. *J. Magn. Reson. Imaging* **2007**, *26*, 94–99. [CrossRef]
50. Ferreira, C.R.; Carvalho, J.P.; Soares, F.A.; Siqueira, S.A.C.; Carvalho, F.M. Mucinous Ovarian Tumors Associated with Pseudomyxoma Peritonei of Adenomucinosis Type: Immunohistochemical Evidence That They Are Secondary Tumors. *Int. J. Gynecol. Cancer* **2008**, *18*, 59–65. [CrossRef]
51. Fadare, O.; Parkash, V. Pathology of Endometrioid and Clear Cell Carcinoma of the Ovary. *Surg. Pathol. Clin.* **2019**, *12*, 529–564. [CrossRef]
52. Watson, P.; Bützow, R.; Lynch, H.T.; Mecklin, J.-P.; Järvinen, H.J.; Vasen, H.F.A.; Madlensky, L.; Fidalgo, P.; Bernstein, I. The Clinical Features of Ovarian Cancer in Hereditary Nonpolyposis Colorectal Cancer. *Gynecol. Oncol.* **2001**, *82*, 223–228. [CrossRef]
53. Matias-Guiu, X.; Stewart, C.J.R. Endometriosis-Associated Ovarian Neoplasia. *Pathology* **2018**, *50*, 190–204. [CrossRef]
54. Tanaka, Y.O.; Yoshizako, T.; Nishida, M.; Yamaguchi, M.; Sugimura, K.; Itai, Y. Ovarian Carcinoma in Patients with Endometriosis. *Am. J. Roentgenol.* **2000**, *175*, 1423–1430. [CrossRef] [PubMed]

55. Tanaka, Y.O.; Okada, S.; Yagi, T.; Satoh, T.; Oki, A.; Tsunoda, H.; Yoshikawa, H. MRI of Endometriotic Cysts in Association with Ovarian Carcinoma. *Am. J. Roentgenol.* **2010**, *194*, 355–361. [CrossRef] [PubMed]
56. van Niekerk, C.C.; Bulten, J.; Vooijs, G.P.; Verbeek, A.L.M. The Association between Primary Endometrioid Carcinoma of the Ovary and Synchronous Malignancy of the Endometrium. *Obstet. Gynecol. Int.* **2010**, *2010*, 465162. [CrossRef]
57. Matsuura, Y.; Robertson, G.; Marsden, D.E.; Kim, S.-N.; Gebski, V.; Hacker, N.F. Thromboembolic Complications in Patients with Clear Cell Carcinoma of the Ovary. *Gynecol. Oncol.* **2007**, *104*, 406–410. [CrossRef]
58. Savvari, P.; Peitsidis, P.; Alevizaki, M.; Dimopoulos, M.-A.; Antsaklis, A.; Papadimitriou, C.A. Paraneoplastic Humorally Mediated Hypercalcemia Induced by Parathyroid Hormone-Related Protein in Gynecologic Malignancies: A Systematic Review. *Onkologie* **2009**, *32*, 517–523. [CrossRef] [PubMed]
59. Avesani, G.; Caliolo, G.; Gui, B.; Petta, F.; Panico, C.; La Manna, V.; Moro, F.; Testa, A.C.; Scambia, G.; Manfredi, R. Pearls and Potential Pitfalls for Correct Diagnosis of Ovarian Cystadenofibroma in MRI: A Pictorial Essay. *Korean J. Radiol.* **2021**, *22*, 1809. [CrossRef]
60. Tang, Y.Z.; Liyanage, S.; Narayanan, P.; Sahdev, A.; Sohaib, A.; Singh, N.; Rockall, A. The MRI Features of Histologically Proven Ovarian Cystadenofibromas—An Assessment of the Morphological and Enhancement Patterns. *Eur. Radiol.* **2013**, *23*, 48–56. [CrossRef] [PubMed]
61. Jung, D.C.; Kim, S.H.; Kim, S.H. MR Imaging Findings of Ovarian Cystadenofibroma and Cystadenocarcinofibroma: Clues for the Differential Diagnosis. *Korean J. Radiol.* **2006**, *7*, 199. [CrossRef]
62. Chen, J.; Wang, J.; Chen, X.; Wang, Y.; Wang, Z.; Li, D. Computed Tomography and Magnetic Resonance Imaging Features of Ovarian Fibrothecoma. *Oncol. Lett.* **2017**, *14*, 1172–1178. [CrossRef]
63. Cho, Y.J.; Lee, H.S.; Kim, J.M.; Joo, K.Y.; Kim, M.-L. Clinical Characteristics and Surgical Management Options for Ovarian Fibroma/Fibrothecoma: A Study of 97 Cases. *Gynecol. Obstet. Invest.* **2013**, *76*, 182–187. [CrossRef]
64. Shinagare, A.B.; Meylaerts, L.J.; Laury, A.R.; Mortele, K.J. MRI Features of Ovarian Fibroma and Fibrothecoma with Histopathologic Correlation. *Am. J. Roentgenol.* **2012**, *198*, W296–W303. [CrossRef] [PubMed]
65. Zhang, H.; Zhang, G.-F.; Wang, T.-P.; Zhang, H. Value of 3.0 T Diffusion-Weighted Imaging in Discriminating Thecoma and Fibrothecoma from Other Adnexal Solid Masses. *J. Ovarian Res.* **2013**, *6*, 58. [CrossRef] [PubMed]
66. Chung, B.M.; bin Park, S.; Lee, J.B.; Park, H.J.; Kim, Y.S.; Oh, Y.J. Magnetic Resonance Imaging Features of Ovarian Fibroma, Fibrothecoma, and Thecoma. *Abdom. Imaging* **2015**, *40*, 1263–1272. [CrossRef] [PubMed]
67. Agostinho, L.; Horta, M.; Salvador, J.C.; Cunha, T.M. Benign Ovarian Lesions with Restricted Diffusion. *Radiol. Bras.* **2019**, *52*, 106–111. [CrossRef]
68. Tanaka, Y.O.; Tsunoda, H.; Kitagawa, Y.; Ueno, T.; Yoshikawa, H.; Saida, Y. Functioning Ovarian Tumors: Direct and Indirect Findings at MR Imaging. *RadioGraphics* **2004**, *24* (Suppl. 1), S147–S166. [CrossRef]
69. Chen, H.; Liu, Y.; Shen, L.; Jiang, M.; Yang, Z.; Fang, G. Ovarian Thecoma-Fibroma Groups: Clinical and Sonographic Features with Pathological Comparison. *J. Ovarian Res.* **2016**, *9*, 81. [CrossRef]
70. Thomassin-Naggara, I.; Darai, E.; Bazot, M. Gynecological Pelvic Infection: What Is the Role of Imaging? *Diagn. Interv. Imaging* **2012**, *93*, 491–499. [CrossRef]
71. Revzin, M.V.; Mathur, M.; Dave, H.B.; Macer, M.L.; Spektor, M. Pelvic Inflammatory Disease: Multimodality Imaging Approach with Clinical-Pathologic Correlation. *RadioGraphics* **2016**, *36*, 1579–1596. [CrossRef]
72. Tukeva, T.A.; Aronen, H.J.; Karjalainen, P.T.; Molander, P.; Paavonen, T.; Paavonen, J. MR Imaging in Pelvic Inflammatory Disease: Comparison with Laparoscopy and US. *Radiology* **1999**, *210*, 209–216. [CrossRef]
73. Bonde, A.; Andreazza Dal Lago, E.; Foster, B.; Javadi, S.; Palmquist, S.; Bhosale, P. Utility of the Diffusion Weighted Sequence in Gynecological Imaging: Review Article. *Cancers* **2022**, *14*, 4468. [CrossRef]
74. Takeuchi, M.; Matsuzaki, K.; Sano, N.; Furumoto, H.; Nishitani, H. Malignant Brenner Tumor with Transition from Benign to Malignant Components. *J. Comput. Assist. Tomogr.* **2008**, *32*, 553–554. [CrossRef] [PubMed]
75. Moon, W.J.; Koh, B.H.; Kim, S.K.; Kim, Y.S.; Rhim, H.C.; Cho, O.K.; Hahm, C.K.; Byun, J.Y.; Cho, K.S.; Kim, S.H. Brenner Tumor of the Ovary: CT and MR Findings. *J. Comput. Assist. Tomogr.* **2000**, *24*, 72–76. [CrossRef] [PubMed]
76. Euscher, E.D. Germ Cell Tumors of the Female Genital Tract. *Surg. Pathol. Clin.* **2019**, *12*, 621–649. [CrossRef] [PubMed]
77. Makani, S.; Kim, W.; Gaba, A.R. Struma Ovarii with a Focus of Papillary Thyroid Cancer: A Case Report and Review of the Literature. *Gynecol. Oncol.* **2004**, *94*, 835–839. [CrossRef]
78. Taylor, E.C.; Irshaid, L.; Mathur, M. Multimodality Imaging Approach to Ovarian Neoplasms with Pathologic Correlation. *RadioGraphics* **2020**, *41*, 289–315. [CrossRef]
79. Elsherif, S.; Bourne, M.; Soule, E.; Lall, C.; Bhosale, P. Multimodality Imaging and Genomics of Granulosa Cell Tumors. *Abdom. Radiol.* **2020**, *45*, 812–827. [CrossRef]
80. Zhang, H.; Zhang, H.; Gu, S.; Zhang, Y.; Liu, X.; Zhang, G. MR Findings of Primary Ovarian Granulosa Cell Tumor with Focus on the Differentiation with Other Ovarian Sex Cord-Stromal Tumors. *J. Ovarian Res.* **2018**, *11*, 46. [CrossRef]
81. Fotopoulou, C.; Savvatis, K.; Braicu, E.-I.; Brink-Spalink, V.; Darb-Esfahani, S.; Lichtenegger, W.; Sehouli, J. Adult Granulosa Cell Tumors of the Ovary: Tumor Dissemination Pattern at Primary and Recurrent Situation, Surgical Outcome. *Gynecol. Oncol.* **2010**, *119*, 285–290. [CrossRef]
82. Lagoo, A.S.; Robboy, S.J. Lymphoma of the Female Genital Tract: Current Status. *Int. J. Gynecol. Pathol.* **2006**, *25*, 1–21. [CrossRef]

83. Slonimsky, E.; Korach, J.; Perri, T.; Davidson, T.; Apter, S.; Inbar, Y. Gynecological Lymphoma. *J. Comput. Assist. Tomogr.* **2018**, *42*, 435–440. [CrossRef]
84. Crawshaw, J.; Sohaib, S.A.; Wotherspoon, A.; Shepherd, J.H. Primary Non-Hodgkin's Lymphoma of the Ovaries: Imaging Findings. *Br. J. Radiol.* **2007**, *80*, e155–e158. [CrossRef] [PubMed]
85. Agnes, A.; Biondi, A.; Ricci, R.; Gallotta, V.; D'Ugo, D.; Persiani, R. Krukenberg Tumors: Seed, Route and Soil. *Surg. Oncol.* **2017**, *26*, 438–445. [CrossRef] [PubMed]
86. Lerwill, M.F.; Young, R.H. Metastatic Tumors of the Ovary. In *Blaustein's Pathology of the Female Genital Tract*; Springer: New York, NY, USA, 2008; pp. 929–998.
87. Koyama, T.; Mikami, Y.; Saga, T.; Tamai, K.; Togashi, K. Secondary Ovarian Tumors: Spectrum of CT and MR Features with Pathologic Correlation. *Abdom. Imaging* **2007**, *32*, 784–795. [CrossRef] [PubMed]
88. Khunamornpong, S.; Suprasert, P.; Pojchamarnwiputh, S.; Na Chiangmai, W.; Settakorn, J.; Siriaunkgul, S. Primary and Metastatic Mucinous Adenocarcinomas of the Ovary: Evaluation of the Diagnostic Approach Using Tumor Size and Laterality. *Gynecol. Oncol.* **2006**, *101*, 152–157. [CrossRef]
89. Xu, Y.; Yang, J.; Zhang, Z.; Zhang, G. MRI for Discriminating Metastatic Ovarian Tumors from Primary Epithelial Ovarian Cancers. *J. Ovarian Res.* **2015**, *8*, 61. [CrossRef]
90. Kurokawa, R.; Nakai, Y.; Gonoi, W.; Mori, H.; Tsuruga, T.; Makise, N.; Ushiku, T.; Abe, O. Differentiation between Ovarian Metastasis from Colorectal Carcinoma and Primary Ovarian Carcinoma: Evaluation of Tumour Markers and "Mille-Feuille Sign" on Computed Tomography/Magnetic Resonance Imaging. *Eur. J. Radiol.* **2020**, *124*, 108823. [CrossRef]
91. Talerman, A. Germ Cell Tumors of the Ovary. In *Blaustein's Pathology of the Female Genital Tract*; Springer: New York, NY, USA, 2002; pp. 967–1034.
92. Jezierska, M.; Gawrychowska, A.; Stefanowicz, J. Diagnostic, Prognostic and Predictive Markers in Pediatric Germ Cell Tumors—Past, Present and Future. *Diagnostics* **2022**, *12*, 278. [CrossRef]
93. Heo, S.H.; Kim, J.W.; Shin, S.S.; Jeong, S.I.; Lim, H.S.; Choi, Y.D.; Lee, K.H.; Kang, W.D.; Jeong, Y.Y.; Kang, H.K. Review of Ovarian Tumors in Children and Adolescents: Radiologic-Pathologic Correlation. *RadioGraphics* **2014**, *34*, 2039–2055. [CrossRef]
94. bin Park, S.; Kim, J.K.; Kim, K.-R.; Cho, K.-S. Imaging Findings of Complications and Unusual Manifestations of Ovarian Teratomas. *RadioGraphics* **2008**, *28*, 969–983. [CrossRef]
95. Saleh, M.; Bhosale, P.; Menias, C.O.; Ramalingam, P.; Jensen, C.; Iyer, R.; Ganeshan, D. Ovarian Teratomas: Clinical Features, Imaging Findings and Management. *Abdom. Radiol.* **2021**, *46*, 2293–2307. [CrossRef]
96. Outwater, E.K.; Siegelman, E.S.; Hunt, J.L. Ovarian Teratomas: Tumor Types and Imaging Characteristics. *RadioGraphics* **2001**, *21*, 475–490. [CrossRef] [PubMed]
97. Nakayama, T.; Yoshimitsu, K.; Irie, H.; Aibe, H.; Tajima, T.; Nishie, A.; Asayama, Y.; Matake, K.; Kakihara, D.; Matsuura, S.; et al. Diffusion-Weighted Echo-Planar MR Imaging and ADC Mapping in the Differential Diagnosis of Ovarian Cystic Masses: Usefulness of Detecting Keratinoid Substances in Mature Cystic Teratomas. *J. Magn. Reson. Imaging* **2005**, *22*, 271–278. [CrossRef] [PubMed]
98. Poncelet, E.; Delpierre, C.; Kerdraon, O.; Lucot, J.-P.; Collinet, P.; Bazot, M. Value of Dynamic Contrast-Enhanced MRI for Tissue Characterization of Ovarian Teratomas: Correlation with Histopathology. *Clin. Radiol.* **2013**, *68*, 909–916. [CrossRef] [PubMed]
99. Kido, A.; Togashi, K.; Konishi, I.; Kataoka, M.L.; Koyama, T.; Ueda, H.; Fujii, S.; Konishi, J. Dermoid Cysts of the Ovary with Malignant Transformation: MR Appearance. *Am. J. Roentgenol.* **1999**, *172*, 445–449. [CrossRef]
100. Verguts, J.; Amant, F.; Moerman, P.; Vergote, I. HPV Induced Ovarian Squamous Cell Carcinoma: Case Report and Review of the Literature. *Arch. Gynecol. Obstet.* **2007**, *276*, 285–289. [CrossRef]
101. Yamaoka, T.; Togashi, K.; Koyama, T.; Fujiwara, T.; Higuchi, T.; Iwasa, Y.; Fujii, S.; Konishi, J. Immature Teratoma of the Ovary: Correlation of MR Imaging and Pathologic Findings. *Eur. Radiol.* **2003**, *13*, 313–319. [CrossRef]
102. Laufer, M.; Goldstein, D. Benign and Malignant Ovarian Masses. In *Pediatric and Adolescent Gynecology*; Lippincott Williams & Wilkins: Philadelphia, PA, USA, 2005; p. 685.
103. Kitajima, K.; Hayashi, M.; Kuwata, Y.; Imanaka, K.; Sugimura, K. MRI Appearances of Ovarian Dysgerminoma. *Eur. J. Radiol. Extra* **2007**, *61*, 23–25. [CrossRef]
104. Shaaban, A.M.; Rezvani, M.; Elsayes, K.M.; Baskin, H.; Mourad, A.; Foster, B.R.; Jarboe, E.A.; Menias, C.O. Ovarian Malignant Germ Cell Tumors: Cellular Classification and Clinical and Imaging Features. *RadioGraphics* **2014**, *34*, 777–801. [CrossRef]
105. Schwartz, N.; Timor-Tritsch, I.E.; WANG, E. Adnexal Masses in Pregnancy. *Clin. Obstet. Gynecol.* **2009**, *52*, 570–585. [CrossRef]
106. van Holsbeke, C.; Amant, F.; Veldman, J.; de Boodt, A.; Moerman, P.; Timmerman, D. Hyperreactio Luteinalis in a Spontaneously Conceived Singleton Pregnancy. *Ultrasound Obstet. Gynecol.* **2009**, *33*, 371–373. [CrossRef]
107. Cathcart, A.M.; Nezhat, F.R.; Emerson, J.; Pejovic, T.; Nezhat, C.H.; Nezhat, C.R. Adnexal Masses during Pregnancy: Diagnosis, Treatment, and Prognosis. *Am. J. Obstet. Gynecol.* **2022**. [CrossRef] [PubMed]
108. Barbieri, M.; Somigliana, E.; Oneda, S.; Ossola, M.W.; Acaia, B.; Fedele, L. Decidualized Ovarian Endometriosis in Pregnancy: A Challenging Diagnostic Entity. *Hum. Reprod.* **2009**, *24*, 1818–1824. [CrossRef] [PubMed]
109. Takeuchi, M.; Matsuzaki, K.; Nishitani, H. Magnetic Resonance Manifestations of Decidualized Endometriomas during Pregnancy. *J. Comput. Assist. Tomogr.* **2008**, *32*, 353–355. [CrossRef] [PubMed]
110. Bourgioti, C.; Preza, O.; Panourgias, E.; Chatoupis, K.; Antoniou, A.; Nikolaidou, M.E.; Moulopoulos, L.A. MR Imaging of Endometriosis: Spectrum of Disease. *Diagn. Interv. Imaging* **2017**, *98*, 751–767. [CrossRef]

111. Thomassin-Naggara, I.; Fedida, B.; Sadowski, E.; Chevrier, M.-C.; Chabbert-Buffet, N.; Ballester, M.; Tavolaro, S.; Darai, E. Complex US Adnexal Masses during Pregnancy: Is Pelvic MR Imaging Accurate for Characterization? *Eur. J. Radiol.* **2017**, *93*, 200–208. [CrossRef]
112. Bourgioti, C.; Konidari, M.; Moulopoulos, L.A. Imaging of Gynecologic Malignancy in a Reproductive Age Female. *Radiol. Clin. N. Am.* **2020**, *58*, 413–430. [CrossRef]
113. Nougaret, S.; Nikolovski, I.; Paroder, V.; Vargas, H.A.; Sala, E.; Carrere, S.; Tetreau, R.; Hoeffel, C.; Forstner, R.; Lakhman, Y. MRI of Tumors and Tumor Mimics in the Female Pelvis: Anatomic Pelvic Space–Based Approach. *RadioGraphics* **2019**, *39*, 1205–1229. [CrossRef]
114. Dhage-Ivatury, S.; Sugarbaker, P.H. Update on the Surgical Approach to Mucocele of the Appendix. *J. Am. Coll. Surg.* **2006**, *202*, 680–684. [CrossRef]
115. Van Hooser, A.; Williams, T.R.; Myers, D.T. Mucinous Appendiceal Neoplasms: Pathologic Classification, Clinical Implications, Imaging Spectrum and Mimics. *Abdom. Radiol.* **2018**, *43*, 2913–2922. [CrossRef]
116. Carr, N.J.; Cecil, T.D.; Mohamed, F.; Sobin, L.H.; Sugarbaker, P.H.; González-Moreno, S.; Taflampas, P.; Chapman, S.; Moran, B.J. A Consensus for Classification and Pathologic Reporting of Pseudomyxoma Peritonei and Associated Appendiceal Neoplasia. *Am. J. Surg. Pathol.* **2016**, *40*, 14–26. [CrossRef]
117. Chira, R.I.; Nistor-Ciurba, C.C.; Mociran, A.; Mircea, P.A. Appendicular Mucinous Adenocarcinoma Associated with Pseudomyxoma Peritonei, a Rare and Difficult Imaging Diagnosis. *Med. Ultrason.* **2016**, *18*, 257. [CrossRef] [PubMed]
118. Nishino, M.; Hayakawa, K.; Minami, M.; Yamamoto, A.; Ueda, H.; Takasu, K. Primary Retroperitoneal Neoplasms: CT and MR Imaging Findings with Anatomic and Pathologic Diagnostic Clues. *RadioGraphics* **2003**, *23*, 45–57. [CrossRef] [PubMed]
119. Kransdorf, M.J.; Bancroft, L.W.; Peterson, J.J.; Murphey, M.D.; Foster, W.C.; Temple, H.T. Imaging of Fatty Tumors: Distinction of Lipoma and Well-Differentiated Liposarcoma. *Radiology* **2002**, *224*, 99–104. [CrossRef] [PubMed]
120. Hoarau, N.; Slim, K.; da Ines, D. CT and MR Imaging of Retroperitoneal Schwannoma. *Diagn. Interv. Imaging* **2013**, *94*, 1133–1139. [CrossRef]
121. Isobe, K.; Shimizu, T.; Akahane, T.; Kato, H. Imaging of Ancient Schwannoma. *Am. J. Roentgenol.* **2004**, *183*, 331–336. [CrossRef] [PubMed]
122. Yu, Y.; Wu, J.; Ye, J.; Chen, M. Radiological Findings of Malignant Peripheral Nerve Sheath Tumor: Reports of Six Cases and Review of Literature. *World J. Surg. Oncol.* **2016**, *14*, 142. [CrossRef] [PubMed]

Disclaimer/Publisher's Note: The statements, opinions and data contained in all publications are solely those of the individual author(s) and contributor(s) and not of MDPI and/or the editor(s). MDPI and/or the editor(s) disclaim responsibility for any injury to people or property resulting from any ideas, methods, instructions or products referred to in the content.

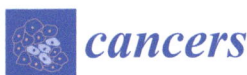

Article

Standardization of Body Composition Status in Patients with Advanced Urothelial Tumors: The Role of a CT-Based AI-Powered Software for the Assessment of Sarcopenia and Patient Outcome Correlation

Antonella Borrelli [1], Martina Pecoraro [1], Francesco Del Giudice [2], Leonardo Cristofani [1], Emanuele Messina [1], Ailin Dehghanpour [1], Nicholas Landini [1], Michela Roberto [1], Stefano Perotti [1], Maurizio Muscaritoli [3], Daniele Santini [1], Carlo Catalano [1] and Valeria Panebianco [1,*]

[1] Department of Radiological Sciences, Oncology and Pathology, Sapienza University of Rome, 00161 Rome, Italy
[2] Department of Maternal Infant and Urologic Sciences, Sapienza University of Rome, 00161 Rome, Italy
[3] Department of Translational and Precision Medicine, Sapienza University of Rome, 00161 Rome, Italy
* Correspondence: valeria.panebianco@uniroma1.it

Simple Summary: Artificial Intelligence (AI)-driven software that utilizes Computed Tomography (CT) images has the capability to automatically assess body composition and diagnose sarcopenia. Our research indicates that combining standardized CT staging methods with sarcopenia analysis could assist in identifying patients with advanced urothelial tumors who may benefit from customized nutritional therapies, ultimately resulting in improved outcomes and quality of life. The AI tool can represent a means to increase the clinical value of CT imaging reports and to promote the development of precision medicine.

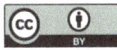

Abstract: Background: Sarcopenia is a well know prognostic factor in oncology, influencing patients' quality of life and survival. We aimed to investigate the role of sarcopenia, assessed by a Computed Tomography (CT)-based artificial intelligence (AI)-powered-software, as a predictor of objective clinical benefit in advanced urothelial tumors and its correlations with oncological outcomes. Methods: We retrospectively searched patients with advanced urothelial tumors, treated with systemic platinum-based chemotherapy and an available total body CT, performed before and after therapy. An AI-powered software was applied to CT to obtain the Skeletal Muscle Index (SMI-L3), derived from the area of the psoas, long spine, and abdominal muscles, at the level of L3 on CT axial images. Logistic and Cox-regression modeling was implemented to explore the association of sarcopenic status and anthropometric features to the clinical benefit rate and survival endpoints. Results: 97 patients were included, 66 with bladder cancer and 31 with upper-tract urothelial carcinoma. Clinical benefit outcomes showed a linear positive association with all the observed body composition variables variations. The chances of not experiencing disease progression were positively associated with Δ_SMI-L3, Δ_psoas, and Δ_long spine muscle when they ranged from ~10–20% up to ~45–55%. Greater survival chances were matched by patients achieving a wider Δ_SMI-L3, Δ_abdominal and Δ_long spine muscle. Conclusions: A CT-based AI-powered software body composition and sarcopenia analysis provide prognostic assessments for objective clinical benefits and oncological outcomes.

Keywords: Artificial Intelligence software; Sarcopenia; Computed Tomography; Urogenital Tumors; Oncology

1. Introduction

Cancer cachexia is a complex condition where there is a progressive reduction in skeletal muscle mass that cannot be fully restored by traditional nutritional intervention, resulting in a gradual decline in bodily functions. The loss of muscle mass and malnutrition are common conditions found in cancer patients, with an incidence ranging from 25% to 60% depending on the type of cancer, stage of disease, and type of treatment [1]. The low muscle mass represents one of the criteria for malnutrition diagnosis according to Global Leadership Initiative on Malnutrition (GLIM) guidelines [2]. Despite affecting about half of patients at diagnosis as described in the PreMIO observational study conducted on over 1000 patients suffering from different solid tumors [3], malnutrition is often underestimated and not fully considered by urogenital oncologists. Standardization of the sarcopenia definition is an urgent issue in oncology [4] indeed no screening tests to assess sarcopenia and/or the risk of malnutrition are usually requested at disease diagnosis. Cachexia has been shown to be a significant poor prognostic factor for relapse-free survival of patients affected with urothelial tumors. [5] Currently, there is no standard method for diagnosing sarcopenia in genitourinary tumor [6] patients, particularly for urothelial tumors, [7] differently from other diagnostic procedures [8–13]. A Computed Tomography (CT)-based imaging for the assessment of muscle mass is a very accurate tool for the detection of sarcopenia in oncological patients. However, the need of tracing manually the muscle groups to calculate body composition parameters is a costly and time-consuming limitation [14]. On the other hand, the development and progressive implementation of a dedicated CT imaging-based artificial intelligence (AI)-powered software has allowed for automated quantification of muscle mass by assessing skeletal muscle cross-sectional area (SMA) at the level of the third lumbar vertebra (L3), providing an ease calculation of another key body composition variable, the skeletal muscle index (SMI) obtained by normalizing the SMA to the patient's height (m^2) [15]. Indeed, AI gives an opportunity to automate the process of sarcopenia assessment [16], providing meaningful clinical measurements that can be considered independent imaging biomarkers for overall survival, as it is carried out for other tumors [17]. Based on the hypothesis that sarcopenia is associated with poorer patients' oncological outcomes, the objective of the study was to verify if sarcopenia, evaluated using a CT-based AI-powered software, can predict objective clinical benefit in terms of tumor response rate to systemic chemotherapy, for advanced urothelial tumors. Additionally, the study aimed, as a secondary endpoint, to establish a correlation between sarcopenia and cancer outcomes.

2. Materials and Methods

2.1. Study Design

This was a retrospective single-center observational study that received formal approval from the Institutional Review Board, with a waiver of informed consent. The study was conducted in accordance with the guidelines for good clinical practice with ethical principles as reported in the latest version of the Declaration of Helsinki.

The medical records data were collected for 97 patients with a histologically confirmed diagnosis of urothelial tumors before the initiation and after 4–6 cycles of chemotherapy (at the first oncological reassessment) from January 2018 to January 2021 at our institution. The data collected included gender, age, height, weight, body mass index, number of drugs taken (not related to cancer treatment), ECOG Performance Status (PS), and clinical- and radiological stages.

Inclusion criteria were the following: age > 18 years, diagnosis of advanced urothelial tumor, availability of CT scan before and after treatment, and follow-up of at least 60 months.

Exclusion criteria were as follows: Patients with a life expectancy lower than 3 months or affected by any chronic inflammatory pathology in active status, with no long-term clinical information available, unsuitable for chemotherapy treatment, or with any contraindication to perform CT examinations.

As per institutional protocols, the staging CT scans were performed at both baselines and after 6 months of treatment.

2.2. Image Acquisition and Analysis

Images were acquired on a multidetector CT scanner (Somatom Sensation 64; Siemens Healthineers, Erlangen, Germany). Scanning parameters were as follows: tube voltage, 120 kVp; tube current, 100–250 mAs; pitch, 1.2; and collimation, 0.625–0.75 mm. Images were reconstructed using a 1-mm slice thickness on axial, coronal, and sagittal planes, using both soft tissue kernel (B31f) and lung kernel (B75f) reconstruction.

The CT acquisition protocol used was the standard for urothelial tumors and it included: A pre-contrast phase, a corticomedullary phase (data acquisition 25–35 s after contrast media injection); a nephrographic phase (80–100 s); an excretory phase (10–16 min).

The Quantib body composition® software (Rotterdam, Netherlands) was used to measure body composition quantitatively [18]. This software analyzed CT images of patients taken during staging CT examinations stored in our institutional picture archiving and communication system (PACS) selecting just the non-contrast phase. The software focused on the L3 vertebral body level and automatically segmented the images to determine the areas of the abdominal, psoas, and long spine muscles. Finally, the software generated in a few minutes a form displaying the relevant values, as shown in Figure 1.

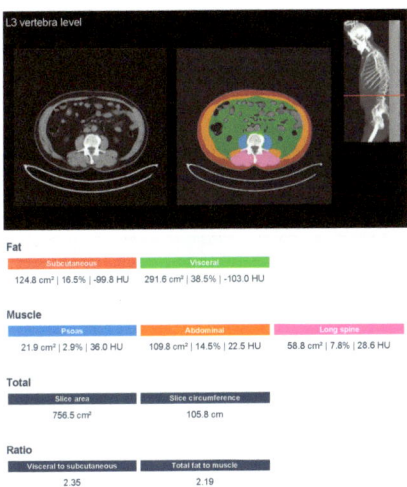

Figure 1. Case example of the automatic segmentation performed by the software at the level of the third lumbar vertebra.

Manual corrections were not made, and patients with grossly incorrect segmentations were excluded from the study. There was no specific definition for what constituted an incorrect segmentation; all segmentations were considered either of high quality or had only a small portion of the muscle volume accurately delineated. Minor errors were permitted without any additional correction.

2.3. Sarcopenia and Response to Therapy Definition

The SMA was obtained by summing the muscle areas of the psoas muscle, abdominal muscle, and long spine muscle.

The SMI was obtained by normalizing the SMA by the patients' squared height. According to the literature, an SMI cut-off value for the sarcopenia definition was set at <55 cm^2/m^2 for men and <39 cm^2/m^2 for women [19]. The body mass index (BMI) was calculated as generally obtained (weight/height^2) before and after therapy.

The RECIST 1.1 criteria [20] were used to identify and classify patients' responses to therapy. Complete response (CR) was defined as the disappearance of all target lesions for a period of at least one month; partial response (PR) as at least a 30% decrease in the sum of the maximum diameter of target lesions, taking as reference the baseline sum of the longest diameter (LD); stable disease (SD) as neither sufficient shrinkage to qualify for PR nor sufficient increase to qualify for PD, taking as reference the smallest sum LD since the treatment started; progressive disease (PD) as at least a 20% increase in the sum of the LD of target lesions, taking as reference the smallest sum LD recorded since the treatment started or the appearance of one or more new lesions. Overall survival (OS) was defined as the time between diagnosis and last contact or date of death. Clinical benefit rate (CBR) was defined as the percentage of advanced-stage patients who achieve complete response, partial response, or at least six months of stable disease as a result of therapy [21].

2.4. Statistical Analysis

Statistical analyses along with reporting and interpretation of the results were conducted according to the previously described methodology [22] and consisted of four separate analytical steps [23,24].

Initially, descriptive statistics were used to summarize pertinent study information. The association between sarcopenia and clinical variables was tested by Fisher's exact test or Mann–Whitney U test.

Second, a set of regression analyses was performed to assess the initial degree of correlation between CT scan AI-based Quantib Body Composition® SMI-L3 and each single anthropomorphic sarcopenia-related measures (i.e., CT-defined subcutaneous and visceral fat as well as psoas, abdominal and long spine muscle). This was tested both at baseline and repeated with the same data after the first cycle of systemic chemotherapy administration. Moreover, a multivariable linear regression model was developed including those clinic-demographic and tumor-related features commonly associated with clinical and survival outcomes (i.e., age at diagnosis, gender, ECOG performance status, number of medications taken unrelated to cancer therapy, as well as tumor location and stage) in order to identify which association was more significantly correlated with the computed SMI-L3 and the sarcopenia pre-established cut-off criteria [25].

Third, the clinical benefit outcome measured at the end of the systemic therapy was defined by the presence of partial/complete radiological response (RaR) as well as the confirmation of the stable disease in contrast with the documented progression of advanced urothelial carcinomas. Given the known association of sarcopenia status with male or female gender, a set of bivariable logistic regression was modeled between each computed sarcopenia-related feature adjusted for gender status and the dichotomized clinical benefit outcome. Additionally, a multivariable logistic model by clinical and demographic confounders was further performed to identify sarcopenia-related predictors independently associated with clinical benefit endpoint.

As the fourth analytic step, we investigated the association of SMI-L3 both as a continuous and dichotomized covariate with OS using univariable Cox regression analysis. Univariable survival estimates were plotted using the Kaplan–Meier method. The log-rank test was used to assess the difference in OS between sub-groups. A multivariate Cox proportional hazards model was also developed by adjusting for previously mentioned confounders also associated with survival outcomes. Finally, sarcopenia status variation as a function SMI-L3 variation (Δ_SMI-L3) as well as any AI-computed subcutaneous/visceral fat or muscular anthropometric variations were forced, using locally weighted scatter plot smoother (LOWESS) function, against the multivariable-adjusted predicted probability models for clinical benefit and survival assessment. This was meant to graphically depict the influence of body composition variations on the pre-established endpoints at the moment of primary disease diagnosis. Statistical analysis was performed using Stata version 17.1 (Stata Corporation, College Station, TX, USA) with statistical significance set as $p < 0.05$.

3. Results

3.1. Demographic, Tumor- and Sarcopenia-Related Characteristics of the Study Population

We retrospectively reviewed the medical records of 97 patients with a histologically confirmed diagnosis of an advanced urothelial tumor of the upper urinary tract (33; 34.1%) (Figure 2) and urothelial tumor of the urinary bladder (64; 65.9%) (Figure 2) [26].

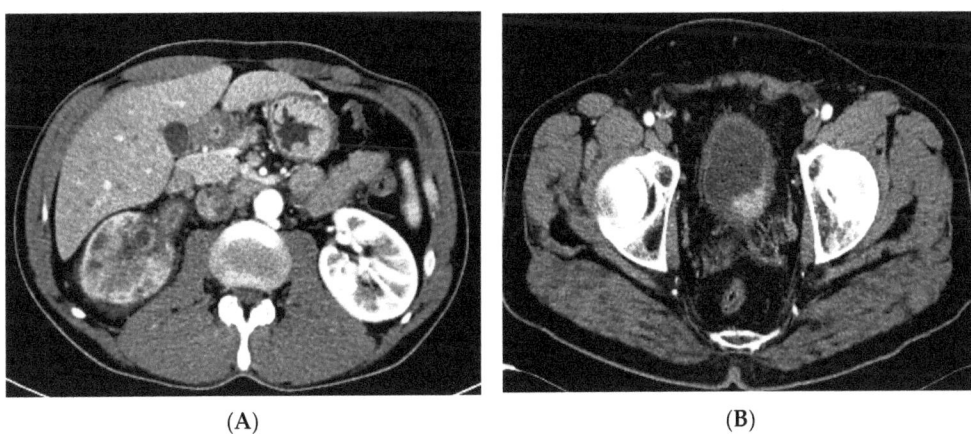

(A)　　　　　　　　　　　　　　　(B)

Figure 2. (**A**) Computed tomography (CT) image of a 75-year-old men with advanced right Upper Tract Urothelial Tumor (SMI value = 40.54 cm^2/m^2; (**B**) CT image of 72-year-old men with advanced Bladder Tumor on left posterior wall. (SMI value = 44.86 cm^2/m^2).

The median age of non-sarcopenic vs. sarcopenic patients was 73 (Interquartile range [IQR], 64–76) vs. 69 (IQR, 64–74) before and 73 (IQR, 66–76) vs. 68 years (IQR, 64–74) after therapy.

There were no differences in the distribution of the clinical and demographical factors among the non-sarcopenic and sarcopenic patients both at baseline and after therapy.

The SMI-L3 variable (cm^2/m^2), as well as the additional variables, were significantly different before and after therapy ($p < 0.001$) (Table 1).

Table 1. Patients' population demographic characteristics and disease outcome according to the body composition status at baseline and after systemic chemotherapy.

Variables	No Sarcopenic Status, Baseline (By SMI-L3 Cut-Off)	Sarcopenic Status, Baseline (By SMI-L3 Cut-Off)	*p*-Value *	No SARCOPENIC Status, after CHT (By SMI-L3 Cut-Off)	Sarcopenic Status, after CHT (By SMI-L3 Cut-Off)	*p*-Value *
Sample size, n (%)	46 (47.4)	51 (52.6)		45 (46.4)	52 (53.6)	
		Demographics and tumor-related features				
Age y, median (IQR)	73 (64–76)	69 (64–74)	0.414	73 (66–76)	68 (64–74)	0.126
Age y, n (%)						
<70 y	19 (41.3)	30 (58.8)	0.105	17 (37.8)	32 (61.5)	0.025
≥70 y	27 (58.7)	21 (42.2)		28 (62.2)	20 (38.5)	
Gender, n (%)						
Male	36 (78.3)	34 (66.7)	0.259	11 (24.4)	16 (30.8)	0.506
Female	10 (27.7)	17 (33.3)		34 (75.6)	36 (69.2)	

Table 1. Cont.

Variables	No Sarcopenic Status, Baseline (By SMI-L3 Cut-Off)	Sarcopenic Status, Baseline (By SMI-L3 Cut-Off)	p-Value *	No SARCOPENIC Status, after CHT (By SMI-L3 Cut-Off)	Sarcopenic Status, after CHT (By SMI-L3 Cut-Off)	p-Value *
ECOG PS, n (%)						
<2	39 (84.8)	40 (78.4)	0.447	38 (84.4)	41 (78.8)	0.603
≥2	7 (15.2)	11 (21.6)		7 (15.6)	11 (21.2)	
n. of Medications, n (%)						
<6	36 (78.3)	42 (82.4)	0.620	34 (75.6)	44 (84.6)	0.311
≥6	10 (21.7)	9 (17.6)		11 (24.4)	8 (15.4)	
Primary location n (%)						
BCa	24 (52.2)	37 (72.5)	0.049	24 (53.3)	37 (71.2)	0.096
UTUC	21 (45.7)	12 (23.5)		20 (44.4)	13 (25.0)	
Concomitant	1 (2.2)	2 (3.9)		1 (2.2)	2 (3.8)	
Oncologic stage, n (%)						
III	22 (47.8)	17 (33.3)	0.155	22 (48.9)	17 (32.7)	0.146
IV	24 (52.2)	34 (66.7)		23 (51.1)	35 (67.3)	
Anthropometric measures						
Height, m	1.70 (1.66–1.75)	1.70 (1.62–1.75)	0.753	1.70 (1.64–1.73)	1.70 (1.64–1.75)	0.677
Weight, kg	77 (70–85.25)	70 (60–75)	0.001	77 (70–80.25)	70 (60–80)	0.005
BMI, kg/m^2	26.3 (24.85–27.75)	24.2 (21.9–26.5)	0.001	26.3 (25.3–29.3)	23.5 (21.7–26.4)	0.007
SMA, cm^2	179.7 (167.8–194)	135.8 (114.8–155.2)	<0.0001	173.1 (157.2–193)	133.7 (116–154.4)	<0.0001
SMI-L3, (cm^2/m^2)	62 (57.8–67.1)	48.6 (43.1–53)	<0.0001	59.9 (57.3–63.8)	47.9 (43.4–50.9)	<0.0001
Subcutaneous fat, (cm^2/m^2)	184.2 (133.6–221.8)	135.2 (108.4–178.6)	0.003	178.7 (130.7–215.1)	143.1 (108.4–183.2)	0.002
Visceral fat, (cm^2/m^2)	207 (153.7–255.7)	103 (67.9–175.7)	<0.0001	182.6 (140–218.4)	137 (64.5–181.6)	<0.0001
Psoas muscle, (cm^2/m^2)	21.7 (19.4–24.6)	16.5 (13.3–20)	<0.0001	20.8 (18–22.8)	16.1 (13.5–19)	<0.0001
Abdominal muscle, (cm^2/m^2)	100.6 (89.6–109.2)	71.5 (59.1–82.2)	<0.0001	93.4 (86.6–106.9)	71.6 (59.7–80.9)	<0.0001
Long spine muscle, (cm^2/m^2)	60.3 (54.8–64.1)	45.5 (40.8–55)	<0.0001	57.9 (51.4–62.8)	46.4 (40.7–55.2)	<0.0001
Δ_SMI-L3, mean (SD)	−1.86 (5.78)					
Δ_Subcutaneous fat mean (SD)	0.25 (24.93)					
Δ_Visceral fat, mean (SD)	−4.93 (42.17)					
Δ_ Psoas muscle, mean (SD)	−0.85 (2.56)					
Δ_ Abdominal muscle, mean (SD)	−3.02 (10.74)					

Table 1. Cont.

Variables	No Sarcopenic Status, Baseline (By SMI-L3 Cut-Off)	Sarcopenic Status, Baseline (By SMI-L3 Cut-Off)	p-Value *	No SARCOPENIC Status, after CHT (By SMI-L3 Cut-Off)	Sarcopenic Status, after CHT (By SMI-L3 Cut-Off)	p-Value *
Δ_ Long spine muscle, mean (SD)	−1.06 (3.39)					
Clinical outcomes						
Clinical Benefit, n (%)						
SD/PR/CR	30 (65.2)	25 (49)	0.151	29 (64.4)	26 (50.0)	0.217
PD	16 (34.8)	26 (51)		16 (35.6)	26 (50.0)	
Survival n (%)						
Deceased	37 (80.4)	23 (45.1)	0.001	35 (77.8)	25 (48.1)	0.003
Survivors	9 (19.6)	28 (54.9)		10 (22.2)	27 (51.9)	

* p-values according to Fisher's Exact test or Mann-Whitney U test when appropriate (bold p-value means that it is statistically significant). CHT, chemotherapy; PS, performance status; BCa, bladder cancer; UTUC, Upper tract Urothelial Carcinoma; BMI, body mass index; SMA, skeletal muscle area; SMI, skeletal muscle mass index; SD, stable disease; PR, partial response; CR, complete response; PD, progression disease.

3.2. Correlation between AI Skeletal Muscle Index (SMI-L3) and Anthropomorphic Sarcopenia-Related Variables Pre-/Post-Systemic Treatment

At baseline, out of 97 patients, 34 (66.7%) males and 17 (33.3%) females met the definition criteria calibrated on the CT-defined AI software SMI-L3 and were considered as affected by sarcopenic status.

At univariable linear regression modeling, we found an increasingly positive and constant association between SMI-L3 and each anthropometric sarcopenia-related feature. The coefficient correlation of determination (r^2) was especially relevant when assessing SMI-L3 and the abdominal muscle area (r^2: 0.726, d.f.: 95, value: 0.450, 95% CI: 0.394–0.507, p < 0.0001), followed by the long spine and psoas area (r^2: 0.599, d.f.: 95, value: 0.740, 95% CI: 0.617–0.863, p < 0.0001 and r^2: 0.463, d.f.: 95, value: 1.471, 95% CI:1.149 –1.794, p < 0.0001). At multivariable linear regression, the goodness of fit statistics for the SMI-L3 model reached the highest degree of correlation (r^2: 0.857) and the correlations were confirmed with the visceral fat area as well as with the psoas, long spine, and abdominal muscle area (cm^2/m^2) independently from demographic and clinical confounders (Figure S1A,B).

After the first cycle of systemic therapy administration, the observed correlations remained stable and highly significant at both unilinear regression with the muscle-skeletal components (i.e., abdominal, psoas, and long spine muscle area [cm^2/m^2]) reaching the highest degree of correlation with SMI-L3 also when adjusted with clinic confounders (r^2: 0.874) (Figure 2A,B).

3.3. Baseline and Early Predictors of Clinical Benefit Measured at the Completion of Systemic Therapy

In total, all patients received a median number of 5 cycles of platinum-based chemotherapy which was mainly represented by Gemcitabine plus Cisplatin (GC) (53, 54.6%) or Carboplatin (44, 45.4%) for patients with renal insufficiency or frailty. The CT scan performed after 4–6 cycles, at the first oncological reassessment, revealed that the overall number of subjects with SMI-L3 defined sarcopenia status was 52 (53.6%). Among these, sarcopenic patients who exhibited disease progression were 26 (50%) while the remaining was associated with both complete/partial RaR (26, 50%). Among the non-sarcopenic group, after chemotherapy, 16 (35.6%) had progression of disease while 29 (64.4%) had complete/partial response. At univariable logistic regression adjusted by gender, baseline predictors for clinical benefit outcomes were represented by the sole abdominal, psoas muscle area, and subcutaneous fat area (aOR: 0.97, 95% CI: 0.95–0.99, aOR: 0.90, 95% CI: 0.82–0.99 and aOR: 0.99, 95% CI: 0.98–1, respectively). However, although not statistically significant, both SMI-L3 and its derived sarcopenia-related cut-off demonstrated an overlapping trend toward significance in line with the other individual aforementioned predictors (aOR: 0.96, 95% CI: 0.92–1.1 and aOR: 2.33, 95% CI: 0.99–5.52) (Table S1A). Notably, at this baseline assessment, none of these anthropometric features resulted independently able to induce relevant clinical benefit outcomes except from some expected clinical variables. Interestingly, after the first oncological reassessment of disease sarcopenic status both by SMI-L3 coefficient and its standardized cut-off, was found independently predicting clinical benefits (OR: 0.93, 95% CI: 0.88–0.98 and OR: 2.31, 95% CI: 1.15–5.78) (Table S1B). Finally, the trajectory of the LOWESS functions depicting the predicted probability for RaR clinical benefit outcomes showed an almost linear positive association with all the observed body composition variables variations between pre-/post-systemic treatment. (Figure 3). This was especially true for Δ_SMI-L3 (Figure 3A) and Δ_psoas (Figure 3C) and Δ_long spine muscle area (cm^2/m^2) (Figure 3F) where the chances of not experiencing disease progression increased from the ~10–20% up to ~45–55%.

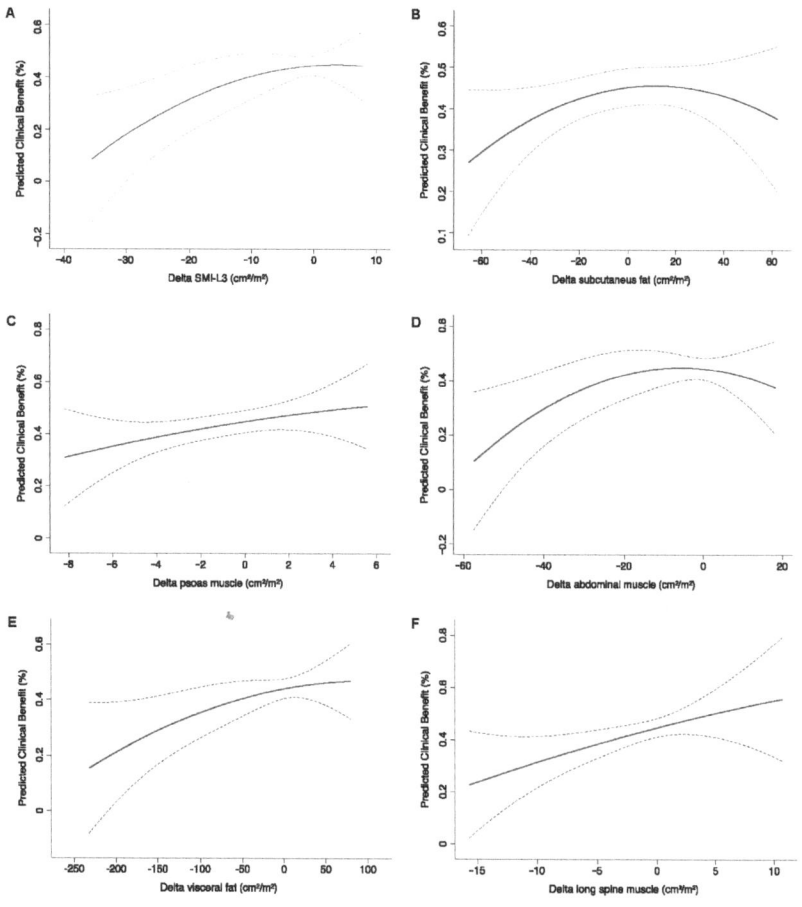

Figure 3. LOWESS functions depicting the predicted probability for RaR clinical benefit outcomes (**A–F**).

3.4. Baseline and Early Determinates for Overall Survival

Within a median follow-up time of 17.43 months (IQR 1.6–80.9), months, 37 (38.1%) subjects were deceased by any cause. In the sarcopenic cohort, 28 patients (75.8%) were recorded as having passed away, while 9 patients (24.3%) were recognized as survivors. SMI-L3 variation (Δ-SMI-L3) was significantly discordant across the two sub-groups ranging from a median value of −1.857 (standard deviation [SD] 5.784), respectively. The univariable effect of sarcopenia and other subgroups on OS has been depicted in Kaplan–Meier plots shown in Figure 4.

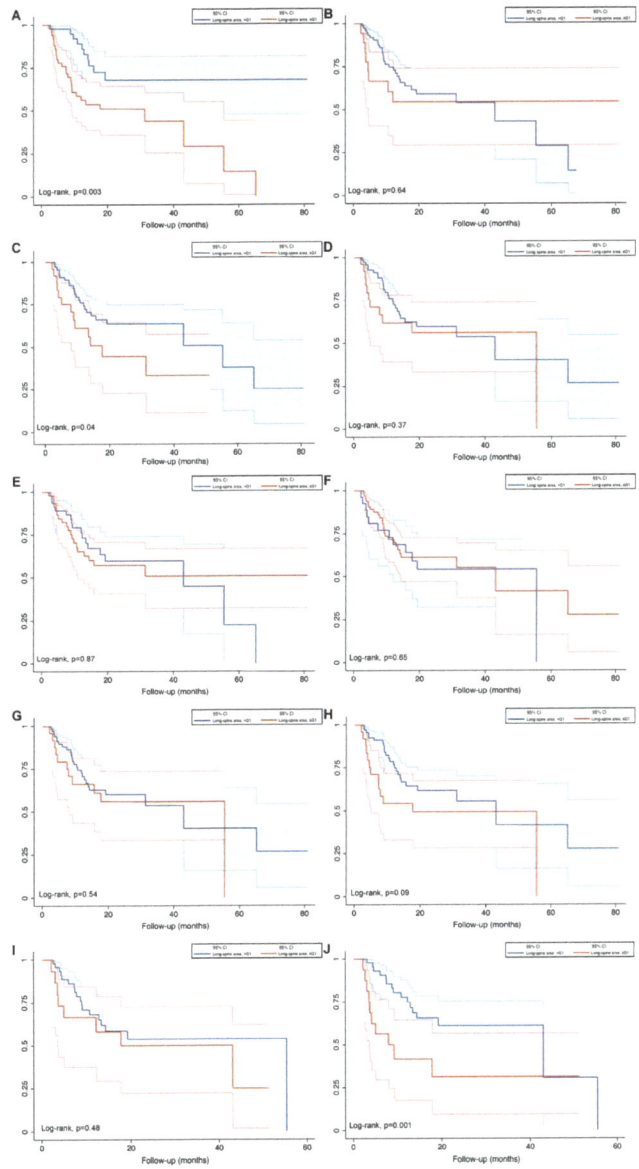

Figure 4. The effect of sarcopenia on OS depicted by Kaplan-Meier plots (**A–J**).

As expected, at univariable Cox regression modeling before and after chemotherapy, higher registered values of sarcopenic and anthropometric measures had been associated with reduced OS. This was also independently true at multivariable assessment for SMI-L3 and the subsequent sarcopenia definition at baseline (HR: 0.95, 95% CI: 0.92–0.99 and HR: 3.80, 95% CI: 1.72–8.41) (Table S2A). and after the first cycle of therapy (HR: 0.94, 95% CI: 0.91–0.98 and HR: 3.29, 95% CI: 1.51–7.17) (Table S2B).

Moreover, when implementing the LOWESS function to model Δ-SMI-L3 on the predicted survival probability derived from the multivariable Cox regression model (Figure 5), greater survival chances were matched by those patients achieving wider Δ_SMI-L3 over the course of follow-up (10–20% vs. 50–60%) (Figure 5A). This was noted especially for Δ_abdominal (Figure 5D) and long spine muscle area (Figure 5F) (cm^2/m^2) which varied from ~20–30% up to ~50–55% when a consistent muscular mass was gained.

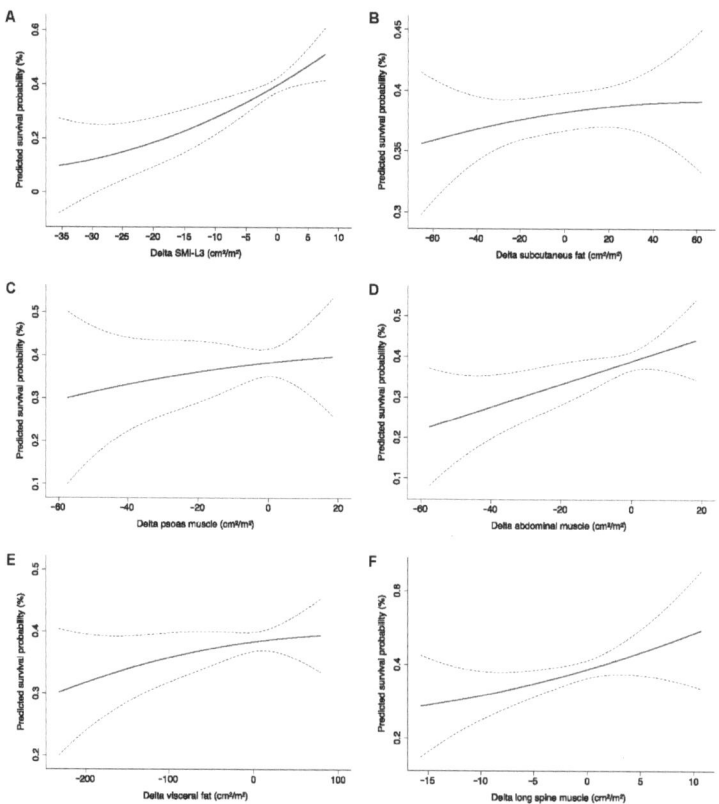

Figure 5. LOWESS function to model Δ-SMI-L3 for the predicted survival probability derived from multivariable Cox regression model (**A–F**).

4. Discussion

Accurate prediction of individual cancer patient's response to chemotherapy remains a goal in the field of oncology.

The development of sarcopenia is a result of tumor progression and systemic inflammation caused by the tumor, so its presence indicates tumor aggressiveness. In addition, sarcopenic patients are characterized by poor general health and physical performance, which can contribute to a worse prognosis for cancer-bearing patients. The effectiveness of sarcopenia as a prognostic biomarker can be attributed to its distinctive hybrid nature [27].

Several studies have investigated the association between sarcopenia, assessed by AI tools and oncological outcomes, [28]; including patients with breast, [29] gastric [30], endometrial [31] and cervical cancer [32]. Focusing on genitourinary tumors [33], Wu et al. (2019) [34] used transfer learning to train a convolutional neural network (CNN) model on a then expanded dataset of pre- and post-treatment CT scans of 123 bladder cancer patients undergoing neoadjuvant chemotherapy; in another study [35] sarcopenia in metastatic renal carcinoma, according to SMI thresholds after segmentation by the deep learning algorithm, had statistically significant correlation with lower overall survival compared to non-sarcopenic patients [36].

However, to date, there are no studies that have analyzed sarcopenia in advanced urothelial tumors through artificial intelligence software. In this setting, our primary endpoint was to confirm the role of sarcopenia, assessed using a CT based AI-powered software, as a prognostic predictor of objective clinical benefit in terms of tumor response rate to systemic therapy, in advanced urothelial tumors and correlate sarcopenia status with oncological outcomes. As anticipated, we discovered a strong connection between sarcopenia and aging, which is widely recognized as a current health concern among older adults [37,38]. Our results also showed that the number of drugs taken (unrelated to the cancer treatment) and consequently the presence of comorbidities in patients were not statistically significant factors. This finding is in contrast with previous research; Pacifico et al. [39] in a systematic review discovered that individuals with multiple comorbidities, such as cardiovascular diseases, dementia, diabetes [40], and respiratory diseases, had the highest prevalence of sarcopenia [41]. Our outcome is likely a result of the insignificant impact of comorbidities on the sarcopenia status of patients who have advanced cancer.

In this study we found that sarcopenia, assessed by the CT-based AI-powered software is a negative prognostic factor in advanced urothelial cancers; indeed, overall survival was significantly different between the sarcopenic and non-sarcopenic groups. Our data are in line with Yumioka's and Shimizu's studies, which demonstrated how sarcopenia is a predictive factor of overall survival in patients affected by urothelial carcinoma and treated with gemcitabine and cis-/carbo-platin [42,43]. Results also confirm recent findings concerning the association of sarcopenia in patients affected by genitourinary tumors and oncologic outcomes [44]. Specifically, sarcopenia has been correlated to a worse prognosis in patients with urothelial carcinoma, including muscle-invasive bladder cancer [45,46] and upper tract urothelial carcinoma by Fukushima et al. in a systematic review of the literature [27]. The findings on genitourinary tumors align with those from systematic reviews and meta-analyses on other types of tumors. It has been shown that pre-treatment sarcopenia is a separate risk factor for both lower overall survival and decreased compliance with adjuvant therapies in pancreatic [47], gastrointestinal [48,49], breast [50], gynecological [51], and hematological [52] cancers. In these prior studies, the presence of sarcopenia was evaluated using commonly accepted methods, such as manually tracing the areas of all muscle groups on CT scans.

It is important to mention that other anthropometric measurements may not be reliable. Indeed, using BMI alone to assess obesity and evaluate outcomes and prognosis in cancer patients is inaccurate since it cannot distinguish between fat and lean mass or between visceral and subcutaneous fat [53].

Although traditional methods of evaluating body composition, such as anthropomorphic measurements, bioelectrical impedance, and dual-energy X-ray absorptiometry, have some drawbacks, computed tomography and magnetic resonance imaging are the benchmark techniques for analyzing body composition. Nevertheless, also these imaging methods demand manual segmentation by an expert reader, which is a time-consuming and labor-intensive task. Consequently, their application in large-scale studies and regular clinical practice is limited [54].

In the present study, we found that integrating a fully automated AI-powered tool into radiological practice, provides an opportunity for innovation to effectively investigate sarcopenia status facilitating the detection of muscle loss and it allows to reduce operator-dependent bias of segmentation in the set of scans routinely acquired for staging and follow-up purposes.

The ability of AI models to analyze large sets of data and extract high-level abstractions beyond manual skills provides impactful information and greatly refines the standard for assessing the risk of muscle depletion in patients with urogenital cancers [55,56] as well as in non-oncological and pediatric patients [57].

This study has several limitations, including its retrospective design and small sample size. Another limitation is the lack of correlation with the patient's nutritional status. Furthermore, this study, like the other retrospective studies previously described, was not designed to show whether sarcopenia is treatable.

Even though our work is focused on advanced-stage urothelial tumors treated with platinum-based systemic chemotherapy, it would be interesting to evaluate how body composition affects other subtypes of urogenital tumors treated with different therapeutic regimens. Finally, the AI tool's performance was not compared to manual muscle area segmentation, as the accuracy of the method has already been established in other studies [58].

Despite its limitations, this study marks the first use of CT AI-based body composition measurement in patients with advanced urothelial tumors. Our findings, supported by further evidence, could lead to the development of standardized pathways that link the radiological staging of cancers with sarcopenia assessment and personalized nutritional therapy. This has the potential to enhance both quality of life and cancer outcomes.

5. Conclusions

The utilization of an easy-to-use CT-based AI tool allowed us to assess the sarcopenia status of patients with advanced urothelial tumors. Indeed, routine CT scans represented an important imaging biomarker on body composition status, which correlated with poorer oncological outcomes. The AI tool can represent a means to increase the clinical value of CT imaging reports and to promote the implementation of precision medicine [59].

Supplementary Materials: The following supporting information can be downloaded at: https://www.mdpi.com/article/10.3390/cancers15112968/s1, Figure S1: Univariable linear regression plots depicting AI-based Quantib Body Composition® Skeletal Muscle Index (SMI-L3) and anthropomorphic sarcopenia-related variables at baseline (A). Multivariable linear regression model assessing SMI-L3, clinic-demographic and anthropomorphic sarcopenia-related variables at baseline (B). Figure S2: Univariable linear regression plots depicting AI-based Quantib Body Composition® Skeletal Muscle Index (SMI-L3) and anthropomorphic sarcopenia-related variables after fist therapy cycle (A). Multivariable linear regression model assessing SMI-L3, clinic-demographic and anthropomorphic sarcopenia-related variables after fist therapy cycle (B). Table S1: Bivariable and Multivariable adjusted Cox regression modeling for anthropometric measures assessing the Odds Ratio for overall survival at baseline (A) and post-systemic treatment (B). Table S2: Bivariable and Multivariable adjusted Cox regression modeling for anthropometric measures assessing the hazard for overall survival at baseline (A) and post-systemic treatment (B).

Author Contributions: Conceptualization, A.B.; Methodology, M.P.; Formal analysis, M.P. and F.D.G.; Resources, A.D.; Data curation, L.C., E.M. and M.R.; Writing—original draft, A.B. and F.D.G.; Writing—review & editing, M.P., N.L., S.P., M.M., D.S. and C.C.; Supervision, V.P. All authors have read and agreed to the published version of the manuscript.

Funding: This research received no external funding.

Institutional Review Board Statement: Ethical review and approval were waived for this study due to its retrospective design.

Informed Consent Statement: Informed consent was obtained from all subjects involved in the study.

Data Availability Statement: The data presented in this study are available upon request from the corresponding author. The data are not publicly available due to restrictions.

Conflicts of Interest: The authors declare no conflict of interest.

References

1. Muscaritoli, M.; Lucia, S.; Farcomeni, A.; Lorusso, V.; Saracino, V.; Barone, C.; Plastino, F.; Gori, S.; Magarotto, R.; Carteni, G.; et al. Prevalence of malnutrition in patients at first medical oncology visit: The PreMiO study. *Oncotarget* 2017, *8*, 79884–79896. [CrossRef] [PubMed]
2. Cederholm, T.; Jensen, G.L.; Correia, M.; Gonzalez, M.C.; Fukushima, R.; Higashiguchi, T.; Baptista, G.; Barazzoni, R.; Blaauw, R.; Coats, A.J.S.; et al. GLIM criteria for the diagnosis of malnutrition—A consensus report from the global clinical nutrition community. *J. Cachexia Sarcopenia Muscle* 2019, *10*, 207–217. [CrossRef]
3. Serinelli, S.; Panebianco, V.; Martino, M.; Battisti, S.; Rodacki, K.; Marinelli, E.; Zaccagna, F.; Semelka, R.C.; Tomei, E. Accuracy of MRI skeletal age estimation for subjects 12–19. Potential use for subjects of unknown age. *Int. J. Legal Med.* 2015, *129*, 609–617. [CrossRef] [PubMed]
4. Taguchi, S.; Nakagawa, T.; Uemura, Y.; Akamatsu, N.; Gonoi, W.; Naito, A.; Kawai, T.; Kume, H.; Fukuhara, H. Comparison of major definitions of sarcopenia based on the skeletal muscle index in patients with urothelial carcinoma. *Future Oncol.* 2021, *17*, 197–203. [CrossRef] [PubMed]
5. Chen, H.-W.; Chen, Y.-C.; Yang, L.-H.; Shih, M.-C.P.; Li, C.-C.; Chueh, K.-S.; Wu, W.-J.; Juan, Y.-S. Impact of cachexia on oncologic outcomes of sarcopenic patients with upper tract urothelial carcinoma after radical nephroureterectomy. *PLoS ONE* 2021, *16*, e0250033. [CrossRef]
6. Richenberg, J.; Løgager, V.; Panebianco, V.; Rouviere, O.; Villeirs, G.; Schoots, I.G. The primacy of multiparametric MRI in men with suspected prostate cancer. *Eur. Radiol.* 2019, *29*, 6940–6952. [CrossRef]
7. Ferro, M.; Babă, D.-F.; de Cobelli, O.; Musi, G.; Lucarelli, G.; Terracciano, D.; Porreca, A.; Busetto, G.M.; Del Giudice, F.; Soria, F.; et al. Neutrophil percentage-to-albumin ratio predicts mortality in bladder cancer patients treated with neoadjuvant chemotherapy followed by radical cystectomy. *Future Sci. OA* 2021, *7*, FSO709. [CrossRef]
8. Maggi, M.; Panebianco, V.; Mosca, A.; Salciccia, S.; Gentilucci, A.; Di Pierro, G.; Busetto, G.M.; Barchetti, G.; Campa, R.; Sperduti, I.; et al. Prostate Imaging Reporting and Data System 3 Category Cases at Multiparametric Magnetic Resonance for Prostate Cancer: A Systematic Review and Meta-analysis. *Eur. Urol. Focus* 2020, *6*, 463–478. [CrossRef]
9. Panebianco, V.; Sciarra, A.; Marcantonio, A.; Forte, V.; Biondi, T.; Laghi, A.; Catalano, C. Conventional imaging and multiparametric magnetic resonance (MRI, MRS, DWI, MRP) in the diagnosis of prostate cancer. *Q. J. Nucl. Med. Mol. Imaging* 2012, *56*, 331–342.
10. Sciarra, A.; Panebianco, V.; Ciccariello, M.; Salciccia, S.; Lisi, D.; Osimani, M.; Alfarone, A.; Gentilucci, A.; Parente, U.; Passariello, R.; et al. Magnetic Resonance Spectroscopic Imaging (^{1}H-MRSI) and Dynamic Contrast-Enhanced Magnetic Resonance (DCE-MRI): Pattern Changes from Inflammation to Prostate Cancer. *Cancer Investig.* 2010, *28*, 424–432. [CrossRef]
11. Pavone, P.; Laghi, A.; Panebianco, V.; Catalano, C.; Lobina, L.; Passariello, R. MR cholangiography: Techniques and clinical applications. *Eur. Radiol.* 1998, *8*, 901–910. [CrossRef] [PubMed]
12. Di Silverio, F.; Sciarra, A.; Parente, U.; Andrea, A.; Von Heland, M.; Panebianco, V.; Passariello, R. Neoadjuvant Therapy with Sorafenib in Advanced Renal Cell Carcinoma with Vena Cava Extension Submitted to Radical Nephrectomy. *Urol. Int.* 2008, *80*, 451–453. [CrossRef] [PubMed]
13. Sciarra, A.; Panebianco, V.; Cattarino, S.; Busetto, G.M.; De Berardinis, E.; Ciccariello, M.; Gentile, V.; Salciccia, S. Multiparametric magnetic resonance imaging of the prostate can improve the predictive value of the urinary prostate cancer antigen 3 test in patients with elevated prostate-specific antigen levels and a previous negative biopsy. *BJU Int.* 2012, *110*, 1661–1665. [CrossRef] [PubMed]
14. Mourtzakis, M.; Prado, C.M.; Lieffers, J.R.; Reiman, T.; McCargar, L.J.; Baracos, V.E. A practical and precise approach to quantification of body composition in cancer patients using computed tomography images acquired during routine care. *Appl. Physiol. Nutr. Metab.* 2008, *33*, 997–1006. [CrossRef] [PubMed]
15. Sánchez-Torralvo, F.J.; Ruiz-García, I.; Contreras-Bolívar, V.; González-Almendros, I.; Ruiz-Vico, M.; Abuín-Fernández, J.; Barrios, M.; Alba, E.; Olveira, G. CT-Determined Sarcopenia in GLIM-Defined Malnutrition and Prediction of 6-Month Mortality in Cancer Inpatients. *Nutrients* 2021, *13*, 2647. [CrossRef] [PubMed]
16. Bedrikovetski, S.; Seow, W.; Kroon, H.M.; Traeger, L.; Moore, J.W.; Sammour, T. Artificial intelligence for body composition and sarcopenia evaluation on computed tomography: A systematic review and meta-analysis. *Eur. J. Radiol.* 2022, *149*, 110218. [CrossRef]
17. Picchio, M.; Mapelli, P.; Panebianco, V.; Castellucci, P.; Incerti, E.; Briganti, A.; Gandaglia, G.; Kirienko, M.; Barchetti, F.; Nanni, C.; et al. Imaging biomarkers in prostate cancer: Role of PET/CT and MRI. *Eur. J. Nucl. Mol. Imaging* 2015, *42*, 644–655. [CrossRef]
18. Ha, J.; Park, T.; Kim, H.-K.; Shin, Y.; Ko, Y.; Kim, D.W.; Sung, Y.S.; Lee, J.; Ham, S.J.; Khang, S.; et al. Development of a fully automatic deep learning system for L3 selection and body composition assessment on computed tomography. *Sci. Rep.* 2021, *11*, 21656. [CrossRef]
19. Fearon, K.; Strasser, F.; Anker, S.D.; Bosaeus, I.; Bruera, E.; Fainsinger, R.L.; Jatoi, A.; Loprinzi, C.; MacDonald, N.; Mantovani, G.; et al. Definition and classification of cancer cachexia: An international consensus. *Lancet Oncol.* 2011, *12*, 489–495. [CrossRef]
20. Eisenhauer, E.A.; Therasse, P.; Bogaerts, J.; Schwartz, L.H.; Sargent, D.; Ford, R.; Dancey, J.; Arbuck, S.; Gwyther, S.; Mooney, M.; et al. New response evaluation criteria in solid tumours: Revised RECIST guideline (version 1.1). *Eur. J. Cancer* 2009, *45*, 228–247. [CrossRef]

21. Delgado, A.; Guddati, A.K. Clinical endpoints in oncology—A primer. *Am. J. Cancer Res.* **2021**, *11*, 1121–1131.
22. Salciccia, S.; Del Giudice, F.; Gentile, V.; Mastroianni, C.M.; Pasculli, P.; Di Lascio, G.; Ciardi, M.R.; Sperduti, I.; Maggi, M.; De Berardinis, E.; et al. Interplay between male testosterone levels and the risk for subsequent invasive respiratory assistance among COVID-19 patients at hospital admission. *Endocrine* **2020**, *70*, 206–210. [CrossRef] [PubMed]
23. Busetto, G.M.; Giovannone, R.; Antonini, G.; Rossi, A.; Del Giudice, F.; Tricarico, S.; Ragonesi, G.; Gentile, V.; De Berardinis, E. Short-term pretreatment with a dual 5α-reductase inhibitor before bipolar transurethral resection of the prostate (B-TURP): Evaluation of prostate vascularity and decreased surgical blood loss in large prostates: Short-term treatment with dutasteride before B-TURP. *BJU Int.* **2015**, *116*, 117–123. [CrossRef] [PubMed]
24. Giovannone, R.; Busetto, G.M.; Antonini, G.; De Cobelli, O.; Ferro, M.; Tricarico, S.; Del Giudice, F.; Ragonesi, G.; Conti, S.L.; Lucarelli, G.; et al. Hyperhomocysteinemia as an Early Predictor of Erectile Dysfunction: International Index of Erectile Function (IIEF) and Penile Doppler Ultrasound Correlation with Plasma Levels of Homocysteine. *Medicine* **2015**, *94*, e1556. [CrossRef]
25. Caan, B.J.; Feliciano, E.M.C.; Prado, C.M.; Alexeeff, S.; Kroenke, C.H.; Bradshaw, P.; Quesenberry, C.P.; Weltzien, E.K.; Castillo, A.L.; Olobatuyi, T.A.; et al. Association of Muscle and Adiposity Measured by Computed Tomography with Survival in Patients with Nonmetastatic Breast Cancer. *JAMA Oncol.* **2018**, *4*, 798. [CrossRef] [PubMed]
26. Del Giudice, F.; Leonardo, C.; Simone, G.; Pecoraro, M.; De Berardinis, E.; Cipollari, S.; Flammia, S.; Bicchetti, M.; Busetto, G.M.; Chung, B.I.; et al. Preoperative detection of Vesical Imaging-Reporting and Data System (VI-RADS) score 5 reliably identifies extravesical extension of urothelial carcinoma of the urinary bladder and predicts significant delayed time to cystectomy: Time to reconsider the nee: VI-RADS score 5 may avoid deep primary TURBT. *BJU Int.* **2020**, *126*, 610–619. [CrossRef]
27. Fukushima, H.; Takemura, K.; Suzuki, H.; Koga, F. Impact of Sarcopenia as a Prognostic Biomarker of Bladder Cancer. *Int. J. Mol. Sci.* **2018**, *19*, 2999. [CrossRef]
28. Huang, Y.-T.; Tsai, Y.-S.; Lin, P.-C.; Yeh, Y.-M.; Hsu, Y.-T.; Wu, P.-Y.; Shen, M.-R. The Value of Artificial Intelligence-Assisted Imaging in Identifying Diagnostic Markers of Sarcopenia in Patients with Cancer. *Dis. Markers* **2022**, *2022*, 1819841. [CrossRef]
29. Jang, W.; Jeong, C.; Kwon, K.; Yoon, T.I.; Yi, O.; Kim, K.W.; Yang, S.-O.; Lee, J. Artificial intelligence for predicting five-year survival in stage IV metastatic breast cancer patients: A focus on sarcopenia and other host factors. *Front. Physiol.* **2022**, *13*, 977189. [CrossRef]
30. Chung, H.; Ko, Y.; Lee, I.; Hur, H.; Huh, J.; Han, S.; Kim, K.W.; Lee, J. Prognostic artificial intelligence model to predict 5 year survival at 1 year after gastric cancer surgery based on nutrition and body morphometry. *J. Cachexia Sarcopenia Muscle* **2023**, *14*, 847–859. [CrossRef]
31. Kim, S.I.; Chung, J.Y.; Paik, H.; Seol, A.; Yoon, S.H.; Kim, T.M.; Kim, H.S.; Chung, H.H.; Cho, J.Y.; Kim, J.-W.; et al. Prognostic role of computed tomography-based, artificial intelligence-driven waist skeletal muscle volume in uterine endometrial carcinoma. *Insights Imaging* **2021**, *12*, 192. [CrossRef] [PubMed]
32. Han, Q.; Kim, S.I.; Yoon, S.H.; Kim, T.M.; Kang, H.-C.; Kim, H.J.; Cho, J.Y.; Kim, J.-W. Impact of Computed Tomography-Based, Artificial Intelligence-Driven Volumetric Sarcopenia on Survival Outcomes in Early Cervical Cancer. *Front. Oncol.* **2021**, *11*, 741071. [CrossRef] [PubMed]
33. Stangl-Kremser, J.; Mari, A.; Lai, L.Y.; Lee, C.T.; Vince, R.; Zaslavsky, A.; Salami, S.S.; Fajkovic, H.; Shariat, S.F.; Palapattu, G.S. Sarcopenic Obesity and its Prognostic Impact on Urological Cancers: A Systematic Review. *J. Urol.* **2021**, *206*, 854–865. [CrossRef] [PubMed]
34. Wu, E.; Hadjiiski, L.M.; Samala, R.K.; Chan, H.-P.; Cha, K.H.; Richter, C.; Cohan, R.H.; Caoili, E.M.; Paramagul, C.; Alva, A.; et al. Deep Learning Approach for Assessment of Bladder Cancer Treatment Response. *Tomography* **2019**, *5*, 201–208. [CrossRef]
35. Roblot, V.; Giret, Y.; Mezghani, S.; Auclin, E.; Arnoux, A.; Oudard, S.; Duron, L.; Fournier, L. Validation of a deep learning segmentation algorithm to quantify the skeletal muscle index and sarcopenia in metastatic renal carcinoma. *Eur. Radiol.* **2022**, *32*, 4728–4737. [CrossRef]
36. Cheung, H.; Wang, Y.; Chang, S.L.; Khandwala, Y.S.; Del Giudice, F.; Chung, B.I. Adoption of Robot-Assisted Partial Nephrectomies: A Population-Based Analysis of U.S. Surgeons from 2004 to 2013. *J. Endourol.* **2017**, *31*, 886–892. [CrossRef]
37. Cruz-Jentoft, A.J.; Landi, F.; Schneider, S.M.; Zúñiga, C.; Arai, H.; Boirie, Y.; Chen, L.-K.; Fielding, R.A.; Martin, F.C.; Michel, J.-P.; et al. Prevalence of and interventions for sarcopenia in ageing adults: A systematic review. Report of the International Sarcopenia Initiative (EWGSOP and IWGS). *Age Ageing* **2014**, *43*, 748–759. [CrossRef]
38. Papadopoulou, S.K. Sarcopenia: A Contemporary Health Problem among Older Adult Populations. *Nutrients* **2020**, *12*, 1293. [CrossRef]
39. Pacifico, J.; Geerlings, M.A.; Reijnierse, E.M.; Phassouliotis, C.; Lim, W.K.; Maier, A.B. Prevalence of sarcopenia as a comorbid disease: A systematic review and meta-analysis. *Exp. Gerontol.* **2020**, *131*, 110801. [CrossRef]
40. Zhang, X.; Zhao, Y.; Chen, S.; Shao, H. Anti-diabetic drugs and sarcopenia: Emerging links, mechanistic insights, and clinical implications. *J. Cachexia Sarcopenia Muscle* **2021**, *12*, 1368–1379. [CrossRef]
41. Campins, L.; Camps, M.; Riera, A.; Pleguezuelos, E.; Yébenes, J.C.; Serra-Prat, M. Oral Drugs Related with Muscle Wasting and Sarcopenia. A Review. *Pharmacology* **2017**, *99*, 1–8. [CrossRef] [PubMed]
42. Yumioka, T.; Honda, M.; Nishikawa, R.; Teraoka, S.; Kimura, Y.; Iwamoto, H.; Morizane, S.; Hikita, K.; Takenaka, A. Sarcopenia as a significant predictive factor of neutropenia and overall survival in urothelial carcinoma patients underwent gemcitabine and cisplatin or carboplatin. *Int. J. Clin. Oncol.* **2020**, *25*, 158–164. [CrossRef]

43. Shimizu, R.; Honda, M.; Teraoka, S.; Yumioka, T.; Yamaguchi, N.; Kawamoto, B.; Iwamoto, H.; Morizane, S.; Hikita, K.; Takenaka, A. Sarcopenia is associated with survival in patients with urothelial carcinoma treated with systemic chemotherapy. *Int. J. Clin. Oncol.* **2022**, *27*, 175–183. [CrossRef] [PubMed]
44. Nicolazzo, C.; Busetto, G.M.; Del Giudice, F.; Sperduti, I.; Giannarelli, D.; Gradilone, A.; Gazzaniga, P.; de Berardinis, E.; Raimondi, C. The long-term prognostic value of survivin expressing circulating tumor cells in patients with high-risk non-muscle invasive bladder cancer (NMIBC). *J. Cancer Res. Clin. Oncol.* **2017**, *143*, 1971–1976. [CrossRef]
45. Del Giudice, F.; Pecoraro, M.; Vargas, H.A.; Cipollari, S.; De Berardinis, E.; Bicchetti, M.; Chung, B.I.; Catalano, C.; Narumi, Y.; Catto, J.W.F.; et al. Systematic Review and Meta-Analysis of Vesical Imaging-Reporting and Data System (VI-RADS) Inter-Observer Reliability: An Added Value for Muscle Invasive Bladder Cancer Detection. *Cancers* **2020**, *12*, 2994. [CrossRef] [PubMed]
46. Panebianco, V.; Pecoraro, M.; Del Giudice, F.; Takeuchi, M.; Muglia, V.F.; Messina, E.; Cipollari, S.; Giannarini, G.; Catalano, C.; Narumi, Y. VI-RADS for Bladder Cancer: Current Applications and Future Developments. *J. Magn. Reson. Imaging* **2022**, *55*, 23–36. [CrossRef] [PubMed]
47. Basile, D.; Corvaja, C.; Caccialanza, R.; Aprile, G. Sarcopenia: Looking to muscle mass to better manage pancreatic cancer patients. *Curr. Opin. Support. Palliat. Care* **2019**, *13*, 279–285. [CrossRef]
48. Kurk, S.A.; Peeters, P.H.M.; Dorresteijn, B.; De Jong, P.A.; Jourdan, M.; Creemers, G.-J.M.; Erdkamp, F.L.G.; De Jongh, F.E.; Kint, P.A.M.; Poppema, B.J.; et al. Loss of skeletal muscle index and survival in patients with metastatic colorectal cancer: Secondary analysis of the phase 3 CAIRO3 trial. *Cancer Med.* **2020**, *9*, 1033–1043. [CrossRef]
49. Panebianco, V.; Grazhdani, H.; Iafrate, F.; Petroni, M.; Anzidei, M.; Laghi, A.; Passariello, R. 3D CT protocol in the assessment of the esophageal neoplastic lesions: Can it improve TNM staging? *Eur. Radiol.* **2006**, *16*, 414–421. [CrossRef]
50. Iwase, T.; Wang, X.; Shrimanker, T.V.; Kolonin, M.G.; Ueno, N.T. Body composition and breast cancer risk and treatment: Mechanisms and impact. *Breast Cancer Res. Treat.* **2021**, *186*, 273–283. [CrossRef]
51. Ubachs, J.; Ziemons, J.; Minis-Rutten, I.J.G.; Kruitwagen, R.F.P.M.; Kleijnen, J.; Lambrechts, S.; Olde Damink, S.W.M.; Rensen, S.S.; Van Gorp, T. Sarcopenia and ovarian cancer survival: A systematic review and meta-analysis. *J. Cachexia Sarcopenia Muscle* **2019**, *10*, 1165–1174. [CrossRef]
52. Jung, J.; Lee, E.; Shim, H.; Park, J.-H.; Eom, H.-S.; Lee, H. Prediction of clinical outcomes through assessment of sarcopenia and adipopenia using computed tomography in adult patients with acute myeloid leukemia. *Int. J. Hematol.* **2021**, *114*, 44–52. [CrossRef]
53. Cecchini, S.; Cavazzini, E.; Marchesi, F.; Sarli, L.; Roncoroni, L. Computed Tomography Volumetric Fat Parameters versus Body Mass Index for Predicting Short-term Outcomes of Colon Surgery. *World J. Surg.* **2011**, *35*, 415–423. [CrossRef]
54. Wang, B.; Torriani, M. Artificial Intelligence in the Evaluation of Body Composition. *Semin. Musculoskelet. Radiol.* **2020**, *24*, 030–037. [CrossRef]
55. Chung, H.; Jo, Y.; Ryu, D.; Jeong, C.; Choe, S.; Lee, J. Artificial-intelligence-driven discovery of prognostic biomarker for sarcopenia. *J. Cachexia Sarcopenia Muscle* **2021**, *12*, 2220–2230. [CrossRef] [PubMed]
56. Bhinder, B.; Gilvary, C.; Madhukar, N.S.; Elemento, O. Artificial Intelligence in Cancer Research and Precision Medicine. *Cancer Discov.* **2021**, *11*, 900–915. [CrossRef] [PubMed]
57. Somasundaram, E.; Castiglione, J.A.; Brady, S.L.; Trout, A.T. Defining Normal Ranges of Skeletal Muscle Area and Skeletal Muscle Index in Children on CT Using an Automated Deep Learning Pipeline: Implications for Sarcopenia Diagnosis. *Am. J. Roentgenol.* **2022**, *219*, 326–336. [CrossRef] [PubMed]
58. Borrelli, P.; Kaboteh, R.; Enqvist, O.; Ulén, J.; Trägårdh, E.; Kjölhede, H.; Edenbrandt, L. Artificial intelligence-aided CT segmentation for body composition analysis: A validation study. *Eur. Radiol. Exp.* **2021**, *5*, 11. [CrossRef] [PubMed]
59. Ferro, M.; de Cobelli, O.; Musi, G.; del Giudice, F.; Carrieri, G.; Busetto, G.M.; Falagario, U.G.; Sciarra, A.; Maggi, M.; Crocetto, F.; et al. Radiomics in prostate cancer: An up-to-date review. *Ther. Adv. Urol.* **2022**, *14*, 175628722211090. [CrossRef] [PubMed]

Disclaimer/Publisher's Note: The statements, opinions and data contained in all publications are solely those of the individual author(s) and contributor(s) and not of MDPI and/or the editor(s). MDPI and/or the editor(s) disclaim responsibility for any injury to people or property resulting from any ideas, methods, instructions or products referred to in the content.

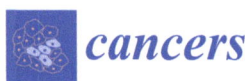

Review

An Update on the Role of MRI in Treatment Stratification of Patients with Cervical Cancer

Amreen Shakur, Janice Yu Ji Lee and Sue Freeman *

Cambridge University Hospitals NHS Foundation Trust, Cambridge CB2 0QQ, UK; amreen.shakur@nhs.net (A.S.); janice.lee1@nhs.net (J.Y.J.L.)
* Correspondence: susan.freeman16@nhs.net

Simple Summary: Magnetic resonance imaging (MRI) has a pivotal role in accurately staging cervical cancer and has been formally incorporated into the 2018 FIGO staging system. MRI can accurately assess tumour size and local and distant invasion as well as lymph node involvement, which is essential for triaging patients into surgical or chemotherapeutic management. In this review, we highlight key MRI findings and pitfalls pertaining to the updated FIGO stages and their implications for treatment selection into surgery or chemoradiation.

Abstract: Cervical cancer is the fourth most common cancer in women worldwide and the most common gynaecological malignancy. The FIGO staging system is the most commonly utilised classification system for cervical cancer worldwide. Prior to the most recent update in the FIGO staging in 2018, the staging was dependent upon clinical assessment alone. Concordance between the surgical and clinical FIGO staging decreases rapidly as the tumour becomes more advanced. MRI now plays a central role in patients diagnosed with cervical cancer and enables accurate staging, which is essential to determining the most appropriate treatment. MRI is the best imaging option for the assessment of tumour size, location, and parametrial and sidewall invasion. Notably, the presence of parametrial invasion precludes surgical options, and the patient will be triaged to chemoradiotherapy. As imaging is intrinsic to the new 2018 FIGO staging system, nodal metastases have been included within the classification as stage IIIC disease. The presence of lymph node metastases within the pelvis or abdomen is associated with a poorer prognosis, which previously could not be included in the staging classification as these could not be reliably detected on clinical examination. MRI findings corresponding to the 2018 revised FIGO staging of cervical cancers and their impact on treatment selection will be described.

Keywords: gynaecological malignancy; cervical malignancy; FIGO staging; MRI

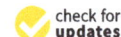

Citation: Shakur, A.; Lee, J.Y.J.; Freeman, S. An Update on the Role of MRI in Treatment Stratification of Patients with Cervical Cancer. *Cancers* 2023, 15, 5105. https://doi.org/10.3390/cancers15205105

Academic Editor: Athina C Tsili

Received: 30 August 2023
Revised: 13 October 2023
Accepted: 16 October 2023
Published: 23 October 2023

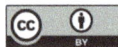

Copyright: © 2023 by the authors. Licensee MDPI, Basel, Switzerland. This article is an open access article distributed under the terms and conditions of the Creative Commons Attribution (CC BY) license (https://creativecommons.org/licenses/by/4.0/).

1. Introduction

Cervical cancer is the fourth most common gynaecological cancer worldwide, with a peak incidence between 25 and 40 years [1]. GLOBOCAN 2020 estimated that, worldwide, there were approximately 604 000 new cases of cervical cancer and 342 000 deaths due to the disease annually. Most new cases (approximately 90%) occur in low- and middle-income countries, where cervical cancer represents the third most common cancer in women.

One of the main risk factors is long-term or persistent infection with human papillomavirus (HPV). Over 70% of newly diagnosed cervical cancers are caused by either the HPV 16 or 18 subtypes. A further 19% of cervical cancers are caused by the HPV types 31, 33, 45, 52, or 58 [2]. HPV is a ubiquitous sexually transmitted infection with a prevalence of 11.7% globally, with a geographic distribution ranging from 2% to 42% [3]. The majority of HPV infections are cleared by women in two years, and only 10% cause a persistent infection.

This knowledge of HPV epidemiology has led the World Health Organisation (WHO) to call for a worldwide HPV eradication program [4]. The WHO global strategy proposes that a 90–70–90 target be met by 2030 for countries to be on the path towards eliminating cervical cancer. This target aims for 90% of girls to be fully vaccinated with the HPV vaccine by 15 years old, 70% of women to be screened with a high-performance test by 35 years of age and again by 45 years of age, and 90% of women affected by a cervical disease (precancer and invasive cancer) to receive treatment [4].

It has been postulated that the median cervical cancer incidence rate will fall by 42% by 2045 and by 97% by 2120 if these 90–70–90 targets are met [4].

Primary prevention through HPV vaccination of adolescent girls has been shown to be the most effective long-term intervention for reducing the risk of cervical cancer. Current guidelines to confer full protection are for two doses to be administered between the ages of 9 and 14 years. In addition to protecting against cervical lesions and cancer, they also reduce the risk of disease in the vulva, vagina, and anus. One study involving 60 million individuals with a follow-up period of 8 years after vaccination found that the prevalence of the various strains of HPV, anogenital warts, and high-grade cervical abnormalities (cervical intraepithelial neoplasia 2 and 3 (CIN2 and CIN3)) all significantly declined in all studied age groups. A separate study also found a significantly reduced risk of HPV-based invasive cervical cancer in the vaccinated population [3].

The Papanicolaou smear test (Pap smear) is a population-based cytological screening test that was effective in reducing the number of cervical cancers. However, the Pap smear required high levels of resources and suffered from variable quality assurance. HPV-based testing has replaced the Pap smear in many countries, including the UK, as it has improved sensitivity, accuracy, and reproducibility. HPV detection has increased the colposcopy referral rate and subsequently improved the detection rate of CIN3 and cervical cancers.

The transformation zone is the junction between the squamous epithelium of the ectocervix and columnar epithelium of the endocervical canal. Metaplasia occurs at the transformation zone, where columnar epithelium is replaced by squamous epithelium, and is the commonest site for cervical intra-epithelial neoplasia (CIN), which can progress to cervical cancer. The transformation zone is easily accessible for assessment by colposcopy using acetic acid. Areas of CIN or cervical cancer are revealed as acetowhite lesions. Under local anaesthetic, the lesion can be biopsied or a large loop excision of the transformation zone (LLETZ) performed.

Cervical cancers are differentiated into different histological types, with the commonest being squamous cell carcinomas, constituting approximately 70–80% of cervical cancers. The glandular histological subtypes include adenocarcinomas, which account for a further approximately 25% of cervical cancers and are typically associated with a poorer prognosis [5]. Rarer subtypes include carcinosarcoma, adenosquamous carcinoma, and adenosarcoma.

2. The Role of Different Imaging Modalities in the Assessment of Cervical Cancer

Transvaginal ultrasound (TVUS) is considered the first-line imaging investigation for patients with gynaecological symptoms and is often more cost-effective and readily available than other imaging modalities, particularly in low-income countries. However, it is not part of routine cervical cancer detection and staging. Recent meta-analyses have shown TVUS to demonstrate comparable sensitivity and specificity for the estimation of tumour volume and presence of parametrial invasion; however, the technique is largely dependent upon operator skill and expertise. TVUS has a limited role in the evaluation of lymph node status, precluding it from becoming the primary imaging modality for cervical cancer assessment. However, TVUS in conjunction with transabdominal ultrasound (which may depict para-aortic lymph nodes or hydronephrosis) may have a role in the assessment of cervical cancer in resource-constrained areas where access to MRI is limited [6,7].

Computed tomography (CT) has fewer contra-indications, is quicker, and is usually more widely available when compared to MRI. The intrinsic lower soft tissue resolution of CT leads to reduced accuracy in the assessment of tumour size and parametrial invasion, although some studies have shown an accuracy of up to 86% in detecting cervical tumours on CT. Tsili et al. found that the relative hypo-enhancement of cervical tumours when compared to the background cervical tissue and the acquisition of thin sections with multiplanar reformats aid in tumour delineation. In comparison, MRI has up to 95% accuracy in the detection of cervical tumours. CT does have a role in the assessment of distant disease and can depict suspicious lymph nodes with a reported accuracy of 86% as well as identifying ureteric/pelvic sidewall involvement and distant metastases [8,9].

The role of F-fluorodeoxyglucose (FDG) positron emission tomography-computed tomography (PET/CT) in cervical cancer staging is well established due to its greater sensitivity in showing the presence of lymph node metastases and extra-pelvic disease extension when compared to CT [10]. Current guidelines recommend FDG-PET/CT in patients with stage IB1 disease or above who are eligible for surgical treatment and in patients with stage II–IVA disease to help assess for nodal and distant metastatic disease to guide therapeutic management [10–12].

The International Federation of Gynaecology and Obstetrics (FIGO) staging system is the most utilised classification system for cervical cancer worldwide, and the cervix was the first organ to be assigned a clinical staging system for cancer by FIGO in 1958. The most recent revision took place in 2018, previously having been revised in 2009, when staging was based on clinical evaluation alone [6]. The European Society of Urogenital Radiology (ESUR) recommended the inclusion of MRI into the staging classification in 2010 due to the high soft tissue resolution and accuracy in determining tumour size, parametrial invasion, pelvic sidewall invasion, and lymph node metastases [13]. MRI has also been shown to be cost effective as patients who underwent MRI as the initial imaging procedure for staging required fewer tests and procedures compared with those who underwent clinical staging alone [14]. The main changes in FIGO 2018 therefore relate to the utilisation of imaging to assign staging, which in turn led to the re-categorisation of stage IB into three size ranges and the inclusion of nodal disease as a new stage IIIC.

MRI Protocol for Uterine Cervical Cancer

Patient preparation is key to optimising imaging quality. A partially filled bladder ensures the uterus is in an optimal position, so patients are encouraged to void their bladder approximately half an hour prior to the examination so their bladder is partially filled during examination. Some centres encourage patients to fast for approximately 4–6 hrs prior to the study to reduce bowel peristalsis. An intramuscular injection of an anti-peristaltic agent (Buscopan) is administered before imaging is performed, which reduces motion artefact from bowel peristalsis. Whilst other methods including enemas and pelvic strapping are used for pelvic MRI for other indications, there is no substantial evidence to support their routine use for cervical cancer MRI [15].

A standard MRI protocol (Table 1) for cervical cancer staging involves obtaining a large field of view (FOV) sagittal T2-weighted image (T2WI); this is then used to plan higher-resolution small FOV imaging perpendicular to the long axis of the cervix, important for local staging of the tumour and accurate assessment of the parametrium (Figure 1). The normal zonal anatomy of the cervix is best depicted on T2WI with the central endocervical glands and mucosa demonstrating hyperintense signal intensity, surrounded by a hypointense fibrous stroma and an outer intermediate signal intensity loose stroma, extending to the parametrium [16]. Cervical tumours, when visible, are best depicted on T2WI, where they appear as intermediate signal intensity lesions, which are readily distinguishable from the hypointense cervical stroma. DWI can aid tumour detection when the lesion is isointense to the background cervix.

Table 1. Recommended MRI sequences for staging of cervical cancer.

Sequence and Plane	Rationale
Large FOV Axial T1WI	Extra pelvic disease, lymph nodes, bone marrow signal
Large FOV Axial T2WI	Extra pelvic disease, para-aortic nodal involvement, hydronephrosis
Small FOV Sagittal T2WI	Accurate tumour size, local staging (e.g., vaginal, bladder, rectal invasion)
Small FOV Axial oblique T2WI	Local staging, parametrial and pelvic sidewall involvement
Sagittal and axial oblique DWI and ADC maps (corresponding to sagittal and axial oblique T2WI)	Identifying small isointense tumours, unsuspected bone metastases

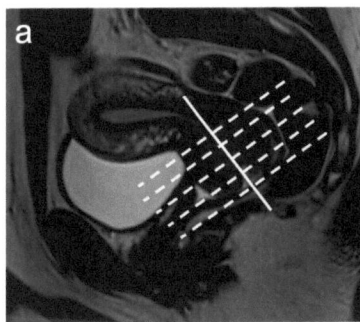 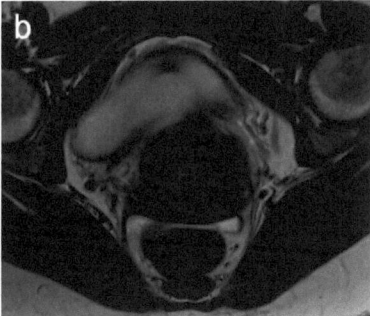

Figure 1. Sagittal T2WI (a) highlights the long axis of the cervix (solid white line) and the perpendicular axis to the cervix (dashed white lines) from which the (b) axial-oblique sequences are obtained.

ESUR guidelines recommend a large FOV axial T1-weighted image (T1WI) and T2WI obtained from the renal hila to the pubic symphysis to assess extra pelvic diseases, such as lymph node enlargement, bone involvement, and hydronephrosis [17,18].

Diffusion-weighted imaging (DWI) is a functional imaging technique that is sensitive to the microscopic motion of water molecules. With derived apparent diffusion coefficient (ADC) maps, it can be used to evaluate the molecular function and micro-architecture of biological tissue [19,20]. Different tissues have characteristic diffusion properties, and in tissues that are highly cellular, the diffusion of water molecules is relatively more restricted. This manifests as a high signal on DWI images, with a corresponding low signal on ADC maps. Several studies have demonstrated the added value of DWI both in the detection of tumours on initial staging, particularly those that are small and isointense on T2WI, as well as in detecting cervical cancer recurrence [18,19,21].

DWI should be acquired in the sagittal and axial oblique planes, with corresponding T2WI for anatomical correlation [22]. For accurate analysis, images should be acquired with a minimum of two b values and must be corroborated with the corresponding ADC maps to avoid the potential pitfall of overcalling diffusion restriction in tissues that have an inherently high T2 signal (T2 shine-through phenomenon). The presence of post-biopsy oedema is a common cause of this pitfall [23]. Whilst malignant cells generally demonstrate restricted diffusion, benign entities including blood products, abscesses, and keratin may also exhibit restricted diffusion, highlighting the importance of correlation with T1WI and T2WI to avoid this pitfall [21].

DWI has also emerged as a potential biomarker for assessing treatment response to chemoradiotherapy in cervical cancer. A meta-analysis analysis performed by Harry et al. assessed the role of DWI and ADC in predicting treatment response [24]. They demonstrated a statistically significant correlation between ADC values detected within three weeks of treatment as well as the percentage change in ADC values during this period with overall treatment response. Therefore, a change in ADC values rather than absolute ADC values may serve as a suitable marker in the determination of early response. However, they did not demonstrate a significant relationship between pre-treatment ADC values and treatment response, and therefore cannot be used to determine initial treatment selection [24,25].

DWI facilitates the detection of lymph nodes; however, it is important to note that both physiological and pathological nodes demonstrate diffusion restriction. T1 and T2 weighted imaging can be used to further evaluate the morphology of the lymph node. Suspicious features include a rounded morphology, an irregular border, and the loss of the fatty hilum (Figure 2). Size criteria for lymph node enlargement differ depending upon location. In general, lymph nodes with a short-axis diameter greater than 10 mm are considered suspicious for metastasis; however, in the inguinal region, lymph nodes measuring up to 15 mm can be considered normal, whereas lymph nodes exceeding 8 mm in the obturator region would raise suspicion [26]. Potential pitfalls arise in patients with increased body habitus; limited studies have demonstrated a correlation between normal lymph node size and body mass index (BMI), which can sometimes result in the overcalling of lymph node involvement [27].

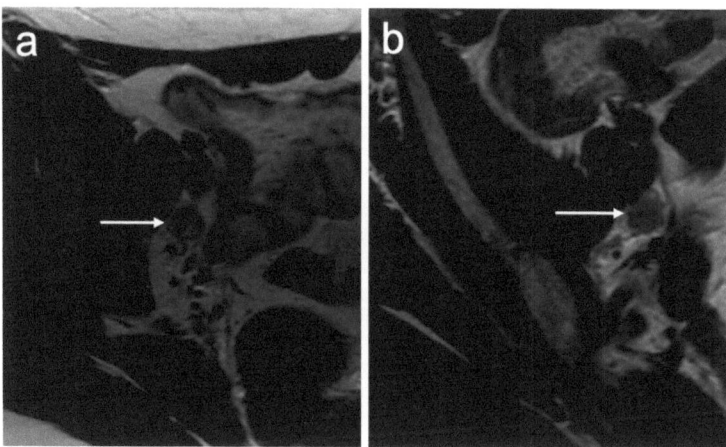

Figure 2. Axial T2WI images demonstrate typical appearances of metastatic lymph nodes with (**a**) a rounded morphology and central necrosis and (**b**) irregular spiculated margins.

According to the latest ESUR recommendations, T2WI and DWI sequences, ideally matched in acquisition plane, field of view, and slice thickness to allow for side-by-side interpretation, are fundamental for the initial staging, the assessment of treatment response, and the detection of recurrence. However, in the same guidelines, the use of contrast-enhanced MRI (CE-MRI) remains optional [15].

A systematic review by Avesani et al. did not find strong evidence to indicate contrast-enhanced (CE) sequences to be helpful in the initial staging or the detection of tumour recurrence and did not find CE-MRI could provide any additional information than that obtained from DWI sequences [28]. Combined chemoradiotherapy is the treatment of choice for large cervical cancers. MRIs are performed pre- and mid-treatment to enable tailored treatment planning and the adjustment of radiotherapy dose to improve local tumour control and minimize the toxic effect of therapy. If initial treatment fails, further therapeutic options are limited. Therefore, the early, accurate prediction of treatment response would profoundly affect the prognosis of patients. Many studies have investigated the potential role of CE-MRI at staging as a predictor of treatment response. Studies have shown that tumours demonstrating lower enhancement (poorly perfused hypoxic tumours are linked to increased aggressiveness, increased risk of metastasis, and treatment failure) had a poorer response to therapy and a lower survival rate. However, the studies did not identify a precise, reproducible value for those parameters, limiting their use in current clinical practice [28].

Some studies have also shown that CE-MRI can improve the sensitivity of depicting small isointense tumours, particularly for patients who may be eligible for fertility-sparing treatment [29]. A potential pitfall can arise in larger/exophytic tumours, where compression of the cervix/vagina can cause surrounding cervical oedema or inflammatory change that can be mistaken for parametrial invasion.

Recently, there has been a growing interest in radiomics and its potential to add value to the discriminatory and prognostic evaluation of cervical cancer when using PET-CT and MRI. Radiomics refers to the technology that uses artificial intelligence and machine learning to extract large quantities of information from a series of medical images and convert them into calculated quantitative data. The extracted features can then be used as alternative markers for underlying gene expression patterns and tumour biological characteristics such as morphology and intra-tumour heterogeneity [30].

Several studies have investigated the use of MRI-based radiomics in cervical cancer with favourable preliminary results. Becker et al. reported that the textural parameter of the ADC map correlates with the differentiation of cervical cancer, which could then be used to predict survival [31]. A study by Wormald et al. found that radiomic features from ADC maps and T2WI could potentially predict recurrence in patients with stage I and II low-volume cancers [32]. Laliscia et al. found that radiomic features from T2WI are useful in predicting the prognosis of locally advanced cervical cancers [33]. Meta-analyses have also been carried out and support the value of MRI-based radiomics models in predicting lymph node metastases and lymph-vascular space invasion status in patients with cervical cancer pre-operatively [34].

More research is needed before radiomics is integrated into routine clinical practice. However, preliminary results are promising and demonstrate that MRI-based radiomic features can be useful in the preoperative prediction and prognosis of patients with cervical cancer.

3. FIGO STAGING with MRI

MRI has a limited role in the detection of cervical cancer and is usually only performed on patients with histological evidence of cervical cancer. Traditionally, the staging system was largely clinically and surgically based. However, the most recent update in 2018 has formally incorporated imaging as part of the criteria, giving added importance to MRI as a way of accurately measuring tumours, which has direct implications on the FIGO stage. MRI has a reported accuracy of 93% compared to 60% with clinical evaluation for accurate tumour measurement, and measurements should be given in three planes: craniocaudal (CC), antero-posterior (AP), and transverse (TS) [35]. MRI can also accurately identify the presence of parametrial and vaginal invasion, nodal involvement, and bladder and bowel invasion [36] (Table 2).

Table 2. FIGO staging 2018.

Stage	Description
Stage I	The carcinoma is strictly confined to the cervix
IA	Invasive carcinoma that can be diagnosed only by microscopy with a maximum depth of invasion <5 mm
IA1	Measured stromal invasion <3 mm in depth
IA2	Measured stromal invasion ≥3 mm and <5 mm in depth
IB	Invasive carcinoma confined to the uterine cervix with measured deepest invasion ≥5 mm
IB1	Tumour measures <2 cm in greatest dimension
IB2	Tumour measures ≥2 cm and <4 cm in greatest dimension
IB3	Tumour measures ≥4 cm in greatest dimension
Stage II	The cervical carcinoma invades beyond the uterus, but has not extended onto the lower third of the vagina or to the pelvic wall
IIA	Involvement limited to the upper two-thirds of the vagina without parametrial invasion
IIA1	Invasive carcinoma <4 cm in greatest dimension
IIA2	Invasive carcinoma ≥4 cm in greatest dimension
IIB	With parametrial invasion but not up to the pelvic wall
Stage III	Involves the lower third of the vagina and/or extends to the pelvic wall and/or causes hydronephrosis or non-functioning kidney and/or involves pelvic and/or paraaortic lymph nodes
IIIA	Involves lower third of the vagina, with no extension to the pelvic wall
IIIB	Extension to the pelvic wall and/or hydronephrosis or non-functioning kidney (unless known to be due to another cause)
IIIC	Involvement of pelvic and/or paraaortic lymph nodes
IIIC1	Pelvic lymph node metastasis only
IIIC2	Paraaortic lymph node metastasis
Stage IV	Spread to adjacent and distant organs
IVA	Rectal or bladder involvement
IVB	Spread to distant organs outside the pelvis

4. FIGO Stage I

A tumour confined to the cervix is considered stage I. Stage IA is a microinvasive disease that is not visible radiologically. Stage IB disease is a tumour that is confined to the cervix with the deepest invasion greater than 5 mm, and in the revised FIGO staging 2018, it is further divided into three subsections: stage IB1 disease is now defined as less than or equal to 2 cm in maximum diameter (Figure 3), stage IB2 is greater than 2 cm and less than or equal to 4 cm (Figure 4), and stage IB3 is greater than 4 cm in maximum diameter (Figure 5). These new subsections reflect the proven better prognosis for tumours under 2 cm and will include those who may be suitable for fertility-sparing treatment.

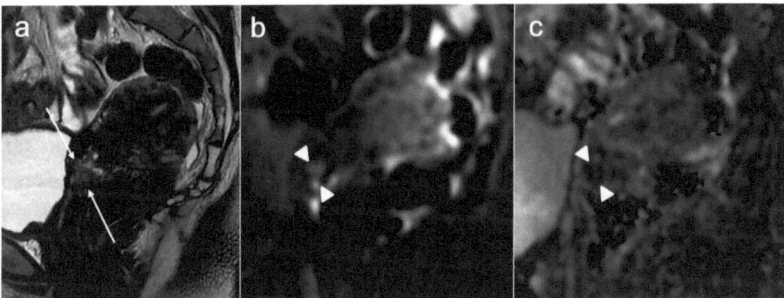

Figure 3. Sagittal T2WI (**a**) demonstrates a 15 mm intermediate signal intensity lesion in the anterior lip of the cervix (arrows). Corresponding DWI (**b**) and ADC map (**c**) show associated restricted diffusion (arrowheads). FIGO stage IB1.

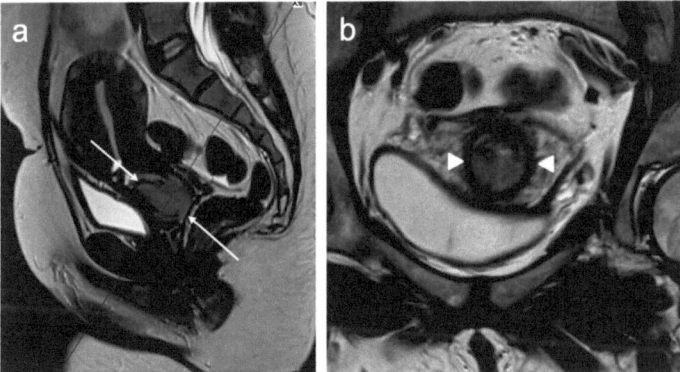

Figure 4. Sagittal T2WI (**a**) shows a well-defined intermediate signal intensity endocervical tumour (arrows); the maximum dimension is 28 mm. (**b**) Axial oblique T2WI through the mass demonstrates an intact low signal intensity stromal ring (arrowheads). FIGO stage IB2.

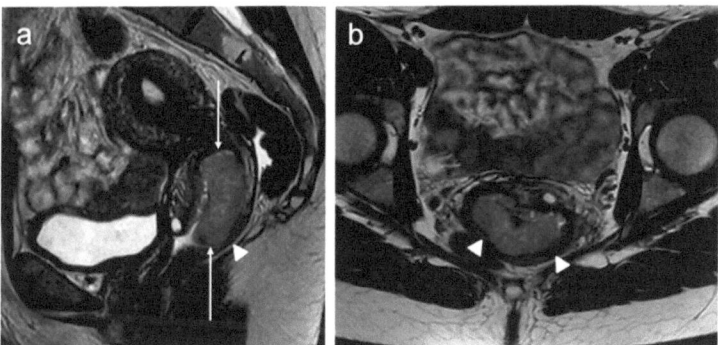

Figure 5. Sagittal T2WI (**a**) demonstrates a large 45 mm intermediate signal intensity lesion confined to the posterior lip of the cervix (arrows). Axial oblique T2WI (**b**) dearly reveals that the posterior vaginal wall is not involved (arrowheads). FIGO stage IB3.

5. FIGO Stage II

A tumour that extends beyond the cervix but without extension to the lower third of the vagina or pelvic sidewall constitutes stage II disease. There has been no change in stage

II between the 2009 and 2018 FIGO classifications. Stage II is further subdivided into IIA and IIB. The stage IIA disease confers involvement of the upper two-thirds of the vagina; this can be challenging to assess radiologically, and vaginal invasion can be overestimated at MRI, particularly at the vaginal fornices, which may be stretched by a bulky exophytic cervical tumour. Overall accuracy for vaginal invasion is reported to be in the range of 86–93% [37]. The vaginal mucosa is normally of high T2 signal intensity, and when there is a loss of this signal in continuity with the primary tumour, vaginal invasion can be reported with confidence. Some centres advocate the use of vaginal gel to improve the accuracy of the involvement of the vagina; however, due to the accurate assessment of the vagina at examination under anaesthesia (EUA), this is not essential [13,38]. Stage IIA is further subdivided depending on the maximum size of the tumour: stage IIA1 comprises tumours measuring less than or equal to 4 cm, and stage IIA2 comprises tumours greater than 4 cm. This distinction relates to prognostication, as tumours that exceed 4 cm are more likely to have nodal metastases and are therefore unlikely to be surgical candidates.

The parametrium is the fatty tissue containing blood vessels and lymphatics surrounding the cervix. Stage IIB disease constitutes parametrial invasion, but the tumour does not extend to the pelvic sidewall. The assessment of the parametrium is best depicted on axial oblique images, where normal cervical stroma is visualised as a low T2 signal ring, which, if intact, has a high negative predictive value (94–100%) for the presence of parametrial invasion [39]. However, when there is an isolated disruption of the stromal ring, parametrial invasion may not be present. The presence of stromal ring disruption and visible nodular or spiculate soft tissue extending into the parametrial soft tissues implies parametrial invasion (Figure 6). It is important to be aware of pitfalls, particularly with regard to post-biopsy cervical oedema, which can mimic parametrial invasion [22]. Whilst increasing the time interval between biopsy and MRI can reduce oedema, an unnecessary delay in imaging is not desirable. The use of DWI can overcome this challenge in distinguishing post-biopsy change from the tumour by identifying restricted diffusion within the tumour [40].

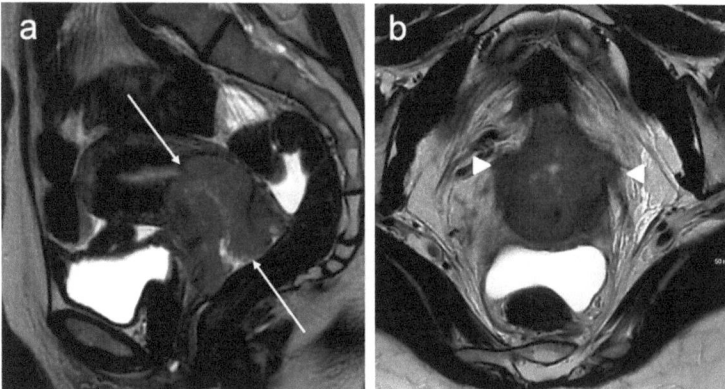

Figure 6. Sagittal T2WI (**a**) shows a large intermediate signal intensity tumour replacing the cervix and extending into the lower uterine segment (arrows). Axial oblique T2WI (**b**) reveals nodular soft tissue extension into the parametria bilaterally (arrowheads) consistent with bilateral parametrial invasion. FIGO stage IIB.

6. FIGO Stage III

Stage III disease denotes further extension of the tumour and has three subsections. Stage IIIA represents an extension to the lower third of the vagina, which is the vaginal tissue below the level of the bladder base, best evaluated on sagittal T2WI or DWI (Figure 7). Stage IIIB is the extension of the tumour to the pelvic sidewall. The pelvic sidewall is bordered by the obturator internus and piriformis muscles and contains the iliac vessels, pelvic ureters, and lateral lymph nodes [41]. On MRI, a tumour within 3 mm of the lateral pelvic wall is considered a sidewall invasion. Stage IIIB also includes the presence of hydronephrosis or a non-functioning kidney (Figure 8); however, it is important to exclude other causes of hydronephrosis, such as endometriosis or urinary tract calculi, to avoid incorrect upstaging. Stage IIIC is a new substage and describes the pattern of abdominopelvic lymph involvement, regardless of primary tumour size and extent. It is further subdivided into IIIC1 (pelvic lymph node involvement, Figure 9) and IIIC2 (para-aortic lymph node involvement, Figure 10). The inclusion of nodal disease relates to prognostication, as patients with lymph node involvement have a significantly reduced 5-year survival rate compared to those without. Wright et al. reported that the five-year survival rate for stage IB1 tumours was accurate for 92% of patients, reducing to 61% for stage IIIC1 and to 38% for stage IIIC2 tumours [42].

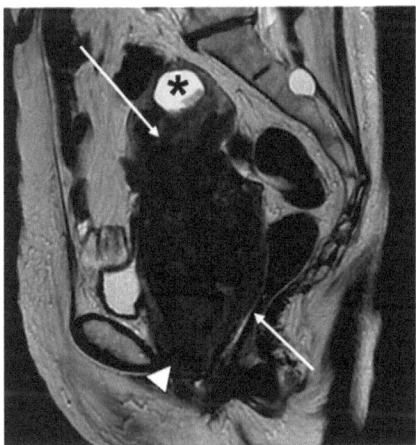

Figure 7. Sagittal T2WI of histologically confirmed cervical cancer demonstrates a large ill-defined intermediate signal intensity tumour replacing the cervix and the lower two thirds of the uterine body (arrows). Fluid distension of the fundal aspect of the endometrial cavity (*) secondary to cervical stenosis. Intermediate signal intensity also extends to and involves the lower third of the vagina (arrowhead). FIGO stage IIIA.

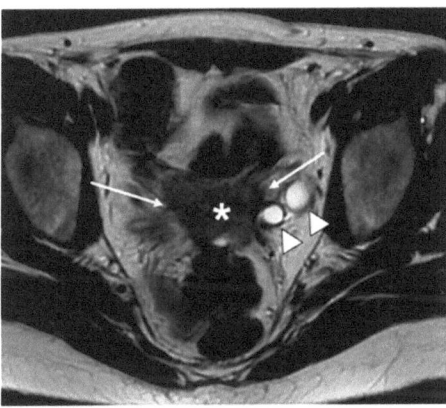

Figure 8. Axial T2WI shows an ill-defined intermediate signal intensity tumour replacing the cervix (*). Spiculated tumour extends into the parametria bilaterally (arrows) and causes a left hydroureter (arrowheads). FIGO stage IIIB.

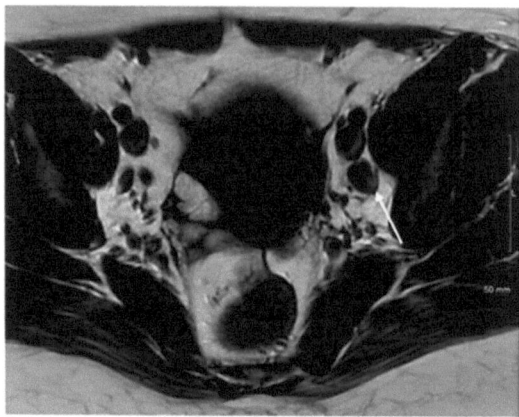

Figure 9. Axial T1WI demonstrating an enlarged left obturator node (arrow). FIGO stage IIIC1.

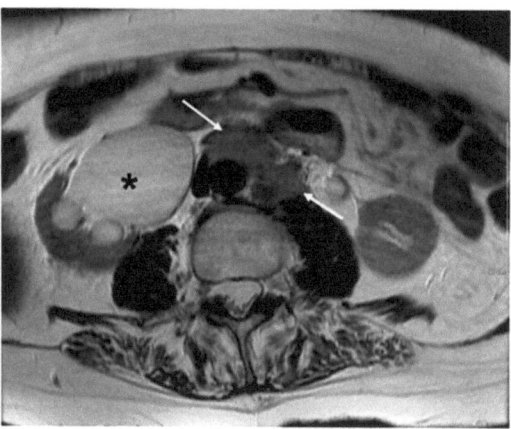

Figure 10. Axial T1WI demonstrating enlarged left para-aortic and pre-aortic nodes (arrows). FIGO stage IIIC2. Right sided hydronephrosis also noted (*).

7. FIGO Stage IV

Stage IV disease is unchanged from 2009 and describes the disease extending into the adjacent organs outside the true pelvis. It is subdivided into two stages: stage IVA describes an extension of the tumour through the bladder wall anteriorly or rectum posteriorly. The tumour must be visualised to project beyond the mucosa into the lumen before describing stage IVA disease (Figure 11). MRI has a reported specificity of 86-88% for bladder/bowel involvement and a high negative predictive value of 96-100%, thereby removing the need for routine cystoscopy/sigmoidoscopy for staging [37]. If there is a loss of fat plane between the cervix and bladder or rectum or abnormal signal intensity of the serosa, this does not constitute stage IVA disease; however, this information should be conveyed to clinicians to prompt further evaluation, and cystoscopy or sigmoidoscopy in these cases would be beneficial. Bullous oedema, which describes the layered appearance of the posterior bladder secondary to urothelial oedema or inflammation, is a common pitfall and should not be mistaken for tumour infiltration. Bullous oedema is often seen in the presence of bladder serosal or muscularis invasion and is commonly seen post-radiotherapy (Figure 11).

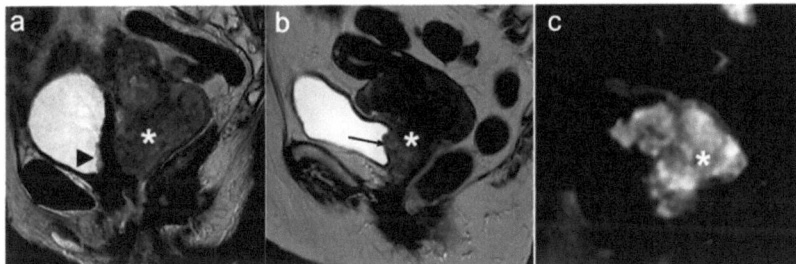

Figure 11. Sagittal T2WI (**a**) showing a heterogeneous intermediate signal intensity bulky cervical tumour (*). Irregular high T2 signal intensity seen along the posterior bladder wall consistent with bullous oedema (arrowhead). No tumour signal intensity is seen protruding into the bladder. Sagittal T2WI (**b**) with corresponding DWI (**c**) of a different patient demonstrating intermediate signal intensity bulky cervical tumour with corresponding diffusion restriction (*). Intermediate tumour signal intensity is seen to disrupt the low signal intensity of the posterior bladder wall and protrudes through the posterior bladder mucosa into the lumen (arrow) consistent with bladder invasion. FIGO stage IVA.

Stage IVB describes metastases to distant organs (e.g., lung, bones, liver) or distant lymph node groups, such as those in the supraclavicular region (Figure 12). Importantly, inguinal nodes are also stage IVB disease, as these represent haematogenous spread.

The benefits of structured reporting have been shown to reduce inter-reader variability, reduce diagnostic errors, and improve communication with fellow clinicians [43]. We demonstrate a sample reporting template, incorporating the pertinent features for FIGO staging (Table 3).

Table 3. Sample structured report for cervical cancer staging.

MR Cervical Cancer Staging	
Uterus size	CC × AP × TS mm
Primary tumour	Not seen (0), Ectocervical (exophytic 1), Endocervical (endophytic 2), Infiltrative (1 predominant expansive or 2 predominant infiltrating)
Size	CC × AP × TS mm
Presence of necrosis	No Yes (diameter)
Parametrial invasion	No Yes: Left/Right/Bilateral (proximal or distal)
Uterine invasion	No Yes: Lower/Mid/Upper
Extension to vagina	No Yes: Upper 1/3/Mid 1/3/Lower 1/3
Hydronephrosis	No Yes: Left/Right/Bilateral
Pelvic sidewall invasion	No Yes: Left/Right/Bilateral
Bladder invasion	No Yes
Rectal invasion	No Yes: Mesorectum/rectal wall
Distant organ invasion	No Yes
Lymph nodes	None, External Iliac, Internal Iliac, Obturator, Inguinal, Para-Aortic (above/below renal hilum)
Additional findings	
FIGO STAGE 2018	IA IB1 IB2 IB3 IIA1 IIA2 IIB IIIA IIIB IIIC IVA IVB

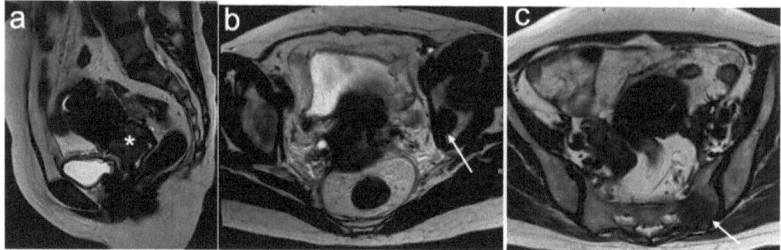

Figure 12. Sagittal T2WI (**a**) demonstrating intermediate signal intensity cervical tumour (*). Axial T2WI at the level of mid pelvis (**b**) and sacrum (**c**) demonstrates focal regions of irregular low signal intensity within the left acetabulum and left sacral ala (arrows) consistent with bone metastases. FIGO stage IVB.

8. Impact of MRI Findings on Treatment Selection

Cervical cancer is managed with curative intent, and the aim of FIGO staging is to risk stratify patients who are eligible for primary surgery and those who will have a better prognosis with chemo-radiation. Surgery is considered for patients where the tumour measures less than 4 cm and is confined to the cervix without parametrial or nodal invasion. For a select cohort of patients desiring the possibility of future pregnancy, fertility-sparing surgery may be an option. In such cases, tumour size, most accurately depicted with MRI, plays a significant role in determining which patients are eligible for fertility-sparing surgery. This is usually reserved for tumours confined to the cervix that measure less than 2 cm (stages IA1, IA2, and IB1) [44].

Fertility-sparing surgery includes cone resection/cone biopsy, simple trachelectomy, or radical trachelectomy [39]. As well as tumour size, other criteria must also be met to be eligible: the distance between the cranial margin of the tumour and internal os should be greater than 1 cm; however, some centres accept a minimum distance of 0.5 cm [45]. MRI has a reported sensitivity of 91% and specificity of 97% in the evaluation of internal os involvement [46]. On sagittal T2WI, the internal os is seen as the narrowest point of the uterine body or the transition point where the low-signal intensity cervical stroma changes to the higher-signal intensity uterine myometrium. The distance between the superior margin of the tumour and the internal os is measured in the sagittal plane [47,48] (Figure 13).

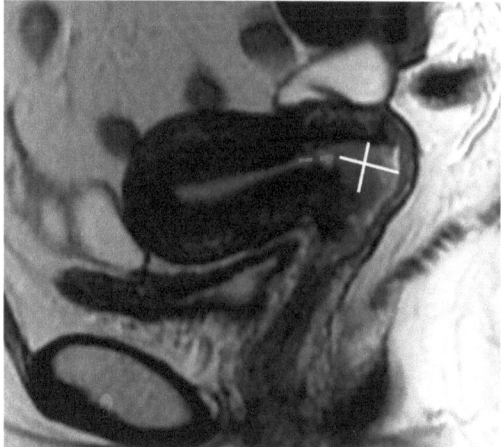

Figure 13. Sagittal T2WI demonstrating cervical tumour margins (white lines) and the distance from the internal cervical os and superior margin of the tumour (red dashed line).

The depth of stromal invasion is also an important consideration and varies between centres, with some only accepting stromal invasion of less than 50% as part of their criteria [44].

Cone resection is the removal of the ectocervix and distal endocervical canal. It is usually performed for stage IA1 tumours without lymphovascular space invasion (LVSI). Simple trachelectomy involves the more extensive removal of the cervix. Radical trachelectomy involves excision of the cervix, vaginal cuff, and parametrium, followed by the creation of an anastomosis between the isthmus and vagina. Trachelectomy can be performed vaginally or abdominally via open or laparoscopic techniques and is the approach for stage IA1 tumours with LVSI, stage IA2, and stage IB1 tumours.

For larger tumours confined to the cervix (exceeding 2 cm) or for patients for whom fertility preservation is not a priority, surgical options include total abdominal hysterectomy with or without bilateral salpingo-oophorectomy and lymphadenectomy via open or laparoscopic routes. Patients with FIGO stages IB2 and IIA1 may also be offered primary chemoradiotherapy if they are considered less favourable surgical candidates [3]. However, a systematic review by Yan et al. demonstrated radical hysterectomy to be superior to chemoradiotherapy for stage IB1, IB2, and IIA1 cancers with regards to overall prognosis [49]

A tumour size of greater than 4 cm (IB3, IIA2), among other factors, increases the risk of lymph node metastases and parametrial invasion [20,21]. Whilst some patients may be considered for surgery, the risk of recurrence and thus the need for adjuvant radiotherapy is greater (which is associated with higher morbidity); therefore, primary chemoradiotherapy is often the preferred treatment option [3].

The standard treatment for locally advanced cervical cancer (stage IIB and above) is chemoradiotherapy, which involves external beam radiation (EBRT) with concurrent chemotherapy, followed by intracavitary brachytherapy. MRI can be used to assess for accurate placement of the brachytherapy applicators (Figure 14) and post-brachytherapy complications (Figures 15 and 16). For patients treated with chemoradiotherapy, interval imaging can be used to monitor disease response (Figure 17). Mid-treatment MRI (after approximately 5 weeks of commencing chemotherapy with EBRT and before intracavitary brachytherapy) can aid dose adjustment in proportion to the residual tumour volume, which can reduce toxicity. Post-treatment MRI is typically performed 3–6 months after chemoradiotherapy, and the reconstitution of the low-signal intensity cervical stroma on T2WI implies a complete response. Post-treatment changes can persist for up to 9 months post-chemoradiotherapy; therefore, distinguishing residual tumours from post-treatment oedema can be challenging as both will appear as intermediate signal intensities on T2W1. The use of DWI can help differentiate the two, as only tumours should demonstrate restricted diffusion [50]. More recently, the application of MRI-guided brachytherapy has been shown to deliver more accurate dosing, which can be individually tailored to the tumour volume, thereby improving overall morbidity [51–53].

At initial staging, whole-body FDG-PET/CT is recommended for patients with stage IB3 and above due to the higher incidence of extra-pelvic disease. PET/CT allows accurate assessment of lymph node involvement and has a reported sensitivity and specificity of 72% and 96%, respectively [12]. PET/CT further optimises patients' triage to the appropriate therapy [10]. For example, patients with para-aortic nodal involvement have been shown to have a survival benefit when treated with extended-field radiotherapy. For bulky lymph nodes, standard EBRT may be insufficient, and these patients may be offered high-dose boost irradiation as part of standard chemoradiation or nodal debulking to reduce the overall dose of radiation required [54].

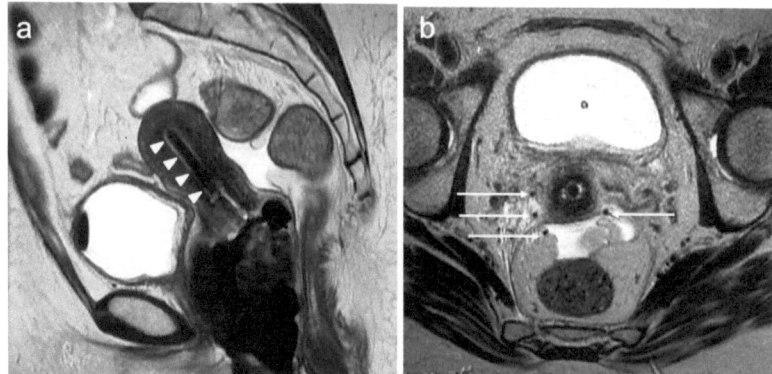

Figure 14. Sagittal T2WI (**a**) demonstrating the brachytherapy applicator appropriately sited within the endometrial cavity (arrowheads). Axial T2WI (**b**) shows several appropriately positioned parametrial needles (arrows).

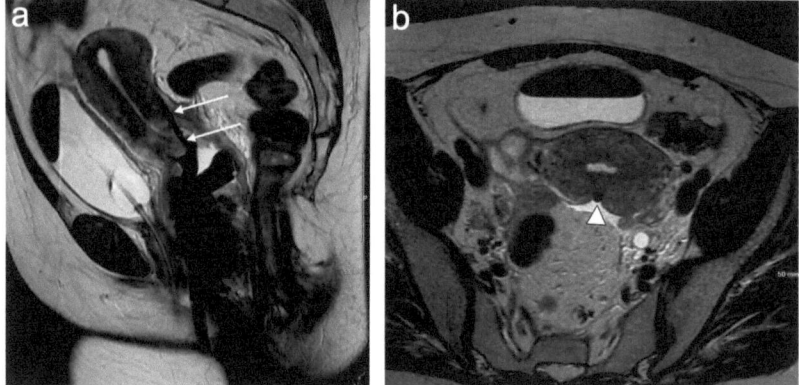

Figure 15. Sagittal T2WI (**a**) and axial T2WI (**b**) demonstrates a malpositioned central brachytherapy applicator which courses through the posterior cervical wall (arrows) with the tip lying posterior to the uterine body (arrowhead).

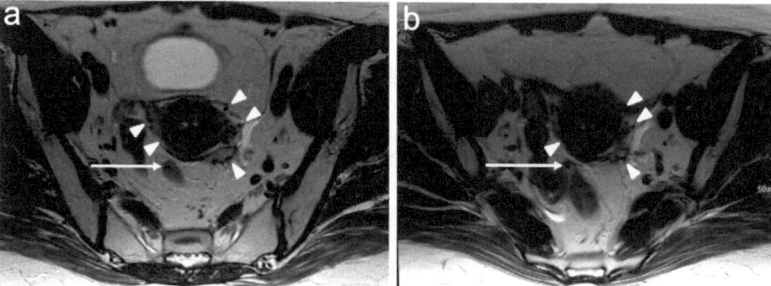

Figure 16. Axial (**a**) and oblique (**b**)T2WI demonstrates a single right sided parametrial needle to be malpositioned, perforating into the sigmoid colon (arrows). The remaining parametrial needles are appropriately sited (arrowheads).

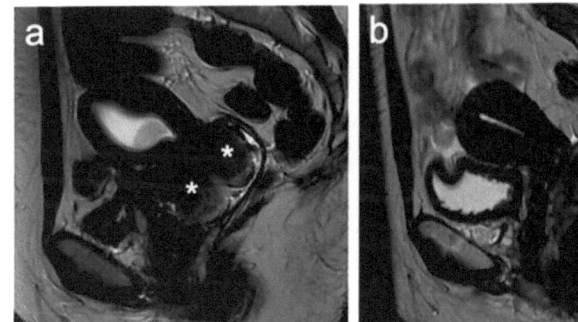
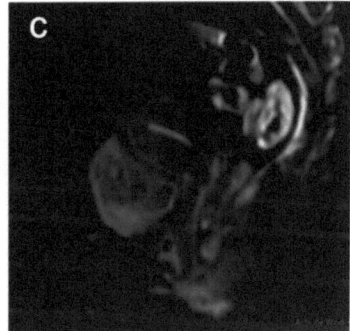

Figure 17. Baseline sagittal T2WI (**a**) shows an intermediate signal intensity bulky, exophytic cervical tumour (*). Sagittal T2WI (**b**) and DWI (**c**) after completion of chemoradiotherapy demonstrates significant reduction in tumour size with no residual abnormal signal intensity or diffusion restriction. This appearance indicates a complete response.

9. Recurrent Cervical Cancer

Recurrent cervical cancer is defined as tumour regrowth or the development of nodal or distant metastases more than six months after the primary lesion has regressed or been resected [55]. Cervical cancer typically recurs early, and in 60–70% of cases, it recurs within 2 years of starting treatment [18]. Recurrence may be loco-regional, including recurrence in the vaginal vault, cervix, uterus, bladder, bowel, or involving pelvic nodal stations. Distant recurrence includes the involvement of extra pelvic nodal stations (e.g., paraaortic, supradiaphragmatic) or distant organ metastases. There is no established role for routine imaging follow-up for patients treated with hysterectomy. Imaging is usually reserved for patients with a clinical suspicion of recurrence, such as those who present with abnormal vaginal discharge or bleeding. The commonest sites of recurrence post-hysterectomy include the vaginal stump and rectovaginal space. After fertility-sparing surgery, patients are imaged with MRI at six months and then annually for 2–3 years. After chemoradiotherapy, patients are reimaged with FDG-PET/CT and MRI at 3–6 months [50]. The protocol is similar to that used in initial staging; however, the axial oblique planes are adjusted to the vaginal vault in the setting of prior hysterectomy. The recurrent tumour has a similar appearance to that of the primary tumour and appears as intermediate signal intensity lesions on T2WI with corresponding diffusion restriction on DWI and ADC maps (Figure 18). Radiotherapy-induced fibrosis usually demonstrates low signal intensity on all sequences. However, in some cases, the signal intensity may be atypical and therefore it can be difficult to differentiate fibrosis from tumour. DWI is helpful in this scenario, as fibrosis does not demonstrate restricted diffusion. Post-contrast imaging is less useful as both fibrosis and tumour can demonstrate enhancement.

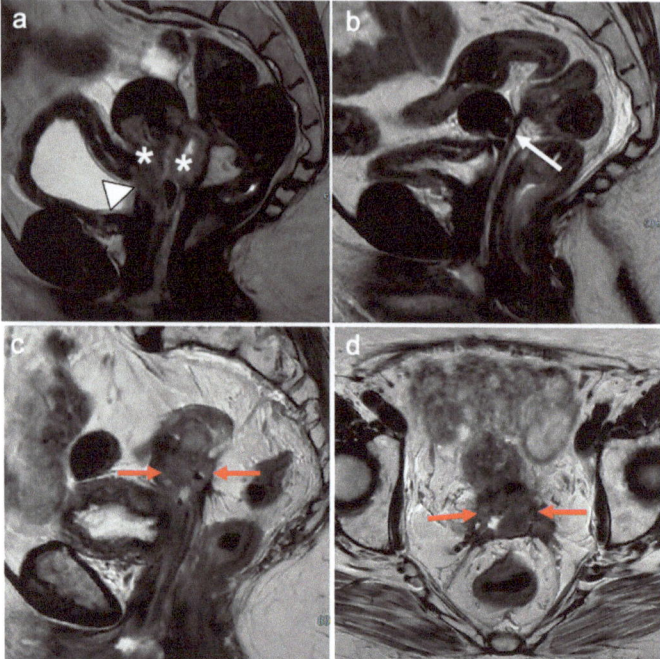

Figure 18. Sagittal T2WI at initial staging (**a**) demonstrates a bulky cervical tumour (*) with bladder involvement (arrow head). 6 month post-treatment (**b**) demonstrates reconstitution of the low signal cervical stroma indicating a complete response. Thin low signal intensity bands extend to the rectum consistent with post treatment fibrosis (white arrow). One year later the patient began experiencing bowel symptoms and subsequent MRI in sagittal (**c**) and axial (**d**) planes demonstrates intermediate signal intensity at the cervix (red arrows), extending to and involving the rectum consistent with recurrence.

10. Conclusions

MRI is integral to the management of cervical cancer, having been formally incorporated into the updated 2018 FIGO staging system. MRI allows the accurate assessment of tumour size, parametrial involvement, and lymph node involvement, which are crucial for triaging patients into those that will be eligible for primary surgery or chemoradiotherapy. MRI has applications for radiotherapy planning and image-guided adaptive brachytherapy. It also has a role in evaluating treatment response and detecting tumour recurrence and possible treatment complications.

Author Contributions: Writing—original draft preparation, A.S.; writing—review and editing, A.S., J.Y.J.L. and S.F. All authors have read and agreed to the published version of the manuscript.

Funding: This research received no external funding.

Informed Consent Statement: Not applicable.

Data Availability Statement: No new data were created or analyzed in this study. Data sharing is not applicable to this article.

Conflicts of Interest: The authors declare no conflict of interest.

References

1. Sung, H.; Ferlay, J.; Siegel, R.L.; Laversanne, M.; Soerjomataram, I.; Jemal, A.; Bray, F. Global Cancer Statistics 2020: GLOBOCAN Estimates of Incidence and Mortality Worldwide for 36 Cancers in 185 Countries. *CA. Cancer J. Clin.* **2021**, *71*, 209–249. [CrossRef] [PubMed]
2. Bosch, F.X.; Lorincz, A.; Muñoz, N.; Meijer, C.J.L.M.; Shah, K.V. The causal relation between human papillomavirus and cervical cancer. *J. Clin. Pathol.* **2002**, *55*, 244–265. [CrossRef] [PubMed]
3. Bhatla, N.; Aoki, D.; Sharma, D.N.; Sankaranarayanan, R. Cancer of the cervix uteri: 2021 update. *Int. J. Gynecol. Obstet.* **2021**, *155*, 28–44. [CrossRef]
4. Global Strategy to Accelerate the Elimination of Cervical Cancer as a Public Health Problem. Available online: https://www.who.int/publications-detail-redirect/9789240014107 (accessed on 22 August 2023).
5. Hu, K.; Wang, W.; Liu, X.; Meng, Q.; Zhang, F. Comparison of treatment outcomes between squamous cell carcinoma and adenocarcinoma of cervix after definitive radiotherapy or concurrent chemoradiotherapy. *Radiat. Oncol. Lond. Engl.* **2018**, *13*, 249. [CrossRef]
6. Alcazar, J.L.; García, E.; Machuca, M.; Quintana, R.; Escrig, J.; Chacón, E.; Mínguez, J.A.; Chiva, L. Magnetic resonance imaging and ultrasound for assessing parametrial infiltration in cervical cancer. A systematic review and meta-analysis. *Med. Ultrason.* **2020**, *22*, 85–91. [CrossRef] [PubMed]
7. Woo, S.; Atun, R.; Ward, Z.J.; Scott, A.M.; Hricak, H.; Vargas, H.A. Diagnostic performance of conventional and advanced imaging modalities for assessing newly diagnosed cervical cancer: Systematic review and meta-analysis. *Eur. Radiol.* **2020**, *30*, 5560–5577. [CrossRef] [PubMed]
8. Pannu, H.K.; Corl, F.M.; Fishman, E.K. CT Evaluation of Cervical Cancer: Spectrum of Disease. *RadioGraphics* **2001**, *21*, 1155–1168. [CrossRef]
9. Tsili, A.C.; Tsangou, V.; Koliopoulos, G.; Stefos, T.; Argyropoulou, M.I. Early-stage cervical carcinoma: The role of multidetector CT in correlation with histopathological findings. *J. Obstet. Gynaecol.* **2013**, *33*, 882–887. [CrossRef]
10. Mirpour, S.; Mhlanga, J.C.; Logeswaran, P.; Russo, G.; Mercier, G.; Subramaniam, R.M. The Role of PET/CT in the Management of Cervical Cancer. *Am. J. Roentgenol.* **2013**, *201*, W192–W205. [CrossRef]
11. Cibula, D.; Raspollini, M.R.; Planchamp, F.; Centeno, C.; Chargari, C.; Felix, A.; Fischerová, D.; Jahnn-Kuch, D.; Joly, F.; Kohler, C.; et al. ESGO/ESTRO/ESP Guidelines for the management of patients with cervical cancer—Update 2023. *Int. J. Gynecol. Cancer* **2023**, *33*, 649–666. [CrossRef]
12. Ruan, J.; Zhang, Y.; Ren, H. Meta-analysis of PET/CT Detect Lymph Nodes Metastases of Cervical Cancer. *Open Med.* **2018**, *13*, 436–442. [CrossRef] [PubMed]
13. Balleyguier, C.; Sala, E.; Da Cunha, T.; Bergman, A.; Brkljacic, B.; Danza, F.; Forstner, R.; Hamm, B.; Kubik-Huch, R.; Lopez, C.; et al. Staging of uterine cervical cancer with MRI: Guidelines of the European Society of Urogenital Radiology. *Eur. Radiol.* **2011**, *21*, 1102–1110. [CrossRef] [PubMed]
14. Hricak, H.; Powell, C.B.; Yu, K.K.; Washington, E.; Subak, L.L.; Stern, J.L.; Cisternas, M.G.; Arenson, R.L. Invasive cervical carcinoma: Role of MR imaging in pretreatment work-up--cost minimization and diagnostic efficacy analysis. *Radiology* **1996**, *198*, 403–409. [CrossRef] [PubMed]
15. Manganaro, L.; Lakhman, Y.; Bharwani, N.; Gui, B.; Gigli, S.; Vinci, V.; Rizzo, S.; Kido, A.; Cunha, T.M.; Sala, E.; et al. Staging, recurrence and follow-up of uterine cervical cancer using MRI: Updated Guidelines of the European Society of Urogenital Radiology after revised FIGO staging 2018. *Eur. Radiol.* **2021**, *31*, 7802–7816. [CrossRef]
16. Gala, F.B.; Gala, K.B.; Gala, B.M. Magnetic Resonance Imaging of Uterine Cervix: A Pictorial Essay. *Indian J. Radiol. Imaging* **2021**, *31*, 454–467. [CrossRef]
17. Salib, M.Y.; Russell, J.H.B.; Stewart, V.R.; Sudderuddin, S.A.; Barwick, T.D.; Rockall, A.G.; Bharwani, N. 2018 FIGO Staging Classification for Cervical Cancer: Added Benefits of Imaging. *RadioGraphics* **2020**, *40*, 1807–1822. [CrossRef]
18. Sala, E.; Rockall, A.G.; Freeman, S.J.; Mitchell, D.G.; Reinhold, C. The Added Role of MR Imaging in Treatment Stratification of Patients with Gynecologic Malignancies: What the Radiologist Needs to Know. *Radiology* **2013**, *266*, 717–740. [CrossRef]
19. Baliyan, V.; Das, C.J.; Sharma, R.; Gupta, A.K. Diffusion weighted imaging: Technique and applications. *World J. Radiol.* **2016**, *8*, 785–798. [CrossRef]
20. Chenevert, T.L.; Stegman, L.D.; Taylor, J.M.; Robertson, P.L.; Greenberg, H.S.; Rehemtulla, A.; Ross, B.D. Diffusion magnetic resonance imaging: An early surrogate marker of therapeutic efficacy in brain tumors. *J. Natl. Cancer Inst.* **2000**, *92*, 2029–2036. [CrossRef]
21. Nougaret, S.; Tirumani, S.H.; Addley, H.; Pandey, H.; Sala, E.; Reinhold, C. Pearls and Pitfalls in MRI of Gynecologic Malignancy With Diffusion-Weighted Technique. *Am. J. Roentgenol.* **2013**, *200*, 261–276. [CrossRef]
22. Otero-García, M.M.; Mesa-Álvarez, A.; Nikolic, O.; Blanco-Lobato, P.; Basta-Nikolic, M.; de Llano-Ortega, R.M.; Paredes-Velázquez, L.; Nikolic, N.; Szewczyk-Bieda, M. Role of MRI in staging and follow-up of endometrial and cervical cancer: Pitfalls and mimickers. *Insights Imaging* **2019**, *10*, 19. [CrossRef] [PubMed]
23. Duarte, A.L.; Dias, J.L.; Cunha, T.M. Pitfalls of diffusion-weighted imaging of the female pelvis. *Radiol. Bras.* **2018**, *51*, 37–44. [CrossRef] [PubMed]
24. Harry, V.N.; Persad, S.; Bassaw, B.; Parkin, D. Diffusion-weighted MRI to detect early response to chemoradiation in cervical cancer: A systematic review and meta-analysis. *Gynecol. Oncol. Rep.* **2021**, *38*, 100883. [CrossRef]

25. Meyer, H.-J.; Wienke, A.; Surov, A. Pre-treatment Apparent Diffusion Coefficient Does Not Predict Therapy Response to Radiochemotherapy in Cervical Cancer: A Systematic Review and Meta-Analysis. *Anticancer Res.* **2021**, *41*, 1163–1170. [CrossRef] [PubMed]
26. Shakur, A.; O'Shea, A.; Harisinghani, M.G. Pelvic Lymph Node Anatomy. In *Atlas of Lymph Node Anatomy*; Harisinghani, M.G., Ed.; Springer International Publishing: Cham, Switzerland, 2021; pp. 93–152, ISBN 978-3-030-80899-0.
27. Keshavarz, E.; Ahangaran, A.; Pouya, E.K.; Maheronnaghsh, R.; Chavoshi, M.; Rouzrokh, P. Effects of Obesity on Axillary Lymph Node Structure: Association of Hilar Fat Deposition and Alterations in Cortex Width. *Maedica* **2020**, *15*, 99–104. [CrossRef]
28. Avesani, G.; Perazzolo, A.; Amerighi, A.; Celli, V.; Panico, C.; Sala, E.; Gui, B. The Utility of Contrast-Enhanced Magnetic Resonance Imaging in Uterine Cervical Cancer: A Systematic Review. *Life* **2023**, *13*, 1368. [CrossRef] [PubMed]
29. Akita, A.; Shinmoto, H.; Hayashi, S.; Akita, H.; Fujii, T.; Mikami, S.; Tanimoto, A.; Kuribayashi, S. Comparison of T2-weighted and contrast-enhanced T1-weighted MR imaging at 1.5 T for assessing the local extent of cervical carcinoma. *Eur. Radiol.* **2011**, *21*, 1850–1857. [CrossRef]
30. Tomaszewski, M.R.; Gillies, R.J. The Biological Meaning of Radiomic Features. *Radiology* **2021**, *298*, 505–516. [CrossRef]
31. Becker, A.S.; Ghafoor, S.; Marcon, M.; Perucho, J.A.; Wurnig, M.C.; Wagner, M.W.; Khong, P.-L.; Lee, E.Y.; Boss, A. MRI texture features may predict differentiation and nodal stage of cervical cancer: A pilot study. *Acta Radiol. Open* **2017**, *6*, 2058460117729574. [CrossRef]
32. Wormald, B.W.; Doran, S.J.; Ind, T.E.J.; D'Arcy, J.; Petts, J.; deSouza, N.M. Radiomic features of cervical cancer on T2-and diffusion-weighted MRI: Prognostic value in low-volume tumors suitable for trachelectomy. *Gynecol. Oncol.* **2020**, *156*, 107–114. [CrossRef]
33. Laliscia, C.; Gadducci, A.; Mattioni, R.; Orlandi, F.; Giusti, S.; Barcellini, A.; Gabelloni, M.; Morganti, R.; Neri, E.; Paiar, F. MRI-based radiomics: Promise for locally advanced cervical cancer treated with a tailored integrated therapeutic approach. *Tumori* **2022**, *108*, 376–385. [CrossRef] [PubMed]
34. Li, L.; Zhang, J.; Zhe, X.; Tang, M.; Zhang, X.; Lei, X.; Zhang, L. A meta-analysis of MRI-based radiomic features for predicting lymph node metastasis in patients with cervical cancer. *Eur. J. Radiol.* **2022**, *151*, 110243. [CrossRef] [PubMed]
35. Subak, L.L.; Hricak, H.; Powell, C.B.; Azizi, L.; Stern, J.L. Cervical carcinoma: Computed tomography and magnetic resonance imaging for preoperative staging. *Obstet. Gynecol.* **1995**, *86*, 43–50. [CrossRef] [PubMed]
36. Salvo, G.; Odetto, D.; Saez Perrotta, M.C.; Noll, F.; Perrotta, M.; Pareja, R.; Wernicke, A.; Ramirez, P.T. Measurement of tumor size in early cervical cancer: An ever-evolving paradigm. *Int. J. Gynecol. Cancer* **2020**, *30*, 1215–1223. [CrossRef] [PubMed]
37. Kido, A.; Nakamoto, Y. Implications of the new FIGO staging and the role of imaging in cervical cancer. *Br. J. Radiol.* **2021**, *94*, 20201342. [CrossRef] [PubMed]
38. Young, P.; Daniel, B.; Sommer, G.; Kim, B.; Herfkens, R. Intravaginal gel for staging of female pelvic cancers--preliminary report of safety, distention, and gel-mucosal contrast during magnetic resonance examination. *J Comput. Assist. Tomogr.* **2012**, *36*, 253–256. [CrossRef] [PubMed]
39. Valentini, A.L.; Gui, B.; Miccò, M.; Giuliani, M.; Rodolfino, E.; Ninivaggi, V.; Iacobucci, M.; Marino, M.; Gambacorta, M.A.; Testa, A.C.; et al. MRI anatomy of parametrial extension to better identify local pathways of disease spread in cervical cancer. *Diagn. Interv. Radiol.* **2016**, *22*, 319–325. [CrossRef]
40. Freeman, S.J.; Aly, A.M.; Kataoka, M.Y.; Addley, H.C.; Reinhold, C.; Sala, E. The revised FIGO staging system for uterine malignancies: Implications for MR imaging. *Radiographics* **2012**, *32*, 1805–1827. [CrossRef] [PubMed]
41. Kostov, S.; Selçuk, I.; Watrowski, R.; Kornovski, Y.; Yalçın, H.; Slavchev, S.; Ivanova, Y.; Dzhenkov, D.; Yordanov, A. Pelvic Sidewall Anatomy in Gynecologic Oncology-New Insights into a Potential Avascular Space. *Diagnostics* **2022**, *12*, 519. [CrossRef]
42. Wright, J.D.; Matsuo, K.; Huang, Y.; Tergas, A.I.; Hou, J.Y.; Khoury-Collado, F.; St Clair, C.M.; Ananth, C.V.; Neugut, A.I.; Hershman, D.L. Prognostic Performance of the 2018 International Federation of Gynecology and Obstetrics Cervical Cancer Staging Guidelines. *Obstet. Gynecol.* **2019**, *134*, 49–57. [CrossRef]
43. Jorg, T.; Halfmann, M.C.; Arnhold, G.; Pinto dos Santos, D.; Kloeckner, R.; Düber, C.; Mildenberger, P.; Jungmann, F.; Müller, L. Implementation of structured reporting in clinical routine: A review of 7 years of institutional experience. *Insights Imaging* **2023**, *14*, 61. [CrossRef] [PubMed]
44. McEvoy, S.H.; Nougaret, S.; Abu-Rustum, N.R.; Vargas, H.A.; Sadowski, E.A.; Menias, C.O.; Shitano, F.; Fujii, S.; Sosa, R.E.; Escalon, J.G.; et al. Fertility-sparing for young patients with gynecologic cancer: How MRI can guide patient selection prior to conservative management. *Abdom. Radiol.* **2017**, *42*, 2488–2512; Erratum in *Abdom. Radiol.* **2017**, *42*, 2966–2973.
45. Halaska, M.; Robova, H.; Pluta, M.; Rob, L. The role of trachelectomy in cervical cancer. *Ecancermedicalscience* **2015**, *9*, 506. [CrossRef]
46. Rockall, A.G.; Qureshi, M.; Papadopoulou, I.; Saso, S.; Butterfield, N.; Thomassin-Naggara, I.; Farthing, A.; Smith, J.R.; Bharwani, N. Role of Imaging in Fertility-sparing Treatment of Gynecologic Malignancies. *Radiographics* **2016**, *36*, 2214–2233. [CrossRef] [PubMed]
47. Moro, F.; Bonanno, G.M.; Gui, B.; Scambia, G.; Testa, A.C. Imaging modalities in fertility preservation in patients with gynecologic cancers. *Int. J. Gynecol. Cancer* **2021**, *31*, 323–331. [CrossRef] [PubMed]
48. Noël, P.; Dubé, M.; Plante, M.; St-Laurent, G. Early cervical carcinoma and fertility-sparing treatment options: MR imaging as a tool in patient selection and as a follow-up modality. *Radiographics* **2014**, *34*, 1099–1119. [CrossRef] [PubMed]

49. Yan, R.N.; Zeng, Z.; Liu, F.; Zeng, Y.Y.; He, T.; Xiang, Z.Z.; Zhang, B.L.; Gong, H.L.; Liu, L. Primary radical hysterectomy vs chemoradiation for IB2-IIA cervical cancer: A systematic review and meta-analysis. *Medicine* **2020**, *99*, e18738. [CrossRef]
50. Ciulla, S.; Celli, V.; Aiello, A.A.; Gigli, S.; Ninkova, R.; Miceli, V.; Ercolani, G.; Dolciami, M.; Ricci, P.; Palaia, I.; et al. Post treatment imaging in patients with local advanced cervical carcinoma. *Front. Oncol.* **2022**, *12*, 1003930. [CrossRef]
51. Pötter, R.; Tanderup, K.; Schmid, M.P.; Jürgenliemk-Schulz, I.; Haie-Meder, C.; Fokdal, L.U.; Sturdza, A.E.; Hoskin, P.; Mahantshetty, U.; Segedin, B.; et al. MRI-guided adaptive brachytherapy in locally advanced cervical cancer (EMBRACE-I): A multicentre prospective cohort study. *Lancet Oncol.* **2021**, *22*, 538–547. [CrossRef]
52. Tanderup, K.; Viswanathan, A.; Kirisits, C.; Frank, S.J. MRI-guided brachytherapy. *Semin. Radiat. Oncol.* **2014**, *24*, 181–191. [CrossRef]
53. Russo, L.; Lancellotta, V.; Miccò, M.; Fionda, B.; Avesani, G.; Rovirosa, A.; Wojcieszek, P.; Scambia, G.; Manfredi, R.; Tagliaferri, L.; et al. Magnetic resonance imaging in cervical cancer interventional radiotherapy (brachytherapy): A pictorial essay focused on radiologist management. *J. Contemp. Brachytherapy* **2022**, *14*, 287–298. [CrossRef] [PubMed]
54. Olthof, E.P.; Wenzel, H.; van der Velden, J.; Spijkerboer, A.M.; Bekkers, R.; Beltman, J.J.; Nijman, H.W.; Slangen, B.; Smolders, R.; van Trommel, N.; et al. Treatment of bulky lymph nodes in locally advanced cervical cancer: Boosting versus debulking. *Int. J. Gynecol. Cancer* **2022**, *32*, 861–868. [CrossRef] [PubMed]
55. Miccò, M.; Lupinelli, M.; Mangialardi, M.; Gui, B.; Manfredi, R. Patterns of Recurrent Disease in Cervical Cancer. *J. Pers. Med.* **2022**, *12*, 755. [CrossRef] [PubMed]

Disclaimer/Publisher's Note: The statements, opinions and data contained in all publications are solely those of the individual author(s) and contributor(s) and not of MDPI and/or the editor(s). MDPI and/or the editor(s) disclaim responsibility for any injury to people or property resulting from any ideas, methods, instructions or products referred to in the content.

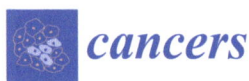

Article

Prediction of the Risk of Malignancy of Adnexal Masses during Pregnancy Comparing Subjective Assessment and Non-Contrast MRI Score (NCMS) in Radiologists with Different Expertise

Camilla Panico [1], Silvia Bottazzi [1], Luca Russo [1], Giacomo Avesani [1,*], Veronica Celli [1], Luca D'Erme [1], Alessia Cipriani [1], Floriana Mascilini [2], Anna Fagotti [2,3], Giovanni Scambia [2,3], Evis Sala [1,3] and Benedetta Gui [1]

[1] Department of Diagnostic Imaging, Oncological Radiotherapy and Haematology, Fondazione Policlinico Universitario A. Gemelli IRCCS, 00168 Rome, Italy; camilla.panico@policlinicogemelli.it (C.P.); silvia.bottazzi01@icatt.it (S.B.); luca.russo@guest.policlinicogemelli.it (L.R.); veronica.celli@guest.policlinicogemelli.it (V.C.); luca.derme01@icatt.it (L.D.); alessia.cipriani03@icatt.it (A.C.); evis.sala@policlinicogemelli.it (E.S.); benedetta.gui@policlinicogemelli.it (B.G.)
[2] Department of Woman and Child Health and Public Health, Fondazione Policlinico Universitario A. Gemelli IRCCS, 00168 Rome, Italy; floriana.mascilini@policlinicogemelli.it (F.M.); anna.fagotti@policlinicogemelli.it (A.F.); giovanni.scambia@policlinicogemelli.it (G.S.)
[3] Faculty of Medicine and Surgery, Università Cattolica del Sacro Cuore, 00168 Rome, Italy
* Correspondence: giacomo.avesani@policlinicogemelli.it

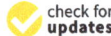

Citation: Panico, C.; Bottazzi, S.; Russo, L.; Avesani, G.; Celli, V.; D'Erme, L.; Cipriani, A.; Mascilini, F.; Fagotti, A.; Scambia, G.; et al. Prediction of the Risk of Malignancy of Adnexal Masses during Pregnancy Comparing Subjective Assessment and Non-Contrast MRI Score (NCMS) in Radiologists with Different Expertise. *Cancers* **2023**, *15*, 5138. https://doi.org/10.3390/cancers15215138

Academic Editor: Athina C Tsili

Received: 18 August 2023
Revised: 18 October 2023
Accepted: 19 October 2023
Published: 25 October 2023

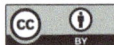

Copyright: © 2023 by the authors. Licensee MDPI, Basel, Switzerland. This article is an open access article distributed under the terms and conditions of the Creative Commons Attribution (CC BY) license (https://creativecommons.org/licenses/by/4.0/).

Simple Summary: Characterising an ovarian mass during pregnancy is essential to avoid unnecessary treatment and, if treatment is required, to plan it accordingly. MRI of the pelvis with post-contrast sequences is indicated when adnexal masses are indeterminate at the US examination. However, the administration of intravenous gadolinium-based contrast agents is a method that should have a limited use in pregnant women. We evaluated the diagnostic accuracy of the Non-Contrast MRI Score (NCMS) in pregnant women, using both a subjective assessment (SA) and the NCMS, between two radiologists with different expertise. Relying on histopathology and imaging follow-up at one year as the gold standard, we found that the expert radiologist correctly classified 90% of the diagnoses using both SA and the NCMS (85.7% sensitivity and 92.3% specificity, with a false positive rate of 7.7% and a false negative rate of 14.3%). The non-expert radiologist correctly identified patients at a lower rate, especially using the SA (60%), with a sensitivity of 85% and a specificity of 46.2%. The analysis of the inter-observer agreement showed a K = 0.47 (95% CI: 0.48–0.94) for the SA (agreement in 71.4% of cases) and a K = 0.8 (95% CI: 0.77–1.00) for the use of the NCMS (agreement in 90% of cases). This study evaluates the diagnostic accuracy of non-contrast MRI scores in pregnant women with indeterminate ovarian masses at the US examination. The NCMS is a reliable tool to predict the risk of malignancy of adnexal masses in these women and extremely useful for inexperienced radiologists.

Abstract: Ovarian cancer represents 7% of all cancers in pregnant women. Characterising an ovarian mass during pregnancy is essential to avoid unnecessary treatment and, if treatment is required, to plan it accordingly. Although ultrasonography (US) is the first-line modality to characterise adnexal masses, MRI is indicated when adnexal masses are indeterminate at the US examination. An MRI risk stratification system has been proposed to assign a malignancy probability based on the adnexal lesion's MRI, but features of the scoring system require the administration of intravenous gadolinium-based contrast agents, a method that might have a limited use in pregnant women. The non-contrast MRI score (NCMS) has been used and evaluated in non-pregnant women to characterise adnexal masses indeterminate at the US examination. Therefore, we evaluated the diagnostic accuracy of the NCMS in pregnant women, analysing 20 cases referred to our specialised institution. We also evaluated the diagnostic agreement between two radiologists with different expertise. The two readers classified ovarian masses as benign or malignant using both subjective assessment (SA), based on the interpretive evaluation of imaging findings derived from personal experience, and the NCMS, which includes five categories where 4 and 5 indicate a high probability of a malignant mass. The expert radiologist correctly classified 90% of the diagnoses, using both SA and the NCMS, relying on a sensitivity of 85.7% and a specificity of 92.3%, with a false positive rate of 7.7% and a false negative rate of 14.3%. The non-expert radiologist correctly identified patients at a lower rate, especially using the SA. The analysis of the inter-observer agreement showed a K = 0.47 (95% CI: 0.48–0.94) for the SA (agreement in 71.4% of cases) and a K = 0.8 (95% CI: 0.77–1.00) for the NCMS (agreement in 90% of cases). Although in pregnant patients, non-contrast MRI is used, our results support the use of a quantitative score, i.e., the NCMS, as an accurate tool. This procedure may help less experienced radiologists to reduce the rate of false negatives or positives, especially in centres not specialised in gynaecological imaging, making the MRI interpretation easier and more accurate for radiologists who are not experts in the field, either.

Keywords: ovarian cancer; MRI; pregnancy

1. Introduction

The incidence of cancer during childbearing is rising due to the increasing age of first pregnancy [1]. Ovarian cancer represents 7% of all cancers in pregnant women [2]. The frequency of adnexal masses in pregnancy differs between different studies—approximately between 0.05% and 2.4% of all pregnancies [3–6]. Most of the masses are benign [3–6], and malignant ones are reported between 1 and 8% [3–6]. Therefore, characterising an ovarian mass during pregnancy is essential to avoid unnecessary treatment and, if treatment is required, to plan it accordingly.

Ultrasound (US) is the first-line modality to characterise adnexal masses, and various diagnostic scores have been proposed and evaluated for sensitivity and specificity to diagnose malignant lesions; the IOTA's (International Ovarian Tumour Analysis) simple rules provide a sensitivity of 92% and a specificity of 69% [6,7]. MRI is indicated when adnexal masses are indeterminate at the US examination [8–10]. The success of the use of MRI was due to its better detection of fat and blood content in lesions.

High rates of MRI were reported in young women (pregnant and non-pregnant) for diagnoses in many body organs. Regarding MRI in pregnancy, the prevalence of 1 gadolinium exposure every 860 pregnancies was detected in a large American study [11]. This prevalence was 4.3-fold greater during the first trimester than during the second trimester and 5.1-fold greater than during the third trimester. In non-pregnant women, the Ovarian–Adnexal Imaging–Reporting–Data System (O-RADS) MRI risk stratification system has been proposed to assign a malignancy probability based on the adnexal lesion's MRI features [12,13]. The score yielded high sensitivity (93%) and specificity (91%) for stratifying the risk of malignancy in adnexal masses [13]. Moreover, Thomassin-Naggara et al. showed that MRI has a high accuracy (>80%) in the characterisation of adnexal masses in pregnancy, especially when evaluating images using the AdnexMR score, in a cohort study of 1340 women [12]. Both these scoring systems require the administration of intravenous gadolinium-based contrast agents (GBCAs) [12,13]. Some clinical studies have shown that, despite gadolinium-based contrast media during pregnancy being relatively safe, with a low incidence of adverse effects, its use should be limited in clinical practice when strictly necessary [14–17]. Recently, the non-Contrast MRI score (NCMS) was proposed [18]. The score includes five categories—from 1 to 5—and does not require the administration of GBCAs (Table 1).

The use of the NCMS, which has already shown promising results in non-pregnant patients, may have an added value in the clinical scenario of pregnancy when the use GBCAs is discouraged.

Table 1. The non-contrast MRI score (NCMS).

Score	Definition	MRI Features
1	No adnexal mass	No adnexal mass present
2	Benign/likely benign	Radiological diagnosis of benign mass (e.g., endometrioma, dermoid, fibroma)
3	Indeterminate	Not classified in another score (it may have a solid component, but it does not reach the criteria for solid tissue *)
4	Suspicious for malignancy	Solid tissue criteria reached *
5	Highly suspicious for malignancy	Solid tissue criteria reached * + lymphadenopathy/peritoneal implants/ascites

* Solid tissue is defined as tissue with a hypointense signal on T1W1, an intermediate signal on T2W1 and corresponding true diffusion restriction. Masses with a score ≥ 4 are considered malignant.

This study aims to investigate the accuracy of non-contrast MRI in the prediction of the risk of malignancy of indeterminate adnexal masses at ultrasonography in pregnancy, comparing subjective assessments (SAs) and NCMSs between radiologists with "different expertise".

Considering the wide range of possible diagnoses, an additional task of the radiologist was to provide diagnostic hypotheses regarding the nature of the mass.

2. Materials and Methods

2.1. Study Design

This is a retrospective monocentric study.

The institutional ethics committee approved this study (approval no. 5681, 5 June 2023).

Inclusion criteria were the following: (1) pregnant women; (2) >18 years old; (3) indeterminate adnexal masses at US examination; (4) availability of MRI and histopathological results or at least one follow-up imaging at one year. Patients with a diagnosis of extra-ovarian mass were excluded.

Our picture archiving and communication system (PACS) was searched to retrieve the MRI examinations of pregnant patients scanned for a US-indeterminate adnexal mass between January 2011 and February 2023. All patients meeting the inclusion criteria were asked to sign informed consent forms to use their clinical data. Only those who gave informed consent were included in the study.

2.2. MRI Protocol

Patients were scanned on different 1.5T MRI scanners from the same vendor (GE Medical Systems, Milwaukee, WI, USA), using a phased-array abdominal coil. The acquisition protocol is reported in Supplementary Table S1.

A gadolinium-based contrast agent was not administered. T2WI fast-spin echo (FSE) sequences were obtained in multiple planes (axial, sagittal and coronal). Axial T1WI gradient-echo or FSE sequences were obtained with and without fat suppression. Axial diffusion-weighted imaging (DWI) was acquired with b values of 0 and 800–1000 s/mm^2. Apparent diffusion coefficient (ADC) maps were derived. In addition, axial T2WIs and axial DWIs of the upper abdomen were acquired to assess the presence of retroperitoneal lymphadenopathy and hydronephrosis.

2.3. Image Interpretation

Two radiologists (reader 1 and reader 2) with different expertise in gynaecological imaging—1 and 7 years, respectively—independently reviewed the images blinded to US examination results. The two readers classified ovarian masses using SA and the NCMS. The lesions were classified according to the SA as benign or malignant. Subjective assessment was based on the interpretive evaluation of imaging findings based on personal experience, expertise and judgment. Then, the readers assigned a score from 1 to 5 following the NCMS (Table 1). The scoring system includes five categories. A score of 1 was assigned in cases where no adnexal masses were found. If a radiological diagnosis of a benign/likely benign mass was made (endometrioma, fibroma, or dermoid), the readers assigned a score of 2. Higher scores (3, 4 and 5) were assigned to masses characterised as indeterminate, suspicious and highly suspicious for malignancy, respectively. If solid tissue was observed, the lesions were scored as 4. Solid tissue was defined as tissue with intermediate signal intensity (SI) on the T2WI, low signal intensity on the T1WI, and diffusion restriction (high SI on the DWI and low SI on ADC maps). A score of 5 was assigned when lymphadenopathy, peritoneal implants, and/or ascites were present. If masses could not be classified in other scores, a score of 3 was given. Masses with an NCMS > 4 and adnexal lesions classified as indeterminate or malignant at the subjective assessment were considered malignant. Masses with an NCMS < 4 and classified as benign at the subjective assessment were considered benign.

2.4. Statistical Analysis

The categorical variables were expressed as absolute numbers and percentages. According to their distribution, continuous variables were described either as a median and interquartile range or as a mean and standard deviation. Sensitivity, specificity, positive predictive value (PPV), negative predictive value (NPV), accuracy, false positive rate and false negative rate were calculated for both the SAs and the NCMSs of reader 1 and reader 2. These values were calculated using the final diagnoses derived from histopathology (when available) or the follow-up imaging results as binary variables (benign or malignant). Borderline diagnoses were considered malignant. The values were presented as percentages (%) and a 95% confidence interval (CI). The inter-observer agreement between reader 1 and reader 2 for NCMSs and SAs was investigated using Cohen's kappa statistic for agreement. Statistical analysis was performed using SPSS software (SPSS Statistics for Mac 24.0, IBM, SPSS Inc., Chicago, IL, USA) [19].

3. Results

Twenty pregnant women were included in this study. Table 2 reports their mean age and range, separated by diagnosis. Information about laterality, dimension and histologic results is included in Supplementary Table S2.

Table 2. Descriptive characteristics of the pregnant patients.

	N	Age = m(range)
All	20	31.3(20–41)
Benign masses	13	30.3(20–37)
Malignant masses	5	32.4(26–41)
Follow-up	2	31.2(25–40)

There was no difference in the diagnostic outcomes performed by the expert radiologist using either a subjective assessment (Table 3a) or the NCMS (Table 3b).

The diagnostic accuracy of the expert radiologist, reported in Table 3c, was the same for the use of SAs and the NCMS, with the following values: sensitivity, 85.7%; specificity, 92.3%; positive predictive value, 85.7%; negative predictive value, 92.3%; false positive rate, 7.7%; false negative rate, 14.3%. The expert radiologist correctly classified 90.0% of cases, using both SA and the NCMS.

Table 3. (a) Diagnostic performance of the expert radiologist using an SA; (b) diagnostic performance of the expert radiologist using the NCMS; (c) diagnostic performance of the expert radiologist based on both SAs and the NCMS.

(a)			
	Subjective Assessment		
Final Diagnosis	Benign	Malignant	Total
Benign	12	1	13
Malignant	1	6	7
Total	13	7	20

(b)			
	NCMS		
Final Diagnosis	Benign (<4)	Malignant (≥4)	Total
Benign	12	1	13
Malignant	1	6	7
Total	13	7	20

(c)		
	Value %	95% Confidence Interval
Sensitivity	85.7	59.8–100
Specificity	92.3	77.8–100
Positive predictive value	85.7	59.8–100
Negative predictive value	92.3	77.8–100
False positive rate	7.7	0–22.2
False negative rate	14.3	0–42.3
Correctly classified	90.0	76.9–100

Different results are shown for the non-expert radiologist with a low rate of correctly identified patients (12/20; 60%), especially for the SA (Table 4a,b), where the specificity was very low (46.2%).

Table 4. (a) Diagnostic performance of the non-expert radiologist using an SA; (b) diagnostic performance of the non-expert radiologist using the NCMS; (c) diagnostic performance of the non-expert radiologist based on SAs; (d) diagnostic performance of the non-expert radiologist based on the NCMS.

(a)			
	Subjective Assessment		
Final Diagnosis	Benign	Malignant	Total
Benign	6	7	13
Malignant	1	6	7
Total	7	13	20

(b)			
	NCMS		
Final Diagnosis	Benign (<4)	Malignant (≥4)	Total
Benign	10	3	13
Malignant	1	6	7
Total	11	9	20

Table 4. Cont.

(c)		
	Value %	95% Confidence Interval
Sensitivity	85.7	59.8–100
Specificity	46.2	19.1–73.3
Positive predictive value	46.2	19.1–73.3
Negative predictive value	85.7	59.8–100
False positive rate	53.8	26.7–80.9
False negative rate	14.3	0–40.2
Correctly classified	60.0	38.5–81.5
(d)		
	Value %	95% Confidence Interval
Sensitivity	85.7	59.8–100
Specificity	76.9	54.0–99.8
Positive predictive value	66.7	35.9–97.5
Negative predictive value	90.9	73.9–100
False positive rate	23.1	0.2–46.0
False negative rate	14.3	0–40.2
Correctly classified	80.0	62.5–97.5

Table 5a shows the inter-observer agreement between the non-expert and expert radiologists regarding the diagnostic outcomes with SAs: they agreed in 71.4% of the cases with a K = 0.47 (95% CI: 0.48–0.94). Table 5b shows the inter-observer agreement between the non-expert and the expert radiologists regarding the diagnostic outcomes with the use of the NMCS: they agreed in 90.5% of cases with a K = 0.8 (95% CI: 0.77–1.00).

Table 5. (a) Diagnosis outcomes with SA: inter-observer agreement between the non-expert and expert radiologists; (b) diagnosis outcomes with the NCMS: inter-observer agreement between the non-expert and the expert radiologists.

(a)				
		Non-Expert		Total
		Benign	Malignant	
Expert	Benign	7	6	13
	malignant	0	7	7
	Total	7	13	20
(b)				
		Non-Expert		Total
		Benign	Malignant	
Expert	Benign	11	2	13
	malignant	0	7	7
	Total	11	9	20

The analytical description of the diagnoses performed by the two radiologists using the NCMS, according to each single score, is reported in Table 6. There were differences for score 3 (6/20 for the non-expert and 3/20 and for the expert) and for the diagnosis of malignant masses (more scores of 4 and 5 by the non-expert). It is interesting to note that the non-expert radiologist tended to overcall on the side of malignancy, with two benign masses classified by the expert radiologist as benign and as malignant by the non-expert one.

Table 6. Analytical description of the diagnoses performed by the two radiologists using the NCMS, according to each single score.

	Score 1	Score 2	Score 3	Score 4	Score 5
Expert	0	11	3	5	2
Non-expert	0	6	6	6	3

4. Discussion

This retrospective study aimed at investigating the accuracy of non-contrast MRI in characterising sonographically indeterminate adnexal masses upon US examination in pregnant women and also in evaluating the diagnostic accuracy of radiologists with different expertise. In our study, the diagnostic accuracy was high using the NCMS (80% of correctly classified diagnoses for the non-expert radiologist and 90% for the expert one). Furthermore, we found that the agreement between the expert and the non-expert radiologists using the SA was low, while it improved with the use of the NCMS, although the non-expert radiologist tended to over-diagnose malignancy.

Sahin et al. used a similar approach to characterise 350 adnexal masses in non-pregnant women, with promising results. An NCMS ≥ 4 was associated with malignancy with an accuracy of 94.2%, a sensitivity of 84.9%, a specificity of 95.9% and a very good positive likelihood ratio [18], when compared to histology or imaging follow-up at one year. These findings were comparable to those from contrast-enhanced studies [11]. The interpretation of images without post-contrast enhancement performed in our study was corroborated by the Sahin study.

Although exposure to MRI in pregnancy is relatively safe for the foetus [20,21], we know that GBCAs pass through the placental barrier and enter foetal circulation, increasing the risk of rheumatological diseases, inflammatory skin diseases and stillbirth or neonatal undesired birth outcomes [14,15,20,21], therefore restricting the use of contrast-enhanced MRIs to very select cases where the benefit outweighs the risk, only if the imaging is essential and cannot be delayed [20,22].

In this context, our study becomes more valuable.

In the literature, only one study characterised sonographically indeterminate adnexal masses in pregnant women with contrast-enhanced MRIs [23]. In this study, 88.9% of cases were correctly classified, and the result was very similar to our expert radiologist's performance (90%) using the NCMS; this finding suggests that contrast is probably not necessary in this delicate scenario. A few other studies have reported data on the prevalence of malignant adnexal masses in pregnancy but not on the diagnostic accuracy of MRIs. Moreover, they are not comparable since they have been carried out in different settings, observing patients with different characteristics, and are not limited to ovarian masses undetermined at the US examination [3,24,25].

Our results highlighted that the diagnostic accuracy was affected by the fact that, in rare cases, there may be subtle differences between a benign and a malignant lesion, causing misinterpretations, thus leading to an increase in false negatives or false positives for both the expert and the non-expert radiologists. One example in our study population, also reported in the literature, was the correct interpretation of decidualised endometrioma [26–32]. During pregnancy, decidual endometrium changes are due to high levels of progesterone, so endometrioma can undergo decidualisation. Even if the decidualisation of ovarian endometrioma is rare, when it occurs, it is difficult to differentiate from ovarian cancer. In fact, the presence of irregular wall thickening in the decidualised endometrioma can mimic the papillary projections of ovarian cancer [26,32]. Supported by the existing literature, our results also suggested that the evaluation of the ADC value is key for the correct diagnosis because it is significantly higher in benign disease than in ovarian cancers [33] (Figures 1 and 2). Another difficult case was the interpretation of a borderline cystadenoma, which was classified as benign using the SA, with a score of three in the NCMS by both the expert and non-expert radiologists due to the presence of multiple thin septations without the detection of macroscopic solid tissue. However, at histopathology, it was classified as malignant. No solid tissue was seen on the MRI images, due to the difficulty of detecting micro-invasive components [34] (Figure 3). On the other hand, the diagnosis of a benign mature cystic teratoma was correctly made by the expert radiologist, while the lesion was misclassified as malignant by the non-expert radiologist (NCMS 5). In fact, the fat component, which is the main sign of a dermoid cyst, was relatively minimal and was not identified by the non-expert radiologist (Figure 4).

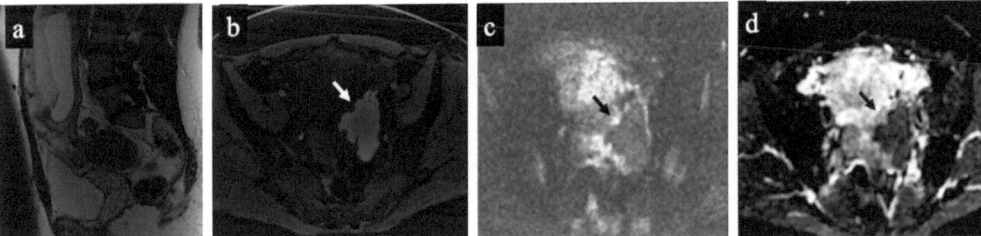

Figure 1. Decidualised endometrioma. MR images of a 37-year-old woman—16 weeks pregnant—with an indeterminate adnexal lesion discovered at the first-trimester US. The sagittal (**a**), axial T1-WI with fat-saturation (**b**), DWI (**c**) and ADC map (**d**) show a unilocular cystic left adnexal mass with haemorrhagic content (high signal intensity on the T1-WI with fat saturation) and some small papillary projections (arrows). Note how the small papillary projections have an intermediate signal on the T2-WI but no corresponding true diffusion restriction (high signal in both DWIs on ADC-map), so they are not considered "solid tissue" according to the NCMS. The lesion was considered indeterminate according to the SA by the non-expert radiologist, who correctly reclassified it as a score of 2 using the NCMS (false positive/true negative).

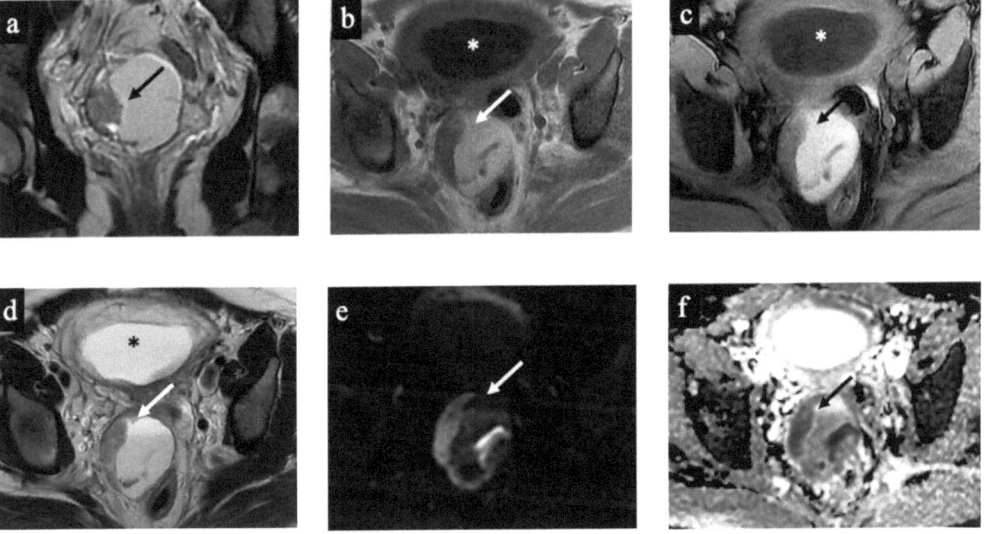

Figure 2. Decidualised endometrioma. MR images of a 34-year-old woman—20 weeks pregnant—with an indeterminate adnexal lesion discovered at the 16-week US. The coronal T2-WI (**a**), axial T1

(**b**), T1-WI with fat-saturation (**c**), T2-WI (**d**), DWI (**e**) and ADC-map images (**f**) show a unilocular cystic right adnexal mass with haemorrhagic content (high signal intensity on the T1-WI, T2-WI, and T1 with fat saturation). This was considered a false positive since both readers misclassified the mass as malignant/score 4 due to the presence of tissue with true diffusion restriction along the lesion's right lateral wall (arrow). Note the gestational sac in the uterine cavity (asterisk).

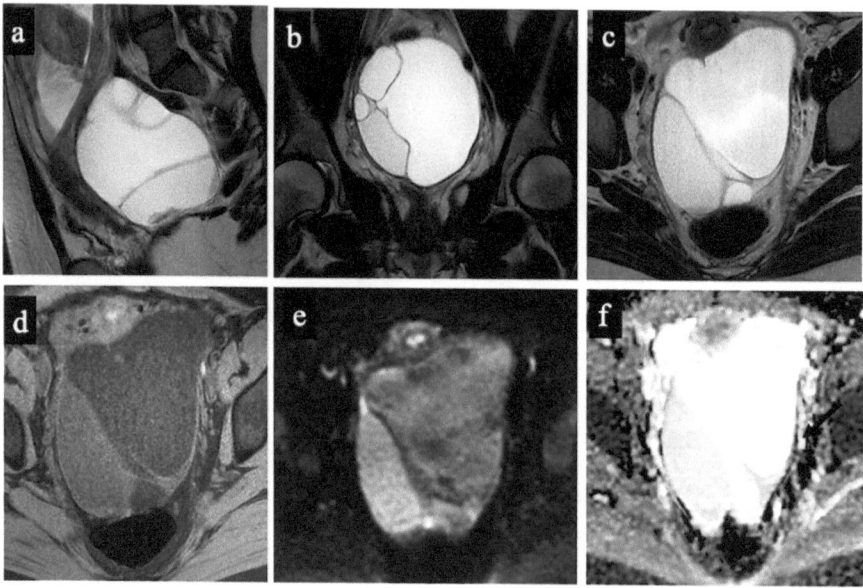

Figure 3. Borderline mucinous cystadenoma. MR images of a 28-year-old woman—17 weeks pregnant—with an indeterminate adnexal lesion discovered at the first-trimester US. The sagittal (**a**), coronal (**b**), and axial T2-WIs (**c**), T1-WI with fat-saturation (**d**), DWI (**e**) and ADC-map images (**f**) show a multilocular cystic left adnexal mass with different signal intensities within the loculi. Both readers considered this lesion as benign/score 3 (probable mucinous cystadenoma) because no solid tissue was found (false negative).

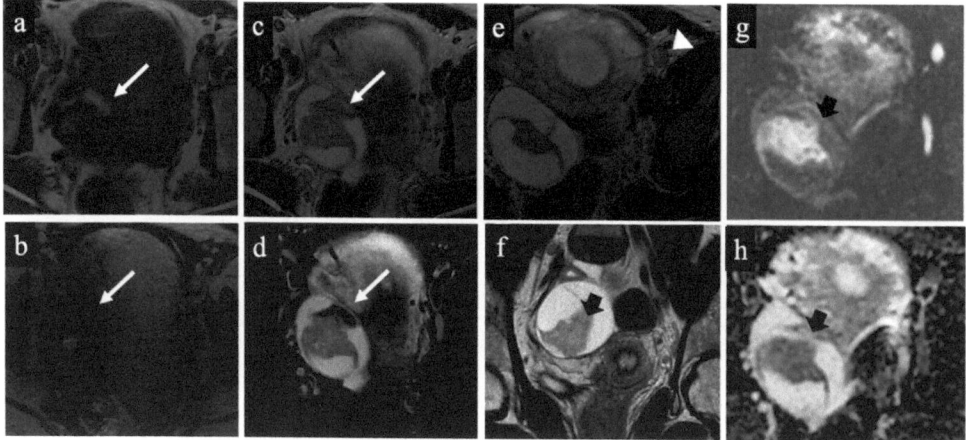

Figure 4. Dermoid cyst. MR images of a 32-year-old woman with an indeterminate adnexal lesion discovered at the first-trimester US. The axial T1-WI (**a**), T1-WI with fat-saturation (**b**), T2-WI (**c**,**e**),

T2-WI with fat-saturation (**d**), coronal T2-WI (**f**), axial DWI (**g**) and ADC-map images (**f**) show a complex right adnexal lesion with fluid and fatty content. Note the drop of the signal of the fatty component, comparing images (**a**)/(**b**) and (**c**)/(**d**) (long arrow). The expert radiologist correctly classified the mass as benign/score 2 (true negative). The subtle fatty content, the left external iliac node with a short axis of 10 mm (arrowhead in image (**e**)), and the presence of tissue with true diffusion restriction within the mass (short arrow in images (**f**–**h**)), tricked the non-expert radiologist who classified it as malignant/score 5 (false positive).

Figures 5 and 6 show two cases of correct diagnoses made by the expert and the non-expert radiologists: one case of a struma ovarii, a multilocular cystic mass without solid tissue that was correctly considered benign/NCMS 2 (true negative), and a case of a low-grade ovarian serous cancer with papillary projections and mural nodules (solid tissue) correctly classified as malignant/score 4 (true positive).

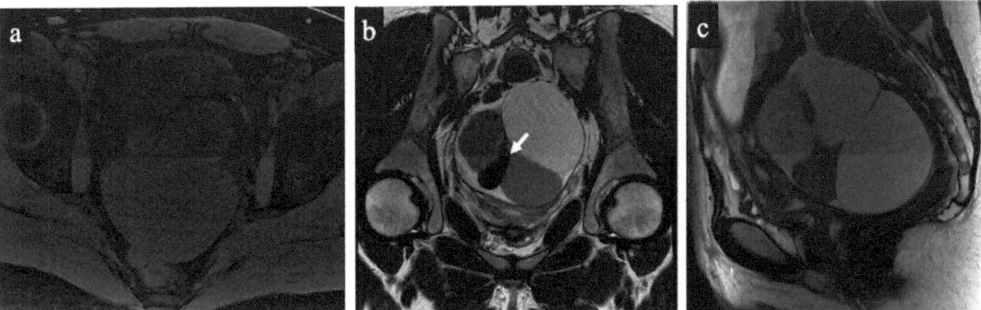

Figure 5. Struma Ovarii. MR images of a 34-year-old woman—16 weeks pregnant—with an indeterminate adnexal mass accidentally discovered at first trimester US. The axial T1 with fat saturation (**a**) and coronal (**b**) and sagittal T2-WI (**c**) images show a multilocular cystic mass with different signal intensities within the loculi. Some loculi have a very low signal intensity on the T2-WI (white arrow in image (**b**)) corresponding to colloid. No solid tissue is seen within the lesion; thus, it was correctly considered as benign/NCMS 2 according to both readers (true negative).

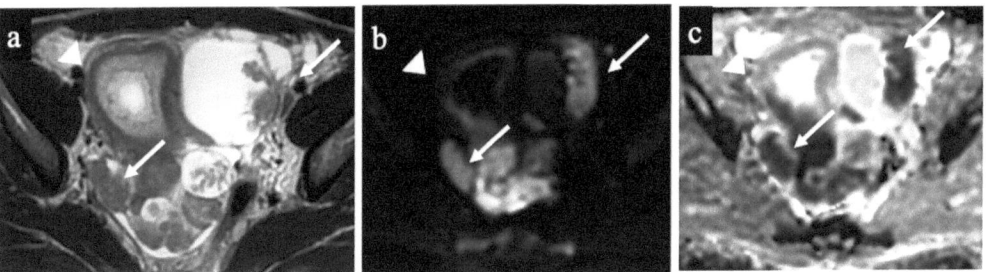

Figure 6. Low-grade ovarian serous cancer. MR images of a 33-year-old woman—7 weeks pregnant—with bilateral indeterminate adnexal lesions discovered at the 6-week US. The axial T2-WI (**a**), DWI (**b**) and ADC-map (**c**) show bilateral adnexal masses with papillary projections and mural nodules (solid tissue) within the lesions (arrows). Solid tissue has an intermediate signal on T2-WIs and corresponding true diffusion restriction. Free pelvic fluid is seen in the pouch of Douglas. No carcinosis was present, so the lesions were correctly classified as malignant/score 4 by both the readers (true positive). Note the gestational sac in the uterine cavity (arrowhead).

The strength of our study was the use of the histopathological results after surgery or the imaging follow-up after one year as the gold standard. Moreover, we evaluated patients with a standard multidisciplinary approach.

Our study has some limitations. First, the retrospective design. Second, the fact that it was performed in a highly specialised institution, and this may provide results that are not easily generalisable to other health institutions. Third, the low number of patients; however, our numbers are not very far from the 31 cases of the only other previous study investigating the diagnostic performance of MRI in pregnant women [23]. Moreover, adnexal masses in pregnancy are rare, and this is the reason for the low number of cases included; multicentric studies may be considered to improve the sample number.

Although in pregnant women, non-contrast MRI is applied, our results support the use of a quantitative score, i.e., the NCMS, as an accurate tool for the characterisation of adnexal masses. This procedure may help less experienced radiologists to reduce the rate of false negatives or positives, especially in centres not specialised in gynaecological imaging, making MRI interpretation easier and more accurate, also for radiologists who are not experts in the field. Nevertheless, it is crucial to emphasise that the patient's overall clinical scenario has a pivotal role; clinical reasoning is the key to the diagnostic process and, together with imaging features, is fundamental for the radiologist to reach an accurate diagnosis.

5. Conclusions

Our study is the first one to evaluate the diagnostic accuracy of NCMSs in pregnant women with indeterminate ovarian masses upon US examination. We found that the NCMS is a reliable tool to predict the risk of malignancy of adnexal masses in pregnant patients. Moreover, the use of the NCMS is particularly useful for less experienced radiologists. Larger, multi-centre prospective studies are necessary to confirm and validate our results.

Supplementary Materials: The following supporting information can be downloaded at: https://www.mdpi.com/article/10.3390/cancers15215138/s1, Supplementary Table S1: MRI protocol. Supplementary Table S2: Characteristics of the masses for each patient included in the study.

Author Contributions: Conceptualisation, C.P., L.R. and S.B.; methodology, L.R. and G.A.; software, L.R. and L.D.; validation, C.P., G.A., E.S. and B.G.; formal analysis, C.P. and F.M.; investigation, L.R. and S.B.; resources, C.P., L.R., V.C., A.C. and S.B.; data curation, C.P., L.R. and S.B.; writing—original draft preparation, C.P., L.R. and S.B.; writing—review and editing, all authors; visualisation, G.A.; supervision, A.F., G.S., E.S. and B.G.; project administration, C.P.; funding acquisition, E.S. All authors have read and agreed to the published version of the manuscript.

Funding: This research received no external funding.

Institutional Review Board Statement: The study was conducted in accordance with the Declaration of Helsinki and approved by the Ethics Committee of Policlinico Gemelli IRCCS (no. 5681, 5 June 2023).

Informed Consent Statement: Informed consent was obtained from all subjects involved in the study.

Data Availability Statement: The data presented in this study are available on request from the corresponding author.

Conflicts of Interest: The authors declare no conflict of interest.

References

1. Gui, B.; Cambi, F.; Miccò, M.; Sbarra, M.; Petta, F.; Autorino, R.; De Vincenzo, R.; Valentini, V.; Scambia, G.; Manfredi, R. MRI in pregnant patients with suspected abdominal and pelvic cancer: A practical guide for radiologists. *Diagn. Interv. Radiol.* **2020**, *26*, 183. [CrossRef] [PubMed]
2. Jha, P.; Pōder, L.; Glanc, P.; Patel-Lippmann, K.; McGettigan, M.; Moshiri, M.; Nougaret, S.; Revzin, M.V.; Javitt, M.C. Imaging cancer in Pregnancy. *Radiographics* **2022**, *42*, 1494–1513. [CrossRef] [PubMed]
3. Leiserowitz, G.S.; Xing, G.; Cress, R.; Brahmbhatt, B.; Dalrymple, J.L.; Smith, L.H. Adnexal masses in pregnancy: How often are they malignant? *Gynecol. Oncol.* **2006**, *101*, 315–321. [CrossRef] [PubMed]

4. Schmeler, K.M.; Mayo-Smith, M.M.; Peipert, J.F.; Weitzen, S.; Manuel, M.D.; Gordinier, M.E. Adnexal Masses in Pregnancy: Surgery Compared with Observation. *Obstet. Gynecol.* **2005**, *105*, 1098–1103. [CrossRef]
5. de Oca, M.K.M.; Dotters-Katz, S.K.; Kuller, J.A.; Previs, R.A. Adnexal Masses in Pregnancy. *Obstet. Gynecol. Surv.* **2021**, *76*, 437–450. [CrossRef]
6. Cathcart, A.M.; Nezhat, F.R.; Emerson, J.; Pejovic, T.; Nezhat, C.H.; Nezhat, C.R. Adnexal masses during pregnancy: Diagnosis, treatment, and prognosis. *Am. J. Obstet. Gynecol.* **2022**, *228*, 601–612. [CrossRef]
7. Lee, S.J.; Oh, H.R.; Na, S.; Hwang, H.S.; Lee, S.M. Ultrasonographic ovarian mass scoring system for predicting malignancy in pregnant women with ovarian mass. *Obstet. Gynecol. Sci.* **2022**, *65*, 1–13. [CrossRef]
8. Kier, R.; McCarthy, S.M.; Scoutt, L.M.; Viscarello, R.R.; Schwartz, P.E. Pelvic masses in pregnancy: MR imaging. *Radiology* **1990**, *176*, 709–713. [CrossRef]
9. Dubernard, G.; Bazot, M.; Barranger, E.; Detchev, R.; David-Montefiore, E.; Uzan, S.; Daraï, E. Accuracy of MR imaging combined with sonography for the diagnosis of persistent adnexal masses during pregnancy: About nine cases. *Gynecol. Obstet. Fertil.* **2005**, *33*, 293–298. [CrossRef]
10. Telischak, N.A.; Yeh, B.M.; Joe, B.N.; Westphalen, A.C.; Poder, L.; Coakley, F.V. MRI of adnexal masses in pregnancy. *AJR Am. J. Roentgenol.* **2008**, *191*, 364–370. [CrossRef]
11. Bird, S.T.; Gelperin, K.; Sahin, L.; Bleich, K.B.; Fazio-Eynullayeva, E.; Woods, C.; Radden, E.; Greene, P.; McCloskey, C.; Johnson, T.; et al. First-Trimester Exposure to Gadolinium-based Contrast Agents: A Utilization Study of 4.6 Million U.S. Pregnancies. *Radiology* **2019**, *293*, 193–200. [CrossRef] [PubMed]
12. Thomassin-Naggara, I.; Poncelet, E.; Jalaguier-Coudray, A.; Guerra, A.; Fournier, L.S.; Stojanovic, S.; Millet, I.; Bharwani, N.; Juhan, V.; Cunha, T.M.; et al. Ovarian-adnexal reporting data system magnetic resonance imaging (O-RADS MRI) score for risk stratification of sonographically indeterminate adnexal masses. *JAMA Netw. Open* **2020**, *3*, e1919896. [CrossRef] [PubMed]
13. Sadowski, E.A.; Thomassin-Naggara, I.; Rockall, A.; Maturen, K.E.; Forstner, R.; Jha, P.; Nougaret, S.; Siegelman, E.S.; Reinhold, C. O-RADS MRI Risk Stratification System: Guide for Assessing Adnexal Lesions from the ACR O-RADS Committee. *Radiology* **2022**, *303*, 35–47. [CrossRef] [PubMed]
14. Ray, J.G.; Vermeulen, M.J.; Bharatha, A.; Montanera, W.J.; Park, A.L. Association Between MRI Exposure During Pregnancy and Fetal and Childhood Outcomes. *JAMA* **2016**, *316*, 952–961. [CrossRef]
15. Perelli, F.; Turrini, I.; Giorgi, M.G.; Renda, I.; Vidiri, A.; Straface, G.; Scatena, E.; D'Indinosante, M.; Marchi, L.; Giusti, M.; et al. Contrast Agents during Pregnancy: Pros and Cons When Really Needed. *Int. J. Environ. Res. Public Health* **2022**, *19*, 16699. [CrossRef]
16. Causa Andrieu, P.I.; Wahab, S.A.; Nougaret, S.; Petkovska, I. Ovarian cancer during pregnancy. *Abdom. Radiol.* **2023**, *48*, 1694–1708. [CrossRef]
17. Committee on Obstetric Practice. Committee Opinion No. 723: Guidelines for Diagnostic Imaging During Pregnancy and Lactation. *Obstet. Gynecol.* **2017**, *130*, e210–e216, Erratum in *Obstet. Gynecol.* **2018**, *132*, 786.
18. Sahin, H.; Panico, C.; Ursprung, S.; Simeon, V.; Chiodini, P.; Frary, A.; Carmo, B.; Smith, S.; Freeman, S.; Jimenez-Linan, M.; et al. Non-contrast MRI can accurately characterize adnexal masses: A retrospective study. *Eur. Radiol.* **2021**, *31*, 6962–6973. [CrossRef]
19. Available online: https://www.ibm.com/spss (accessed on 30 July 2023).
20. Webb, J.A.W.; Thomsen, H.S.; Morcos, S.K. Members of Contrast Media Safety Committee of European Society of Urogenital Radiology (ESUR). The use of iodinated and gadolinium contrast media during pregnancy and lactation. *Eur. Radiol.* **2005**, *15*, 1234–1240. [CrossRef]
21. Cowper, S.E. Nephrogenic fibrosing dermopathy: The first 6 years. *Curr. Opin. Rheumatol.* **2003**, *15*, 785–790. [CrossRef]
22. Food and Drug Administration. FDA Drug Safety Communication: FDA Warns that Gadolinium-Based Contrast Agents (GBCAs) are Retained in the Body; Requires New Class Warnings. Available online: https://www.fda.gov/Drugs/DrugSafety/ucm589213.htm (accessed on 30 July 2023).
23. Thomassin-Naggara, I.; Fedida, B.; Sadowski, E.; Chevrier, M.-C.; Chabbert-Buffet, N.; Ballester, M.; Tavolaro, S.; Darai, E. Complex US adnexal masses during pregnancy: Is pelvic MR imaging accurate for characterization? *Eur. J. Radiol.* **2017**, *93*, 200–208. [CrossRef] [PubMed]
24. Whitecar, P.; Turner, S.; Higby, K. Adnexal masses in pregnancy: A review of 130 cases undergoing surgical management. *Am. J. Obstet. Gynecol.* **1999**, *181*, 19–24. [CrossRef] [PubMed]
25. Hakoun, A.; Al-Shaar1, A.I.; Zaza, J.; Abou-Al-Shaar, H.; Salloum, M.N.A. Adnexal masses in pregnancy: An updated review. *Avicenna J. Med.* **2017**, *7*, 153–157. [CrossRef] [PubMed]
26. Morice, P.; Uzan, C.; Gouy, S.; Verschraegen, C.; Haie-Meder, C. Gynaecological cancers in pregnancy. *Lancet* **2012**, *379*, 558–569. [CrossRef]
27. Rozalli, F.I.; Rahmat, K.; Fadzli, F.; Boylan, C.; Deb, P. Decidualized Ovarian Endometrioma in a Pregnant Woman Mimicking Ovarian Malignancy: Magnetic Resonance Imaging and Ultrasonographic Findings. *Iran. J. Radiol.* **2015**, *12*, e21260. [CrossRef]
28. Miyakoshi, K.; Tanaka, M.; Gabionza, D.; Takamatsu, K.; Miyazaki, T.; Yuasa, Y.; Mukai, M.; Yoshimura, Y. Decidualized ovarian endometriosis mimicking malignancy. *AJR Am. J. Roentgenol.* **1998**, *171*, 1625–1626. [CrossRef]
29. Poder, L.; Coakley, F.V.; Rabban, J.T.; Goldstein, R.B.; Aziz, S.; Chen, L.M. Decidualized endometrioma during pregnancy: Recognizing an imaging mimic of ovarian malignancy. *J. Comput. Assist. Tomogr.* **2008**, *32*, 555–558. [CrossRef]

30. Yin, M.; Wang, T.; Li, S.; Zhang, X.; Yang, J. Decidualized ovarian endometrioma mimicking malignancy in pregnancy: A case report and literature review. *J. Ovarian Res.* **2022**, *15*, 33. [CrossRef]
31. Takeuchi, M.; Matsuzaki, K.; Nishitani, H. Magnetic Resonance Manifestations of Decidualized Endometriomas During Pregnancy. *J. Comput. Assist. Tomogr.* **2008**, *32*, 353–355. [CrossRef]
32. Morisawa, N.; Kido, A.; Kataoka, M.; Minamiguchi, S.; Konishi, I.; Togashi, K. Magnetic Resonance Imaging Manifestations of Decidualized Endometriotic Cysts: Comparative Study with Ovarian Cancers Associated with Endometriotic Cysts. *J. Comput. Assist. Tomogr.* **2014**, *38*, 879–884. [CrossRef]
33. Takeuchi, M.; Matsuzaki, K.; Haradaa, M. Computed diffusion-weighted imaging for differentiating decidualized endometrioma from ovarian cancer. *Eur. J. Radiol.* **2016**, *85*, 1016–1019. [CrossRef] [PubMed]
34. Thomassin-Naggara, I.; Aubert, E.; Rockall, A.; Jalaguier-coudray, A.; Rouzier, R.; Darai, E.; Bazot, M. Adnexal Masses: Development and Preliminary Validation of an MR Imaging Scoring System. *Radiology* **2013**, *267*, 432–443. [CrossRef] [PubMed]

Disclaimer/Publisher's Note: The statements, opinions and data contained in all publications are solely those of the individual author(s) and contributor(s) and not of MDPI and/or the editor(s). MDPI and/or the editor(s) disclaim responsibility for any injury to people or property resulting from any ideas, methods, instructions or products referred to in the content.

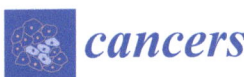

Review

Multiparametric Ultrasound for Diagnosing Testicular Lesions: Everything You Need to Know in Daily Clinical Practice

Carlotta Pozza [1], Marta Tenuta [1], Franz Sesti [1], Michele Bertolotto [2], Dean Y. Huang [3], Paul S. Sidhu [3], Mario Maggi [4], Andrea M. Isidori [1,†] and Francesco Lotti [5,*,†]

1. Department of Experimental Medicine, Sapienza University of Rome, 00161 Rome, Italy; carlotta.pozza@uniroma1.it (C.P.); marta.tenuta@uniroma1.it (M.T.); franz.sesti@uniroma1.it (F.S.); andrea.isidori@uniroma1.it (A.M.I.)
2. Department of Radiology, Ospedale Di Cattinara, University of Trieste, Strada di Fiume 447, 34149 Trieste, Italy; bertolot@units.it
3. Department of Imaging Sciences, Faculty of Life Sciences and Medicine, School of Biomedical Engineering and Imaging Sciences, King's College London, London WC2R 2LS, UK; dean.huang@nhs.net (D.Y.H.); paulsidhu@nhs.net (P.S.S.)
4. Endocrinology Unit, Department of Experimental and Clinical Biomedical Sciences "Mario Serio", University of Florence, 50139 Florence, Italy; mario.maggi@unifi.it
5. Andrology, Female Endocrinology and Gender Incongruence Unit, Department of Experimental and Clinical Biomedical Sciences "Mario Serio", University of Florence, Viale Pieraccini 6, 50139 Florence, Italy
* Correspondence: francesco.lotti@unifi.it or flottimd@yahoo.it
† The authors contributed equally to this work.

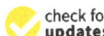

Citation: Pozza, C.; Tenuta, M.; Sesti, F.; Bertolotto, M.; Huang, D.Y.; Sidhu, P.S.; Maggi, M.; Isidori, A.M.; Lotti, F. Multiparametric Ultrasound for Diagnosing Testicular Lesions: Everything You Need to Know in Daily Clinical Practice. *Cancers* **2023**, *15*, 5332. https://doi.org/10.3390/cancers15225332

Academic Editor: Michael J. Spinella

Received: 29 August 2023
Revised: 20 October 2023
Accepted: 24 October 2023
Published: 8 November 2023

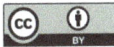

Copyright: © 2023 by the authors. Licensee MDPI, Basel, Switzerland. This article is an open access article distributed under the terms and conditions of the Creative Commons Attribution (CC BY) license (https://creativecommons.org/licenses/by/4.0/).

Simple Summary: Testicular lesions (TLs) are challenging clinical or ultrasound findings. When large, hard palpable lumps, TL management is mainly clinical, requiring conventional color-Doppler ultrasound (CDUS) to confirm that they are solid, vascularized lesions suggesting malignancy. However, when their CDUS characteristics are uncertain or when nonpalpable, multiparametric US (mp-US) (i.e., the combination of CDUS and more recent US techniques such as contrast-enhanced US and sonoelastography) plays a key role in their characterization, aimed at differentiating benign from malignant TL. This is relevant, since TLs are frequent, testicular tumors are the most common malignancies in young men, and the accurate assessment of a TL is critical to define its correct management including testicular salvage and US follow-up or orchiectomy. In this scenario, this narrative and pictorial review reports a practical mp-US "identity card" and iconographic characterization of several benign and malignant TLs, useful to the physician in daily clinical practice.

Abstract: Background: Ultrasonography (US) represents the gold standard imaging method for the assessment of testicular lesions (TL). The gray-scale (GSUS) and color-Doppler (CDUS) ultrasound examination allow sonographers to investigate the size, margins, echotexture, and vascular features of TLs with the aim to differentiate benign from malignant lesions. Recently, the use of contrast-enhanced US (CEUS) and sonoelastography (SE) has led to further improvements in the differential diagnosis of TL. Although GSUS and CDUS are often sufficient to suggest the benign or malignant nature of the TL, CEUS can be decisive in the differential diagnosis of unclear findings, while SE can help to strengthen the diagnosis. The contemporary combination of GSUS, CDUS, CEUS, and SE has led to a new diagnostic paradigm named multiparametric US (mp-US), which is able to provide a more detailed characterization of TLs than single techniques alone. This narrative and pictorial review aimed to describe the mp-US appearance of several TLs. Methods: An extensive Medline search was performed to identify studies in the English language focusing on the mp-US evaluation of TLs. Results: A practical mp-US "identity card" and iconographic characterization of several benign and malignant TLs is provided herein. Conclusions: The mp-US characterization of TL reported herein can be useful in daily clinical practice.

Keywords: ultrasound (US); multi-parametric ultrasound (mp-US); gray-scale ultrasound (GSUS); color-Doppler ultrasound (CDUS); contrast-enhanced ultrasound (CEUS); sonoelastography (SE); testicular lesions; testicular tumors; differential diagnosis

1. Introduction

Ultrasonography (US) represents the gold standard imaging method for scrotal investigation and is widely used to assess a variety of scrotal diseases [1–3]. It is a simple, rapid, and harmless diagnostic tool that is able to provide live images of the scrotal content and, among the imaging techniques, it is the least expensive [1–3]. Over time, the use of US has progressively expanded since it is useful to assess scrotal features related to reproductive health, scrotal pain, masses, and trauma [1–3].

Currently, conventional gray-scale US (GSUS), supplemented by color-Doppler US (CDUS), is considered as being highly sensitive in detecting testicular lesions, however, it has limits in delineating their nature [3]. If performed by an expert operator, scrotal US, together with clinical history and physical examination, may suggest a differential diagnosis among benign and malignant testicular lesions [4]. However, in some cases, it is difficult to discriminate the benign or malignant origin of a testicular lesion, and in case of a "likely" malignant lesion, it is challenging to suggest a possible cancer type. Hence, to date, histology remains the only certain diagnostic tool to define the nature of a testicular lesion [2].

Recently, the use of contrast-enhanced US (CEUS) and sonoelastography (SE) have led to improvements in the differential diagnosis of testicular lesions [2]. This led to a new diagnostic paradigm, the so called "multiparametric US" (mp-US) [5,6], combining conventional techniques (i.e., GSUS and CDUS) with CEUS [7] and SE [8]. Although not entirely diagnostic, mp-US is able to provide a detailed characterization of testicular lesions [4,9,10]. This is relevant in clinical practice, since an accurate mp-US evaluation of a testicular lesion, beside and along with clinical assessment, is critical to define its correct management including testicular US follow-up or orchiectomy [11]. On the one hand, when "palpable" testicular masses are found, they can be malignant in more than 90% of cases, making radical orchiectomy the standard treatment [12]. On the other hand, when nonpalpable testicular lesions are detected, often incidentally during a scrotal US performed for different reasons (e.g., male infertility, varicocele, history of cryptorchidism, scrotal pain or trauma), the clinical management is more cautious. In fact, these lesions are small and mostly benign [13,14], so unnecessary orchiectomy must be avoided, however, they can also be malignant and can grow over time. In this scenario, US is crucial in the follow-up of small lesions, suggesting surgery in the case of growth/modification of small nodules, especially if testicular tumor-related risk factors (e.g., age 15 to 40 years old, family history of testicular tumors, history of contralateral testicular tumor, cryptorchidism or oligo-/azoospermia) are present [1,15]. Hence, either in the case of palpable testicular masses or, especially, in the case of small testicular lesions, US is useful. In particular, mp-US can help in distinguishing benign and malignant lesions with good accuracy, providing a more detailed characterization than CDUS, CEUS, or SE alone.

The role of mp-US for characterizing testicular lesions has been investigated in some retrospective and prospective studies [16–20], mainly focusing on diagnostic accuracy. This review aims to summarize and update these reports, providing an "identity card" description and a wide iconographic characterization of the GSUS, CDUS, CEUS and SE appearance of several common and uncommon benign and malignant testicular lesions.

2. Brief Summary of What to Investigate before Running Mp-US

Clinical history and physical examination are very important to suggest a correct diagnosis when facing a testicular lesion and should be performed before running US.

Anamnesis should investigate testicular malignancy-related risk factors including age (testicular cancer represents the most common malignancy in young men aged 15 to 40 years), family history of testicular tumors, history of contralateral testicular tumor, history of cryptorchidism/orchiopexy, and history of infertility, which represent the main risk factors associated with testicular tumors [1,21]. In addition, previous testicular inflammation (orchitis), torsion, trauma, and other relevant diseases (i.e., Klinefelter syndrome) useful to define a differential diagnosis should be assessed [1–3,21]. Patients should be asked to describe eventual signs (testicular mass/nodule, testicular swelling or enlargement, new onset hydrocele, sometimes revealed by self-examination by the patient) and symptoms (i.e., scrotal pain or heaviness, fever, back pain, new onset gynecomastia), together with the moment of onset and their duration [21]. Performing a physical examination before starting US is always recommended: usually palpable hard and large masses are suggestive of testicular tumors while non-palpable lesions are in most cases benign lesions, however, they still need to be assessed carefully [1–3,21].

3. Mp-US Methodological Standards

Mp-US is increasingly recognized as a valuable problem-solving technique in scrotal pathologies, particularly in differential diagnosis of testicular lesions [9,22]. Mp-US combines conventional techniques (GSUS and CDUS) with CEUS, and SE [9,22], which are relatively recent in evaluating scrotal organs, particularly testicular lesions [2,23].

3.1. Scrotal/Testicular Color-Doppler Ultrasonography (CDUS)

The standardization of the methodology used to perform scrotal color-Doppler ultrasonography (CDUS) is relatively new. A detailed description of the standard operating procedures (SOPs) for performing scrotal CDUS have been reported by the European Academy of Andrology for the entire male genital tract [23–26]. The EAA-proposed SOPs to assess scrotal CDUS and, in particular, testicular lesions, have been reported elsewhere [2,23,25] (see https://www.andrologyacademy.net/eaa-studies (accessed on 20 October 2023)). In particular, testicular US should be performed with a high frequency linear transducer, with the patient in the supine position. A US scan of both testicles should be performed including longitudinal, oblique, and transverse scans, with slow, continuous side-to-side movements that allow for the assessment of the entire parenchyma. The operator should evaluate at GSUS the volume of the testes (using the "ellipsoid" formula [height × width × length × 0.52] for adult testes [27] and the Lambert's empirical formula [height × width × length × 0.71] for pre-pubertal testes [3]), the echogenicity, the echotexture, the possible presence of testicular calcifications or microlithiasis, and vascularization by CDUS, comparing the two sides. Testicular lesions should be accurately evaluated in longitudinal, oblique, and transverse scans. A complete evaluation should include: (1) diameters (length × height × width); (2) position and extension; (3) type (solid, cystic, mixed), homogeneity (homogeneous/inhomogeneous), and echogenicity (hypoechoic, hyperechoic, anechoic); (4) presence of intralesional calcifications; (5) shape (regular or irregular) and margins (clean-cut, smooth, multi-lobed, infiltrating); (6) vascularization pattern (absent, peripheral, intranodular). The images must be stored to be used for the comparison during follow-up. The report must also describe, besides the lesion, the US characteristics of both testicles and must specify the absence of lesions in the contralateral testicle [1–3,23,25].

3.2. Contrast-Enhanced US (CEUS)

The methodological standards for the clinical practice of contrast-enhanced US (CEUS) in non-hepatic applications including scrotum investigation have been reported by the EFSUMB Guidelines [27]. As a result, the assessment of some pathological conditions using CEUS has improved [7,27]. Using time–intensity curves, evaluating the wash-in and wash-out curves may help to distinguish malignant from benign tumors, although CEUS analyses still overlap between different histological types [7]. In addition, CEUS can discriminate non-viable regions in testicular trauma and can identify segmental testicular infarction [7,27].

For CEUS, a dedicated machine-setting with a low mechanical index (0.05–0.08) is needed to avoid early microbubble destruction. US contrast medium (very small-sized organic shells filled with gas with high impedance) should be injected as intravenous bolus and followed immediately by 10 mL of 0.9% saline solution. The entire examination needs to be recorded to perform qualitative and quantitative analyses [7].

3.3. Sonoelastography (SE)

The methodological standards for the clinical practice of sonoelastography (SE) in non-hepatic applications including testicular investigation have been reported by the EFSUMB Guidelines and Recommendations [28]. So far, strain elastography and shear wave elastography, which includes acoustic radiation force impulse-based techniques, and transient elastography are available. The basic principles of SE have been extensively described in previous EFSUMB Guidelines [29], while methodological standardization for different organs including the testis are reported in the updated EFSUMB guidelines [28]. From a methodological point of view, the use of SE to investigate focal testicular lesions can only be recommended in conjunction with other US techniques as there is overlap between benign and malignant neoplasms [28,30].

4. Non-Neoplastic Testicular Lesions

Several non-neoplastic diseases can occur within the testes, and may mimic testicular tumors. Differential diagnosis may be difficult but is imperative to avoid unnecessary surgical interventions. A summary of the clinical characteristics and mp-US features of non-neoplastic testicular lesions is provided in Table 1, and their mp-US appearance is reported in Figures 1–9.

4.1. Intratesticular Cysts

Prevalence: Intratesticular cysts are rare in pediatric patients [31,32] and in young-adult men, while their prevalence in subjects aged >40 years old has been estimated to be 8% to 10% [32].

Clinical history and physical examination: Simple intratesticular cysts are usually asymptomatic. They are often incidentally detected during US as they are usually not palpable [33]. However, they can even be palpable, since their size can range from 2 mm to 2 cm [34]. On palpation, they have a soft or tense-elastic consistency.

GSUS + CDUS: Upon GSUS examination, intratesticular cysts appear as solitary, or less commonly multiple, anechoic lesions, with a thin, clear, hyperechoic wall, and posterior acoustic enhancement [32]. They often occur near the mediastinum and can be simple or complex (if they have internal septa). Usually, they do not contain solid portions. Only when complicated by an infection or an internal hemorrhage can they appear as hypoechoic or mixed echogenicity lesions [33]. In CDUS, they show absent internal vascularization.

SE: Intratesticular cysts generally appear as soft lesions showing a tricolor pattern, blue-green-red [20].

CEUS: CDUS is usually sufficient for the diagnosis of a testicular cyst, and CEUS is not necessary. However, if CEUS is performed, intratesticular cysts show absent contrast enhancement [20].

Differential diagnosis: Complex testicular cysts must be differentiated from cystic teratomas. Complex teratomas tend to have solid, outlying, vascularized masses, rather than fibrous strands [33]. As a corollary, besides teratomas, cystic areas can be found in embryonal carcinomas, yolk sac tumors, and choriocarcinomas, but they are included in the solid lesion (see below).

Table 1. Ultrasound, CDUS, and CEUS characteristics of principal non-neoplastic intratesticular lesions.

	Clinical Presentation	Non-Neoplastic Intratesticular Lesions			
		GS-US	CD-US	CEUS	SE
Simple cyst	Asymptomatic/incidental finding, usually not palpable	Rounded anechoic lesions with thin, clear, hyperechoic wall and posterior acoustic enhancement	Avascular	Unenhanced	Soft lesion with High elastic strain
Epidermoid cyst	Asymptomatic can be palpable	Well-circumscribed rounded lesion with "onion ring" aspect (concentric hypo- and hyper-echoic rings) OR densely calcified mass with acoustic shadow OR cyst with hypoechoic rim and central calcification OR mixed atypical pattern	Avascular	Unenhanced/ Perilesional Rim enhancement	Hard lesion with low/absent elastic strain
Adrenal rest tumor	Patients with congenital adrenal hyperplasia; usually not palpable	Hypoechoic lesions with irregular margins, hyperechogenic foci, typically localized in the mediastinum testis, usually bilateral	Markedly vascularized	Hyperenhanced	Hard lesions with low/absent elastic strain
Sarcoidosis	In the context of a multisystem disease; granulomas in other organs; asymptomatic OR painless/painful mass	Hypoechoic lesions with irregular margins, often bilateral	Possible signs of internal vascularization	Hypoenhanced	Hard lesions with low/absent elastic strain
Segmental infarction	Idiopathic or consequent to surgery, inflammatory events, blood disorders or autoimmune diseases; usually acute painful swollen scrotum OR asymptomatic	Hypoechoic wedge-shaped or roundish area	Avascular OR peripheral rim of low CD	Unenhanced/ perilesional rim enhancement	Soft lesions with high elastic strain
Abscess	Acute scrotal pain and swelling/ fever/high WBC	Complex heterogeneous low reflecting lesion with irregular walls (in rare cases focal hyperechoic spots due to gas bubble)	Avascular/ vascular rim	Unenhanced/ perilesional rim enhancement	Heterogeneous pattern of firmness
Hematoma	History of scrotal trauma	Well-circumscribed hyperechoic lesions which subsequently liquefy over time, becoming complex lesions with septa, cystic components, and fluid levels. Size decrease over time.	Avascular	Unenhanced/ perilesional rim enhancement	Soft lesion with intermediate/ high elastic strain
Idiopathic (diffuse) granulomatous orchitis	In the context of a multisystem disease; asymptomatic OR painless/painful mass	Diffusely hypoechoic testis or hypoechoic areas with ill-defined margins	Markedly vascularized	Hyperenhanced	Heterogeneous pattern of firmness
Infectious (focal) granulomatous orchitis	Acute scrotal pain, testicular enlargement, fever; possible epididymal enlargement, scrotal wall thickening and hydrocele	Single or multiple variable echogenicity areas with blurred margins; appearance depends by the pathologic stages of infection, which include caseous necrosis, granulomas, and healing by fibrosis and calcification	Internal OR peripheral depending on the stage	Unenhanced/ perilesional rim enhancement OR hyperenhanced	Heterogeneous pattern of firmness depending on the stage

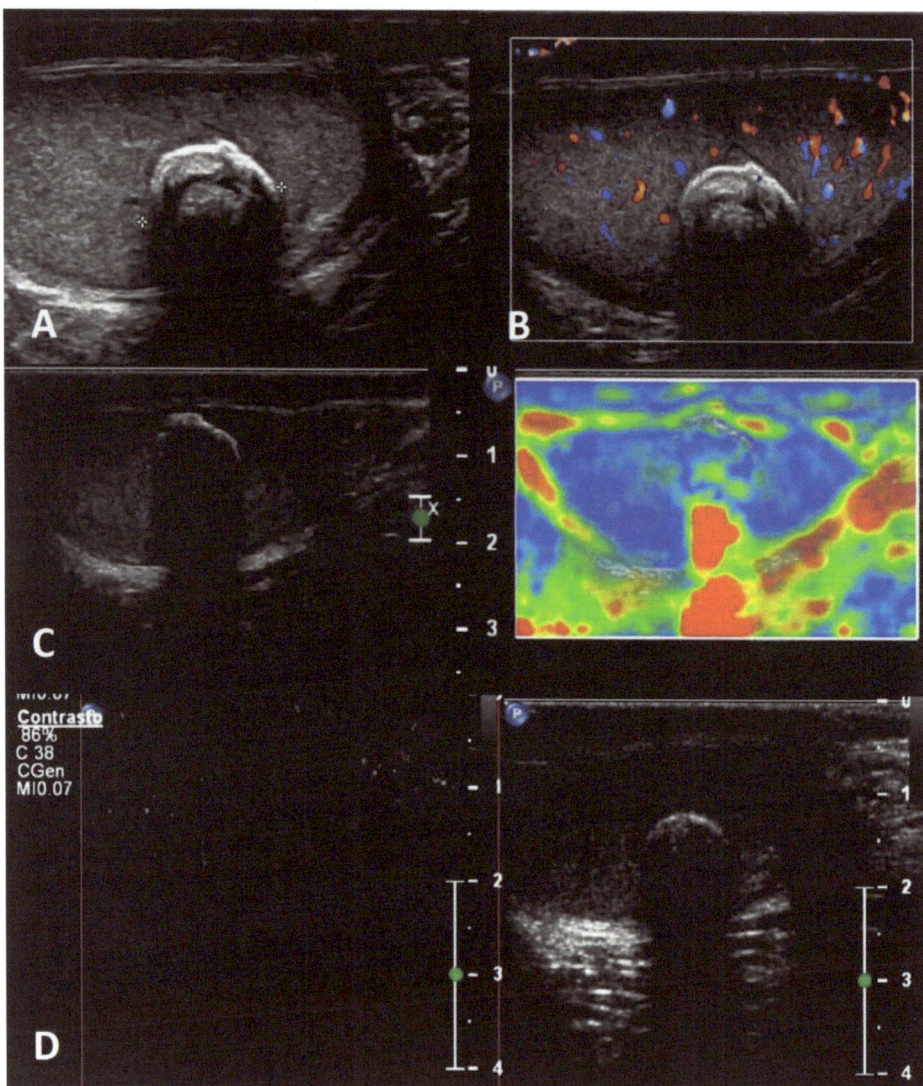

Figure 1. Epidermoid cyst. GSUS demonstrates a well-circumscribed, solid, mixed-reflectivity lesion with high-reflectivity "onion-skin" peripheral rims (panel **A**), avascular in CDUS (panel **B**) in a 17-year-old male patient who was referred for testicular pain. SE shows a mixed elasticity lesion (panel **C**), demonstrated by a blue-green pattern, while contrast-enhanced US demonstrates a clear lack of enhancement within the lesion (panel **D**).

4.2. Epidermoid Cysts

Prevalence: Epidermoid cysts represent 1.5–2.1% of all testicular benign tumors of germ cell origin among men aged 20 to 40 years [35].

Clinical history and physical examination: At physical examination, they are palpable painless non-tender nodules (single or multiple) with sizes ranging from 1 to 3 cm [36,37]. Some epidermoid cysts have a tendency to increase in size over time, hence at clinical history and physical examination, they can be described as a firm nodule growing slowly. Very rarely, in post-pubertal subjects, have they been described as associated with/part of part of invasive testicular germ cell tumors, representing a teratoma [37].

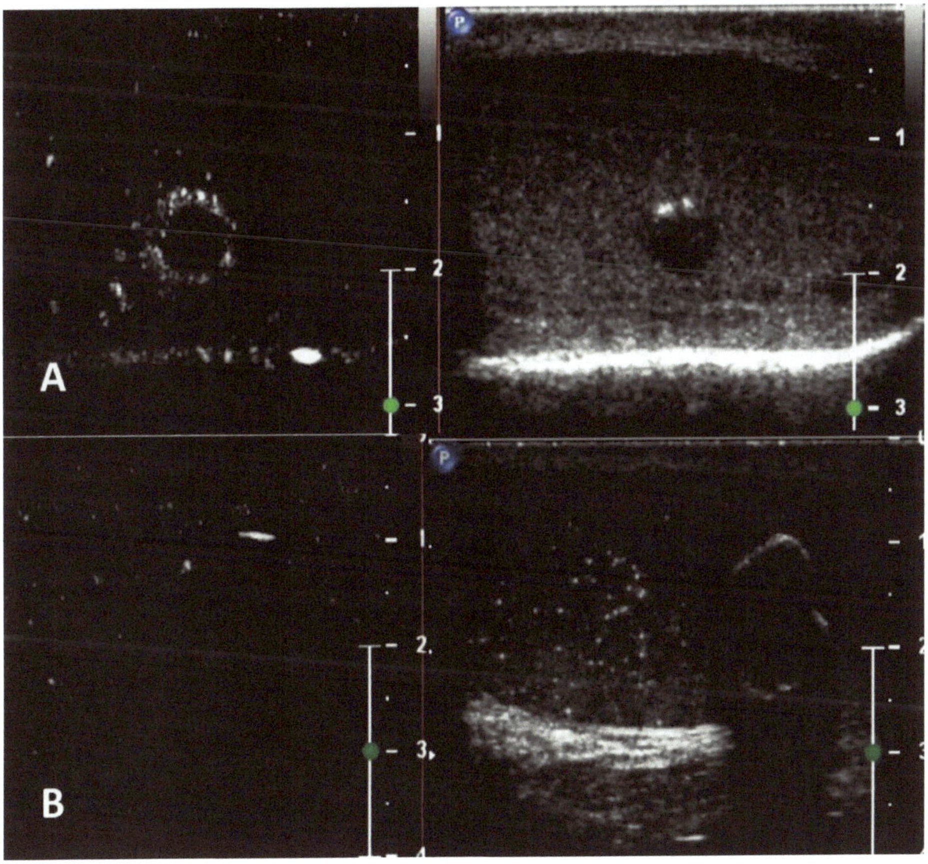

Figure 2. Embryonal carcinoma with internal necrosis (panel **A**) in a 30-year-old man referred for varicocele and atypical epidermoid cyst (panel **B**) in a 16-year-old boy referred for a lump in the testis: both demonstrate in CEUS a lack of vascularity.

GSUS + CDUS: In GSUS, testicular epidermoid cysts show a variable appearance depending on their maturation, compactness, and amount of keratin component. They can be classified into four categories: type 1, well-circumscribed rounded lesions with an "onion-ring" pattern consisting of concentric rings of hypoechogenicity and hyperechogenicity (Figure 1, Panel A); type 2, densely echogenic and calcified masses with a dark acoustic shadow; type 3, "target" appearance lesions consisting of a hypoechoic rim with a central area of increased echogenicity; type 4, mixed pattern lesions [38]. The onion-ring pattern, which corresponds to lamellar layers of keratin, is the most typical, accounting for about 60% of cases [39]. CDUS examination shows absent vascularization within the cyst (Figure 1, Panel B).

SE: Testicular epidermoid cysts demonstrate hard SE properties, showing low/absent elastic strain [38] (Figure 1, Panel C).

CEUS: No contrast enhancement is expected after contrast administration as the lesion is avascular; occasionally it can be present a rim enhancement [38,40] (Figure 1, Panel D).

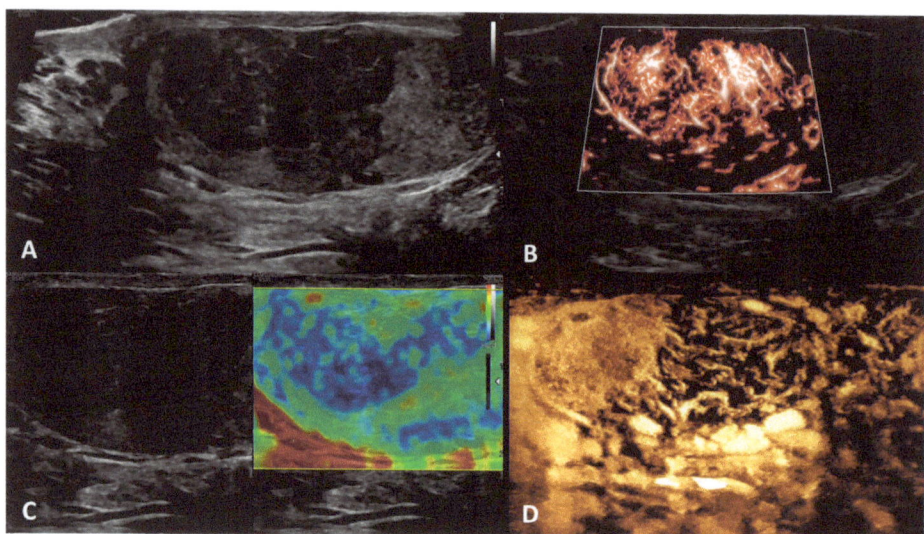

Figure 3. Testicular adrenal rest tumor. GSUS (panel **A**) and CDUS (panel **B**) demonstrated bilateral hypoechoic lesions, highly vascularized, with irregular, lobulated margins in a 28-year-old man with congenital adrenal hyperplasia. In SE, they appeared as hard lesions (panel **C**). TARTs showed increased contrast-enhancement in CEUS (panel **D**).

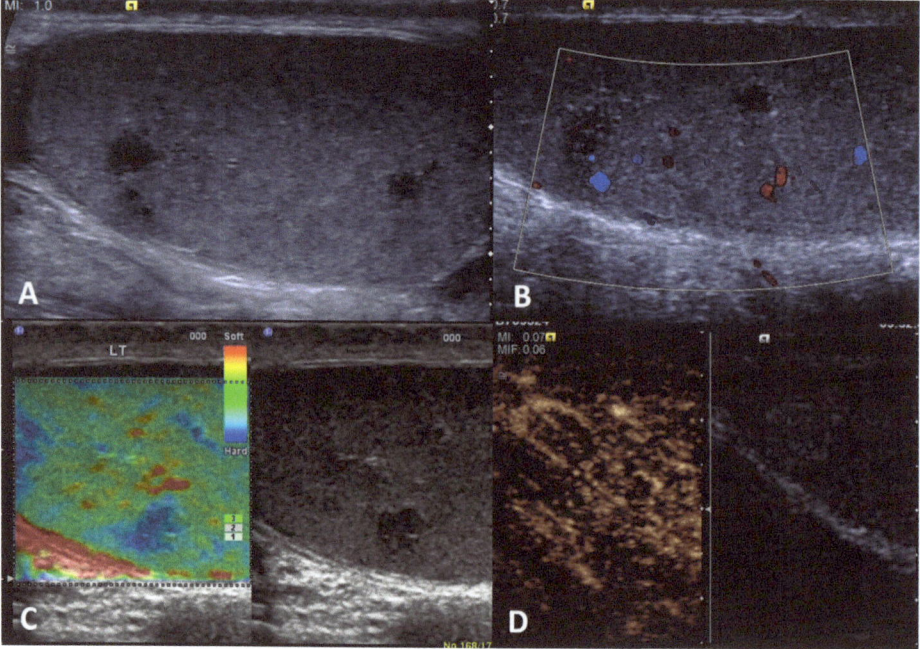

Figure 4. Sarcoidosis. GSUS (panel **A**) and CDUS (panel **B**) demonstrated multiple small hypoechoic lesions with irregular margins and some internal vascular spots. In SE, sarcoidosis granulomas appeared as hard lesions (panel **C**). CEUS can confirm the presence of contrast-enhancement within the lesions (panel **D**).

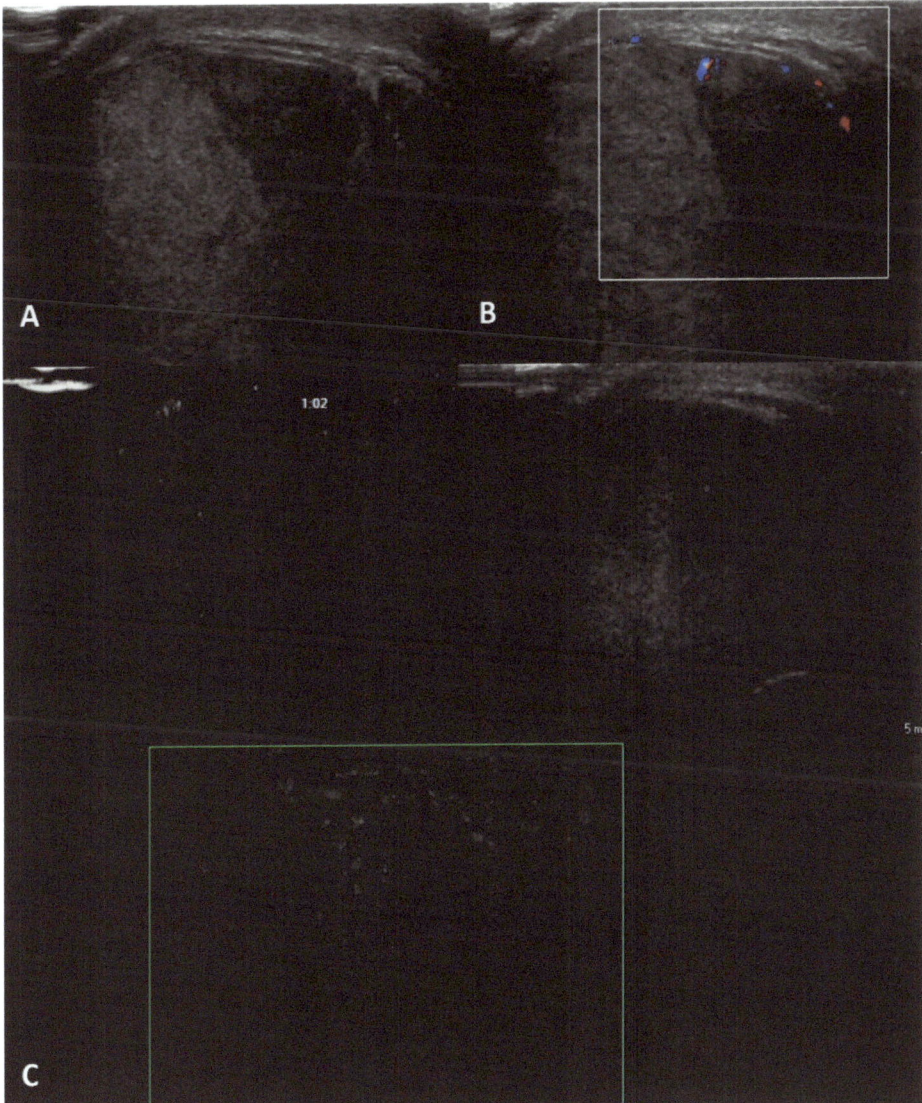

Figure 5. Segmental testicular infarction. GSUS demonstrates hypoechoic lesions, mimicking a tumor (panel **A**) in a 28-year-old patient with a positive personal history of testicular cancer who was performing regular US follow-up. CDUS shows a lack of internal vascularization (panel **B**). CEUS confirmed the absence of vascularity within the lesion (panel **C**).

Differential diagnosis: An atypical epidermoid cyst may be mistaken for a malignant tumor, namely embryonal carcinoma with internal necrosis and calcified margins (Figure 2, Panel A), as they can both appear as avascular lesions in CDUS and CEUS (Figure 2, Panel B) and hard in SE. Serum tumor markers can be helpful in differential diagnosis as well as the meticulous study of the margins, which are usually well-demarcated in epidermoid cyst and irregular in malignant tumors. In this scenario, differential diagnosis is decisive, since while the suspicion of a malignant testicular tumor requires orchiectomy, that of an epidermoid cyst, usually benign, avoids the removal of the entire testicle. However, even if epidermoid cysts show a typical "benign" pattern in US, due to the tendency of an increase in size over time both in pediatric and adult patients, and to the rare association with testicular germ cell tumors, they usually are treated with testis-sparing surgery associated with biopsies of the surrounding parenchyma [37].

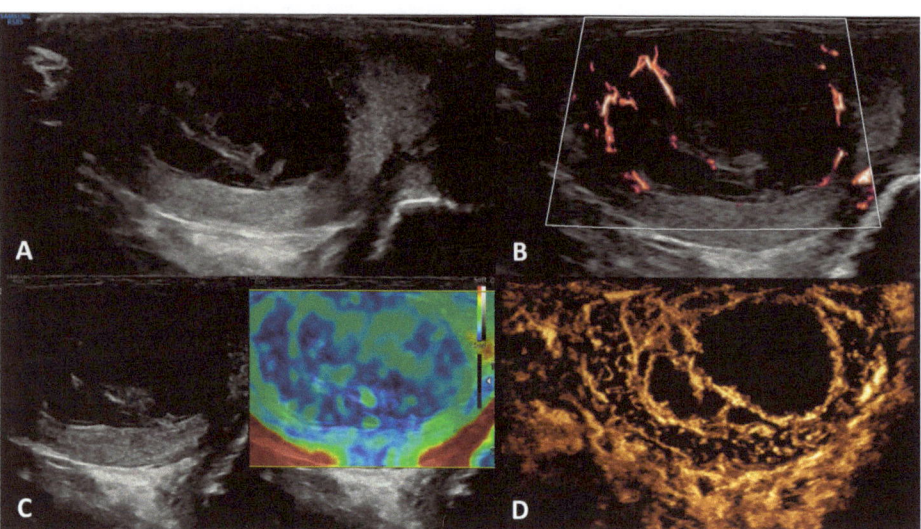

Figure 6. Abscess. GSUS demonstrated a focal, complex, heterogeneous low reflecting lesion with irregular margins (panel **A**). CDUS showed a hypervascular rim surrounding the lesion, with no internal vascular signal (panel **B**). In SE, testicular abscess showed a heterogeneous pattern of firmness (panel **C**). CEUS demonstrated the absence of internal contrast-enhancement with some peripheral enhancement (panel **D**).

4.3. Testicular Adrenal Rest Tumors (TARTs)

Prevalence: TARTs are benign lesions occurring in nearly 40% of patients with congenital adrenal hyperplasia (CAH) [41].

Clinical history and physical examination: TARTs are supposed to originate from an adrenal-like pluripotent stem cell type rising from the urogenital ridge, already present in the gonads during embryogenesis, which undergo adrenal differentiation and increased proliferation under the stimulation of high levels of adrenocorticotropic hormone (ACTH) [41]. Generally, TARTs are bilateral and non-palpable due to their occurrence near or within the mediastinum, and a firm mass can be palpated only when the lesion exceeds 2 cm in diameter [41].

GSUS + CDUS: In GSUS examination, TARTs usually appear as hypoechoic lesions with irregular, lobulated margins, or less frequently as hypoechoic lesions with hyperechogenic foci, and rarely as hyperechogenic lesions [41] (Figure 3, Panel A). CDUS shows markedly increased intralesional blood flow (Figure 3, Panel B).

SE: TARTs usually appear as hard lesions showing low/absent elastic strain [42] (Figure 3, Panel C).

CEUS: TARTs show increased contrast-enhancement in CEUS [43,44] (Figure 3, Panel D).

Differential diagnosis: It is challenging to discriminate TARTs from other tumors based on their US appearance. However, TARTs are typical findings in patients with CAH. Moreover, their size might decrease with proper glucocorticoid treatment. In addition, TARTs are usually bilateral, an uncommon occurrence in malignant tumors. If small, they can be similar to Leydig cell tumors in GS [45]. Hence, the patient's clinical history, the occurrence within the mediastinum, and bilaterality of the lesions can help clinicians in the management and appropriate follow-up of these lesions, often avoiding unnecessary orchiectomy [41].

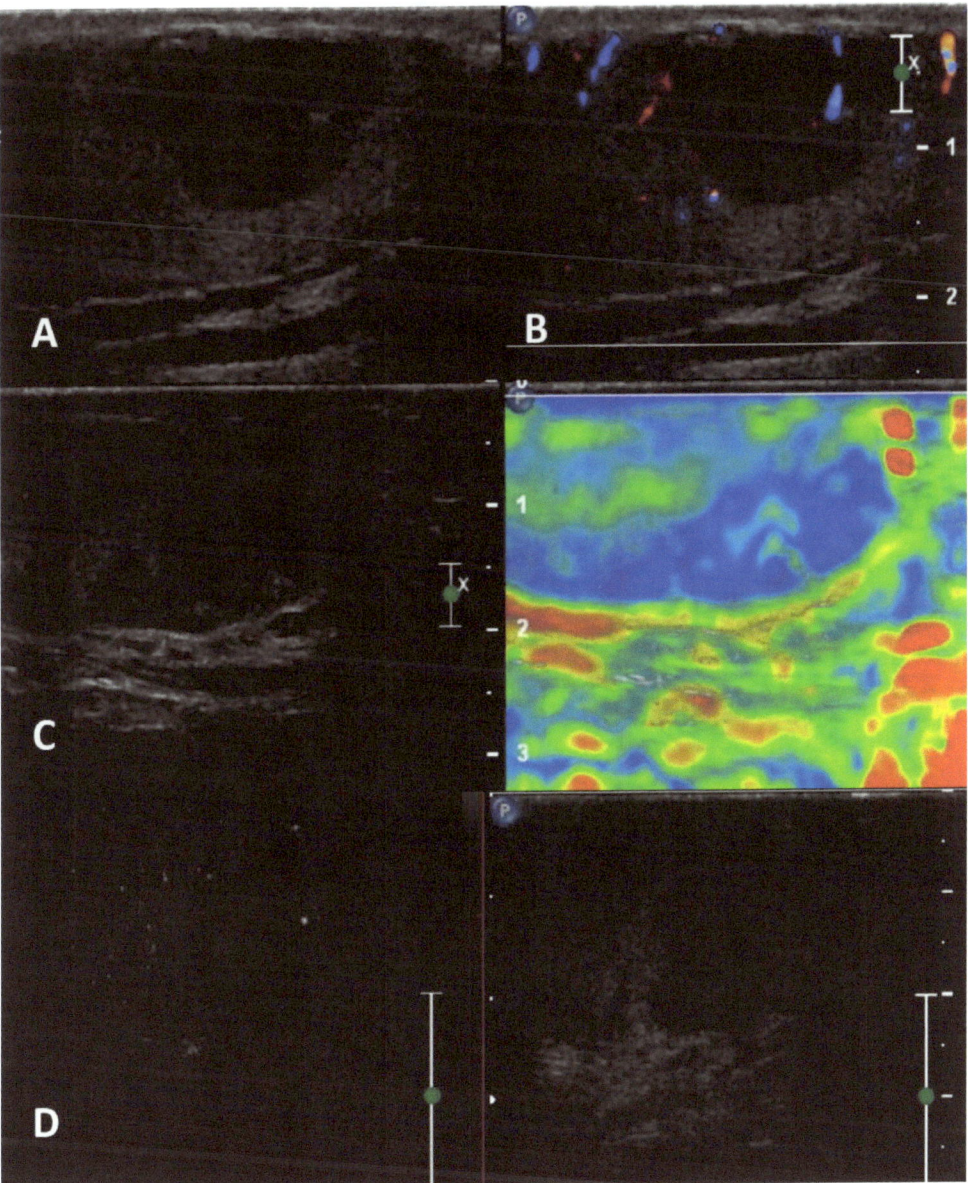

Figure 7. Hematoma. GSUS demonstrated well-circumscribed anechoic lesions with septa and solid components (panel **A**) in a 38-year-old man referred after testicular trauma related to the ball of padel. CDUS showed a lack of internal vascularization (panel **B**). In SE, hematoma showed intermediate/high elastic strain (panel **C**), whereas CEUS confirmed the absence of vascularity within the lesion (panel **D**).

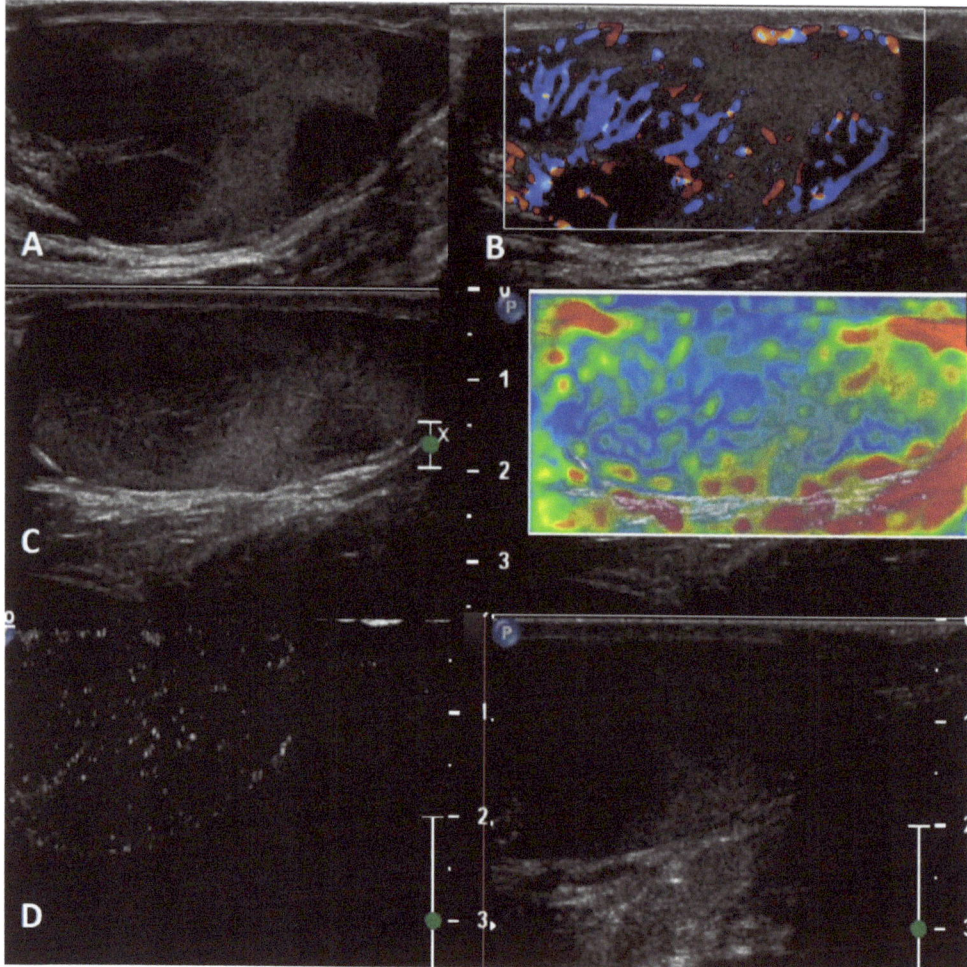

Figure 8. Idiopathic granulomatous orchitis. GSUS demonstrated multiple ill-defined, homogeneous, hypoechoic lesions (panel **A**) in a 24-year-old patient with a positive personal history of testicular cancer (seminoma) diagnosed 6-months earlier during his regular US follow-up. CDUS showed increased internal vascularization (panel **B**). In SE, the testis showed diffuse intermediate elastic strain (panel **C**), whereas CEUS confirmed the hyperenhancement within the lesions (panel **D**).

4.4. Sarcoidosis

Prevalence: Sarcoidosis is a multisystem disease involving the lungs, lymph nodes, kidneys, skin, liver, and spleen, and is characterized by noncaseating granulomas. The reported prevalence of sarcoidosis-related testicular involvement is 4–4.5%, with only 0.5% of symptomatic patients [46].

Clinical history and physical examination: Testicular sarcoidosis is usually asymptomatic, being incidentally detected during the patients' diagnostic work-up [47]. When clinically manifest, testicular sarcoidosis presents as painless or painful nodules [48].

GSUS + CDUS: In GSUS, sarcoidosis appears as single or more typically multiple and bilateral small hypoechoic lesions with irregular margins [4,47] (Figure 4, Panel A). In CDUS, testicular sarcoidosis granulomas can show some internal vascular spots [4,49,50] (Figure 4, Panel B).

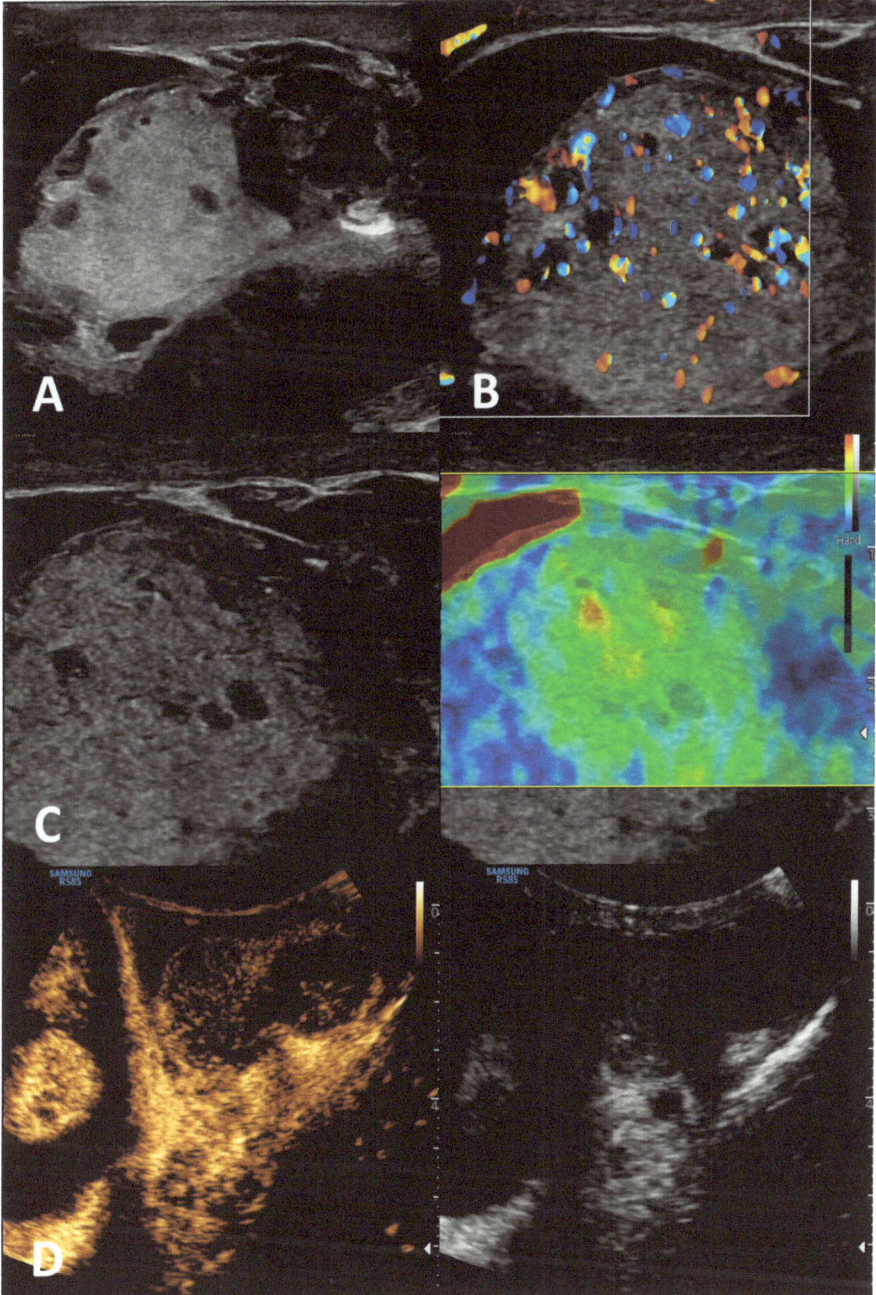

Figure 9. Tuberculous granulomatous orchitis. GSUS demonstrated focal hypoechoic lesions with blurred margins (panel **A**). CDUS showed only peripheric vascularization (panel **B**). In SE, tuberculous granuloma showed intermediate elastic strain (panel **C**). CEUS confirmed the hypoenhanced lesions with peripheral rim (panel **D**).

SE: Sarcoidosis granulomas appear as hard lesions showing low/absent elastic strain [4] (Figure 4, Panel C).

CEUS: CEUS can confirm the presence of contrast-enhancement within the lesions [4,49,50]; however, a hypovascular appearance of the lesions has been described [51] (Figure 4, Panel D).

Differential diagnosis: Differential diagnosis from a testicular neoplasm may be difficult with GS, however, the presence of multiple bilateral lesions involving simultaneously the testis, along with other systemic evidence of sarcoidosis in other organs may suggest the diagnosis [47,48].

4.5. Segmental Testicular Infarction

Prevalence: Segmental testicular infarction is a rare clinical and US entity [52]. Most cases have been reported as idiopathic; it can also occur as a sequela of recent surgery, inflammatory and infective events, blood disorders such as sickle cell disease and polycythemia, or autoimmune diseases such as vasculitis [52,53].

Clinical history and physical examination: Segmental testicular infarction frequently presents with an acute painful, swollen scrotum, especially in men aged 20 to 40 years [54,55]. However, clinically silent cases have been described [52].

GSUS + CDUS: In GSUS evaluation, segmental testicular infarction appears as a hypoechoic wedge-shaped lesion [52], usually involving the upper third of the testicle due to poor collateral vessels [56] (Figure 5, Panel A). CDUS shows absent internal vascularization, and a peripheral rim of low vascular signal may be observed [52] (Figure 5, Panel B).

SE: It appears in SE as a soft lesion showing high elastic strain [4].

CEUS: CEUS can confirm the absence of vascularization within the lesion (Figure 5, Panel C); in cases of subacute testicular infarction, a peripheral hyperenhancing rim can be detected, corresponding to histologic evidence of granulation tissue. During follow-up, the peripheral hyperemic rim diminishes [57].

Differential diagnosis: In some cases, the US appearance of segmental testicular infarction can be round-shaped, resembling a testicular tumor [52]. A helpful US feature to distinguish segmental infarction from a testicular tumor is markedly decreased or absent vascular flow in CDUS imaging or in CEUS. In ambiguous cases, the patient's clinical history and lesion size reduction during follow-up can help the clinician [57].

4.6. Abscess

Prevalence: Testicular abscess is an unusual finding, complicating 3–5% of epididymitis and epididymo-orchitis [58]. It may also occur as a complication of mumps, trauma, or infarction [36].

Clinical history and physical examination: Patients are usually symptomatic, presenting with acute scrotal pain and swelling and frequently with an elevated white blood cell count and fever. Patients often have comorbidities such as diabetes mellitus, human immunodeficiency virus infection, or other immunosuppressive conditions [3].

GSUS + CDUS: GSUS appearance is of a focal, complex, heterogeneous low reflecting lesion with irregular margins [48]. In rare cases, focal hyperechoic spots with posterior shadowing may be present, corresponding to gas bubbles within the abscess cavity [59] (Figure 6, Panel A). In CDUS, a hypervascular rim may surround the lesion, with no internal vascular signal [4] (Figure 6, Panel B).

SE: Testicular abscess shows in SE a heterogeneous pattern of firmness [4] (Figure 6, Panel C).

CEUS: CEUS demonstrates the absence of internal contrast-enhancement with some peripheral enhancement [4,60,61] (Figure 6, Panel D).

Differential diagnosis: In some cases, a testicular abscess can resemble a testicular tumor, although it never shows internal vascularization. Evidence of epididymitis/epididymo-orchitis, reactive hydrocele, and scrotal skin thickening could be present in the case of testicular abscess. Serial US examinations to ensure resolution should be performed.

4.7. Hematoma

Prevalence: Intratesticular hematomas are a possible sequela of a scrotal trauma, which is the third most common cause of acute scrotal pain after epididymo-orchitis and testicular torsion.

Clinical history and physical examination: A history of scrotal trauma is usually related to the detection of hematoma in US, even if not all patients report this event [62].

GSUS + CDUS: Hematomas in US features change in time according to the evolving of blood products [56]. In the acute phase, hematomas appear as well-circumscribed hyperechoic lesions that subsequently liquefy over time, becoming complex lesions with septa, cystic components, and fluid levels [36,58] (Figure 7, Panel A). Typically, the size of the hematomas decreases over time [3]. In CDUS imaging, there is no signal of internal vascularization [58] (Figure 7, Panel B). It is essential to investigate the vascularization of the residual parenchyma to assess its degree of vitality, and CEUS can be helpful in this context [58,59]. Moreover, CEUS can be useful in ambiguous cases to discriminate between intratesticular hematoma and tumor [63].

SE: Intratesticular hematomas show predominantly "soft" SE properties with intermediate/high elastic strain [64] (Figure 7, Panel C).

CEUS: CEUS confirms the absence of vascularity within the lesion. Peripheral rim and internal septa enhancement may be present [64] (Figure 7, Panel D).

Differential diagnosis: Especially when a scrotal trauma does not occur temporally close to US evaluation, hematomas may mimic testicular tumors [62]. However, performing close, serial US evaluations to assess the decrease in the size of the hematomas can help in the differential diagnosis.

4.8. Viral Orchitis and Bacterial Orchitis (Epididymo-Orchitis)

Prevalence: The majority of orchitis originate with a previous epididymitis, later on extending to the testis (44–47% of cases). In this case, the etiology is mainly bacterial [1,2]. Conversely, primary orchitis is mainly viral in origin (mumps orchitis), occurring in 20–30% of infected postpubertal men [1,2,35].

Clinical history and physical examination: Primary orchitis is less common than epididymo-orchitis and is mostly caused by mumps during or after puberty [35]. Epididymo-orchitis usually follows epididymitis, mainly due to urinary tract infections (e.g., *Escherichia coli*) in young boys and sexually transmitted organisms (e.g., *Naisseria gonorrhoeae* and *Chlamydia trachomatis*) in older patients, although urine cultures are positive in only 10–25% of cases [1–3,35]. Clinically, gradual onset of pain (especially in epididymo-orchitis) or acute scrotum can occur. Both primary and secondary orchitis present with painful hemiscrotum and testis enlargement, usually bilateral in the primary form and unilateral in the secondary form, the latter often associated with epididymal enlargement or tenderness or pain [1–3]. Scrotal edema, fever and pyuria may occur.

GSUS + CDUS: The testis appears enlarged, diffusely hypoechoic and inhomogeneous in GSUS and diffusely hyperemic in CDUS [1–4,20].

SE: In SE, orchitis appears with a heterogeneous pattern of firmness [4,20].

CEUS: In CEUS, diffuse vascular hyperenhancement throughout the testis can be observed [4,20].

Differential diagnosis: When an enlarged, hard, hypoechoic, and diffusely hyperemic testis is detected in US, differential diagnosis should be considered with large seminomas or lymphomas. The occurrence of bilateral orchitis in postpubertal boys or of concurrent epididymitis in adult men can help to suggest primary or secondary orchitis, respectively, instead of large malignancies.

4.9. Idiopathic Granulomatous Orchitis

Prevalence: Idiopathic granulomatous orchitis, an inflammatory condition of the testis of unknown etiology, is rarely encountered [65,66]. The condition tends to present in a wide age range (19–84 years), with the highest frequency between 50 and 70 years of age [67].

Clinical history and physical examination: Idiopathic granulomatous orchitis is characterized by the presence of non-specific granulomatous inflammation and admixed multinucleated giant cells [65]. Histologically, there is extensive destruction of seminiferous tubules with tubular or interstitial pattern of granulomatous inflammation and prominent collagen fibrosis. Clinical presentation of diffuse granulomatous orchitis includes scrotal pain and testicular enlargement [68].

GSUS + CDUS: In GSUS, idiopathic granulomatous orchitis appears as diffusely hypoechoic testis or focal hypoechoic areas with ill-defined margins (Figure 8, Panel A) [69]. CDUS often shows hypervascularization (Figure 8, Panel B) [36].

SE: In SE, focal orchitis appears predominantly with a heterogeneous pattern of firmness (Figure 8, Panel C) [8,20].

CEUS: In CEUS, diffuse vascular hyperenhancement throughout the lesions can be observed (Figure 8, Panel D) [70].

Differential diagnosis: In the case of diffuse orchitis, there is a high suspicion of testicular malignancy, and physical examination fails to differentiate the benign from malignant condition [68]. In this scenario, other signs of inflammation such as scrotal wall thickening and hydrocele may help in the differential diagnosis with testicular tumor [41].

4.10. Infectious Granulomatous Orchitis

Prevalence: Infective granulomatous orchitis is very rare and can be caused by tuberculosis, brucellosis, and actinomycosis [69]. Tuberculous orchitis usually results from contiguous extension from the epididymis. Infectious granulomatous orchitis can be acute or chronic. In the acute form, patients present with sudden onset of pain, while in the chronic form, they usually present with unilateral scrotal swelling. In some cases, granulomatous orchitis presents as a single or multiple testicular mass and can be suspicious of malignancy.

Clinical history and physical examination: Clinical presentation of focal granulomatous orchitis includes acute scrotal pain, fever, and testicular enlargement [68]. Epididymal involvement is common in infectious granulomatous orchitis, especially tuberculosis as well as concurrent septated hydrocele, scrotal wall edema, and calcification of the tunica vaginalis.

GSUS + CDUS: In genitourinary tuberculosis, both the GS- and CD-US appearance of the testes can be explained by various pathologic stages of tubercular infection, which include caseous necrosis, granulomas, and healing by fibrosis and calcification [36]. Generally, in GSUS, focal orchitis appears as a single or multiple hypoechoic lesion/s with variable echogenicity and blurred or well-defined margins (Figure 9, Panel A). Vascularization can be internal or peripheral (Figure 9, Panel B).

SE: In SE, focal orchitis can appear as both soft and hard lesions [8,20], depending on the stage of infection (Figure 9, Panel C).

CEUS: In focal orchitis, CEUS can vary from uniform vascular enhancement throughout the lesions [70] to unenhanced lesions with peripheral rim, depending on the stage of the infection (Figure 9, Panel D).

Differential diagnosis: Imaging features of testicular tuberculosis are non-specific and often impossible to distinguish from other more common pathologies such as tumor, infection, inflammation, and infarction [71]. In this scenario, other signs of inflammation such as scrotal wall thickening, hydrocele, and most of all epididymitis, favors the diagnosis of infection [72]. In the suspicion of a tubercular infection, it is mandatory to perform microbiological analysis (e.g., Mantoux test).

5. Neoplastic Testicular Lesions

Testicular cancers are rare tumors, accounting for ~1% of adult neoplasms, but represent the most common malignancies in young men aged 15 to 40 years, with increasing incidence rates in many countries in the last two decades [73–75].

According to the most recent World Health Organization (WHO) histological classification [76], testicular tumors can be distinguished in two main groups: (1) testicular germ cell tumors (TGCTs), which are the most common (~98% of all testicular cancers), in turn divided into two subclasses, seminomatous (s-TGCTs) and non-seminomatous (ns-TGCTs), and (2) stromal cell tumors, which are rare, even if probably underestimated. In addition, malignancies with testicular localization derived from non-testicular neoplasms (non-primary malignant tumors, i.e., hematologic tumors and metastases) must be considered.

Testicular tumors usually present as painless or paucisymptomatic (heaviness, swelling) testicular masses. In some cases, they are incidentally found during US performed for other reasons.

Serum tumor markers must be included in the diagnostic work-up, namely alpha fetoprotein (α-FP), beta subunit of human chorionic gonadotropin (β-hCG), and lactate dehydrogenase (LDH) [77,78]. Overall, the serum tumor markers show low sensitivity (especially in seminoma) and, if negative, the diagnosis of testicular tumor cannot be excluded [79]. Of note, patients with positive β-hCG often have gynecomastia, since β-hCG is very similar to the LH hormone, which has a direct action in stimulating male breast tissue [80,81].

A summary of the clinical characteristics and mp-US features of neoplastic testicular lesions is provided in Table 2, and their mp-US appearance is reported in Figures 10–17.

5.1. Seminomatous TGCTs (s-TGCTs)

Prevalence: s-TGCTs represent 55–60% of TGCTs. The median age at diagnosis is 20–40 years [82]. They are revealed as components of mixed TGCTs in 30% of cases.

Clinical history and physical examination: Patients with s-TGCTs can refer to clinicians for the detection of a testicular firm mass, testicular swelling, testicular pain, or lumbar pain when lymph node metastases are present. However, the diagnosis can be incidental during US performed for other reasons. Infertility [83–85] and cryptorchidism [86,87] are common risk factors for seminomas [15]. Physical examination usually reveals a large, hard testicular mass. However, sometimes they are incidental findings in US, since small lesions (<1.5 cm) are not always palpable, especially if placed in the center of the testicle.

GSUS + CDUS: The US appearance reflects the histological characteristics that consist of a nest of large, round cells with abundant cytoplasm and distinct borders, with fibrous septa containing lymphocyte infiltration. Occasionally, they can include syncytiotrophoblasts. Necrosis, intercellular edema, and hemorrhage can be present, especially in larger tumors [76,88]. Therefore, in GSUS evaluation, classic seminomas usually appear as focal round homogeneous lesions, hypoechoic to the normal surrounding parenchyma [89–91] (Figure 10, Panel A). However, large seminomas can also appear as inhomogeneous lesions with hypo/anechoic internal areas, reflecting tumor necrosis and/or bleeding [92]. Margins can be regular, irregular, or polylobate. Microlithiasis in the affected testicle is common [93,94]. CDUS shows increased peripheral and internal vascularization [89], which is commonly characterized by arborization and branches (Figure 10, Panel B).

SE: Seminomas usually appear as hard lesions showing low/absent elastic strain [8,95,96] (Figure 10, Panel C).

CEUS: Seminomas usually show hyperenhancement of the whole lesion after CEUS administration, apart from necrotic areas. A rapid wash-in and wash-out are distinctive characteristics of seminomas [40] (Figure 10, Panel D).

Table 2. Ultrasound, CDUS, and CEUS characteristics of principal neoplastic intratesticular lesions.

	Clinical Presentation	Serum Tumor Markers	Neoplastic Intratesticular Lesions			
			GS-US	CD-US	CEUS	SE
Leydig cell tumor	Generally asymptomatic; it can produce androgens	Negative	Hypoechoic, homogeneous well-demarcated lesion (possible hyperechoic halo)	Hypervascularized	Homogeneously hyperenhanced (rapid wash-in, delayed wash-out)	Hard lesions with low/absent elastic strain
Sertoli cell tumor	Asymptomatic; they can be a part of multiple neoplasia syndromes such as Carney complex and Peutz–Jegers	Negative	Hypo- or hyper-echoic lesion, with possible calcifications	Hypervascularized	Homogeneously hyperenhanced	Hard lesions with low/absent elastic strain
Seminoma	Testicular swelling, pain, lumbar pain OR asymptomatic; palpable firm testicular mass; possible gynecomastia	possible increase of β-hCG	Hypoechoic homogeneous round or oval lesion, occasionally multinodular or with polycyclic lobulated margins (unfrequently inhomogeneous)	Hypervascularized, with arborization and branches	Homogeneously hyperenhanced (rapid wash-in and wash-out)	Hard lesions with low/absent elastic strain
Embryonal cell carcinoma	Testicular swelling, pain, lumbar pain; palpable firm testicular mass; possible gynecomastia	Can be positive α-FP, β-hCG, LDH(not always)	Hypoechoic heterogeneous lesions with irregular polylobate marginscan present internal cystic areas or calcific margins.	Hypervascularized/avascular	Enhanced/unenhanced OR perilesional rim enhancement	Hard lesions with low/absent elastic strain
Teratoma	Testicular swelling, pain, lumbar pain; palpable firm testicular mass; possible gynecomastia	Can be positive α-FP, β-hCG, LDH(not always)	Heterogeneous lesions, well-circumscribed with cystic areas and internal septa	Hypervascularized in the solid part	Inhomogeneously hyperenhanced	Hard lesions with low/absent elastic strain (depending on liquid amount)
Choriocarcinoma	Testicular swelling, pain, lumbar pain; palpable firm testicular mass; possible gynecomastia	Can be positive β-hCG, (not always)	Heterogeneous lesions with hypo-anechoic areas (hemorrhage, necrosis) and calcifications	Hypervascularized	Hyperenhanced	Hard lesions with low/absent elastic strain
Yolk sac tumors	Testicular swelling, pain, lumbar pain; palpable firm testicular mass	Can be positive α-FP (not always)	Heterogeneous lesions with anechoic areas	Hypervascularized	Hyperenhanced	Hard lesions with low/absent elastic strain
Mixed	Testicular swelling, pain, lumbar pain; palpable firm testicular mass; possible gynecomastia	Can be positive α-FP, β-hCG, LDH(not always)	Different aspect regarding main histological component	Hypervascularized	Homogeneously/inhomogeneously hyperenhanced	Hard lesions with low/absent elastic strain
Burned-out tumor	Lumbar pain, vomit; possible gynecomastia	Can be positive α-FP, β-hCG, LDH(not always)	No testicular nodule; highly echogenic foci or gross calcifications/hypoechoic irregular areas	Hypovascularized	Unenhanced	/

Table 2. Cont.

	Clinical Presentation	Serum Tumor Markers	Neoplastic Intratesticular Lesions			
			GS-US	CD-US	CEUS	SE
Lymphoma	Testicular swelling, pain, and specific lymphoma symptoms; affects men older than 50 years, palpable firm testicular mass	Negative	Hypoechoic lesions with diffuse infiltration or multifocal hypoechoic lesions of various size	Hypervascularized with linear non-branching pattern	Hyperenhanced	Hard lesions with low/absent elastic strain
Leukemia	More frequent in children and young patients; it can be asymptomatic	Negative	Infiltrating pattern with irregular hypoechoic longitudinal striae/focal pattern with irregular hypoechoic nodules	Hypervascularized	Inhomogeneously hyperenhanced	Hard lesions with low/absent elastic strain

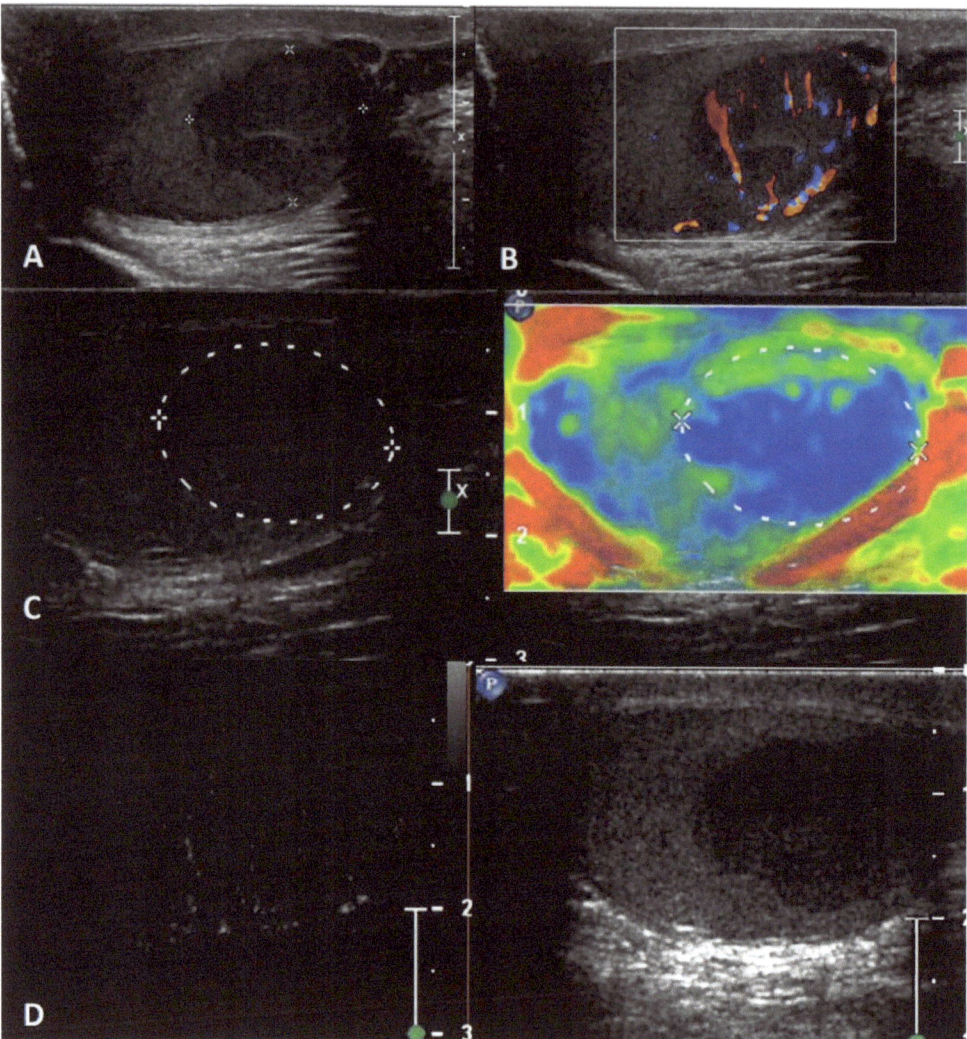

Figure 10. Seminoma. GSUS demonstrated a well-circumscribed homogeneously hypoechoic lesion in a 37-year-old man referred for infertility (panel **A**). CDUS showed increased internal vascularization (panel **B**). In SE, seminoma showed absent elastic strain (panel **C**), whereas CEUS confirmed the hyperenhancement within the lesion (panel **D**).

Differential diagnosis: Several neoplastic and non-neoplastic conditions may mimic testicular seminomas in imaging. Among the non-neoplastic conditions, testicular inflammation including orchitis with or without abscess formation may mimic seminoma. In the acute phase of orchitis, diffuse testicular edema results in the hypoechoic appearance of the testis, which is enlarged compared to the contralateral. Helpful imaging findings to suggest orchitis instead of seminoma include hypoechogenicity (edema) and hypervascularization of the ipsilateral epididymis, reactive hydrocele, associated scrotal edema, and pain [11]. Among the neoplastic conditions, non-seminomatous testicular germ cell tumors (ns-TGCTs) and lymphomas may mimic seminomas. Although seminomas, especially when large, may demonstrate cystic spaces and calcifications, these findings are more commonly encountered in ns-TGCTs. Ns-TGCTs are more likely to have ill-defined margins than seminomas, and age at the diagnosis can help (younger in ns-TGCT, older in seminomas). The US appearance of lymphomas can overlap that of seminomas, but the affected patient population is significantly older [11]. Finally, the imaging appearance of small seminomas can resemble that of Leydig cell tumors (LCTs; see below).

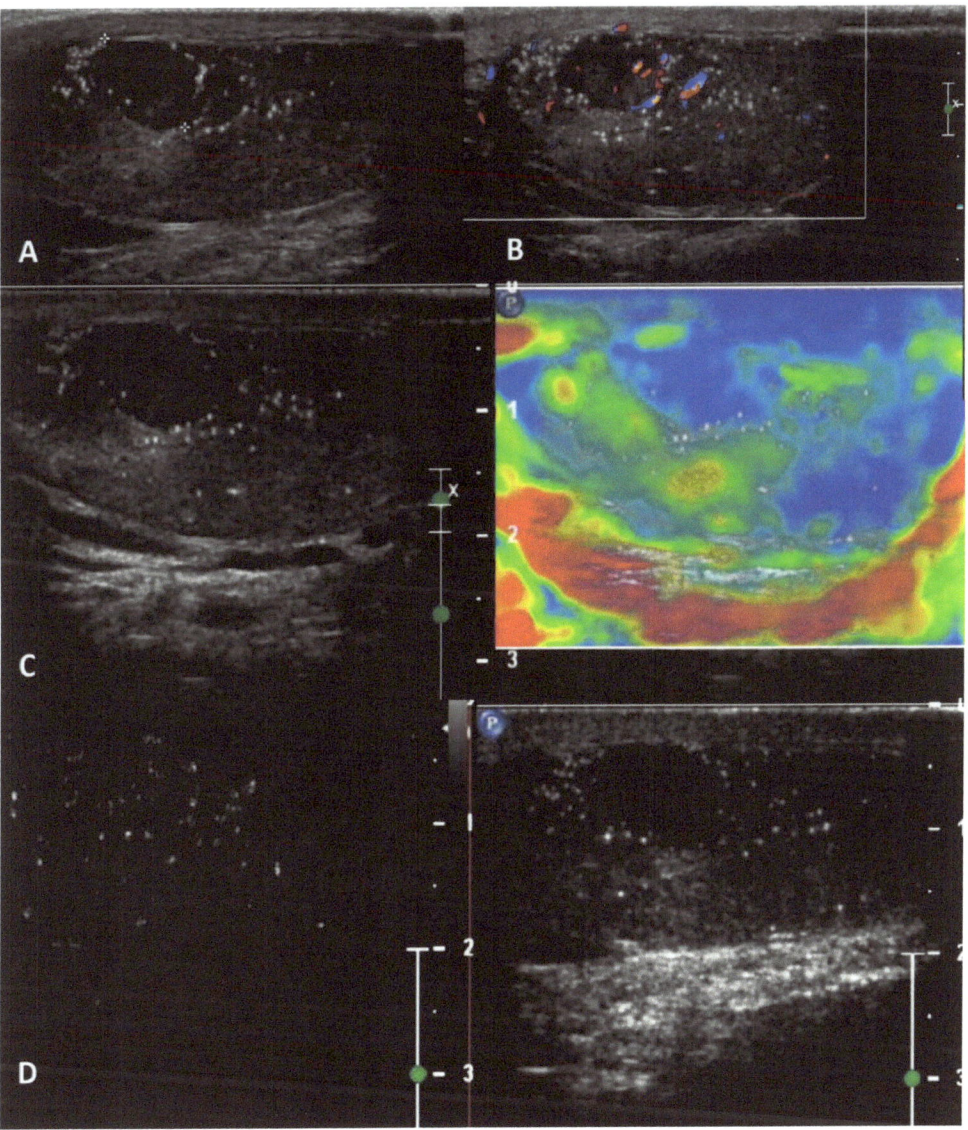

Figure 11. Embryonal carcinoma. GSUS demonstrated a markedly hypoechoic lesion (panel **A**) in a testis with starry sky appearance in a 29-year-old patient referred for testicular pain in the contralateral testis. CDUS showed peripheral and internal vascularization (panel **B**). In SE, the tumor showed absent elastic strain (panel **C**), whereas CEUS confirmed the hyperenhancement within the lesion (panel **D**).

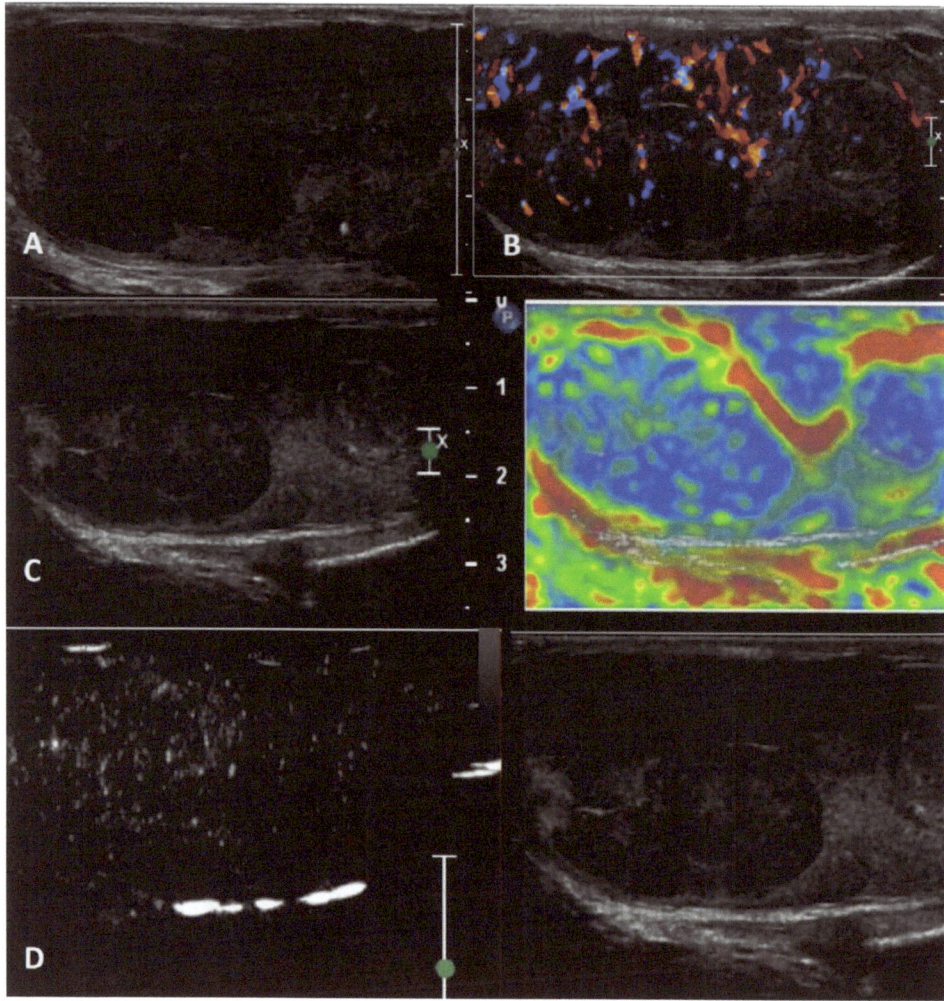

Figure 12. Mixed germ cell tumor. GSUS demonstrated multiple markedly and mild hypoechoic lesions (panel **A**), occupying almost the entire testis of a 26-year-old patient referred for scrotal swelling. CDUS showed peripheral and markedly internal vascularization (panel **B**). In SE, the tumor showed intermediate/absent elastic strain (panel **C**). CEUS demonstrated hyperenhancement of the entire lesion (panel **D**).

5.2. Non-Seminomatous TGCTs (ns-TGCTs)

Prevalence: Ns-TGCTs represent 40–45% of TGCTs. They usually occur in younger patients than s-TGCTs (median age at diagnosis 25 years) [82].

Clinical history and physical examination: Similar to patients with seminomas, those with ns-TGCTs can refer to clinicians for the detection of a testicular mass, testicular swelling, testicular pain, or lumbar pain when lymph node metastases are present. Due to a faster growth of ns-TGCTs, incidental diagnoses are rare, but possible [97,98].

Gynecomastia is a frequent finding [99]. Serum tumor markers, namely β-hCG and α-FP, are frequently positive, especially when distant metastases are present.

Ns-TGCTs are a heterogeneous group of tumors including different malignancies such as embryonal carcinomas, teratomas, choriocarcinomas, yolk sac tumors, and mixed germ cell tumors, whose mp-US characteristics are reported below.

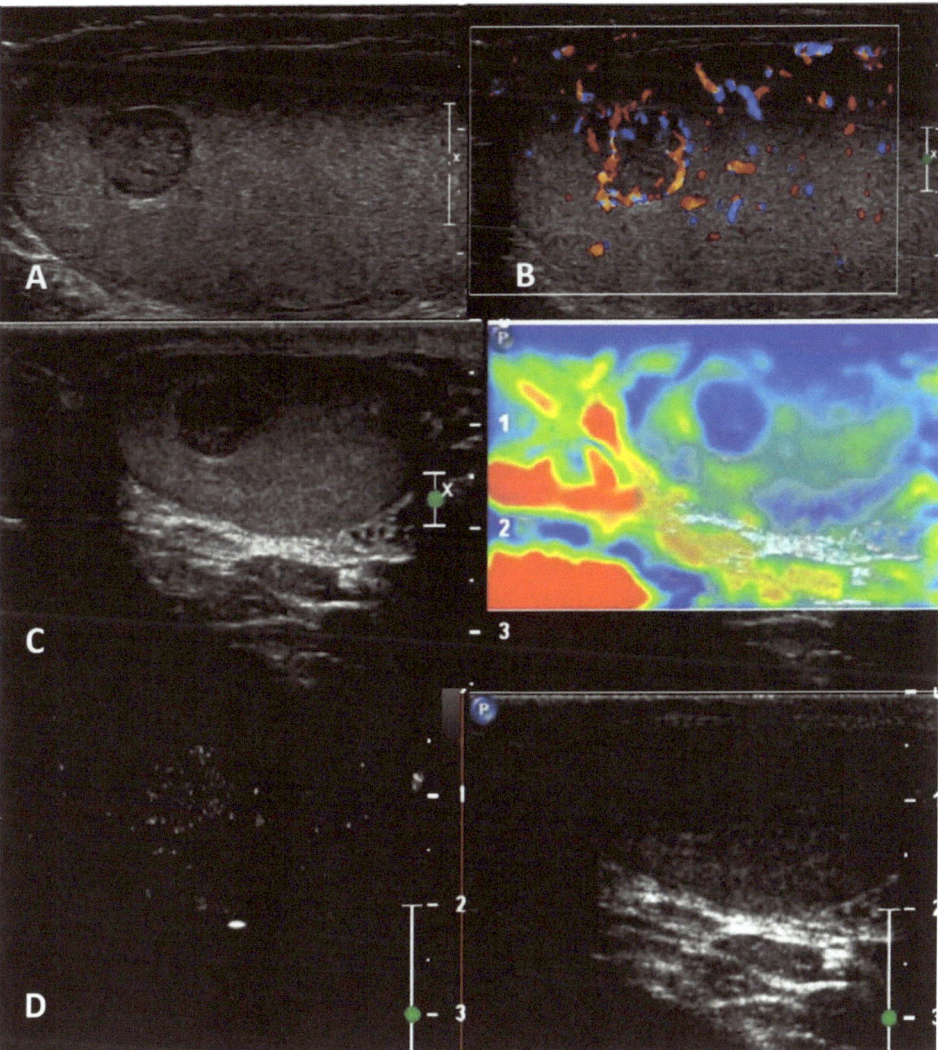

Figure 13. Leydig cell tumor. GSUS demonstrated a well-defined hypoechoic lesion (panel **A**), with a hyperechoic halo in a 34-year-old man referred for primary infertility. CDUS showed peripheral and marked internal vascularization (panel **B**). In SE, the tumor showed an absent elastic strain (panel **C**). CEUS confirmed the hyperenhancement within the lesion (panel **D**).

5.2.1. Embryonal Carcinoma

Prevalence: Embryonal carcinoma accounts for about 3% of TGCTs. It represents the most frequent (80%) component in mixed TGCTs.

Clinical history and physical examination: See above (Section 5.2).

GSUS + CDUS: In GSUS, embryonal carcinoma often appears as an hypoechoic and/or inhomogeneous lesion, frequently with internal calcifications [70] (Figure 11, Panel

A). US features may reflect histological features, which consist of significant anaplasia and necrotic areas. Sometimes, these tumors may appear as hypoechoic lesions with calcified margins [100] that may mimic an epidermoid cyst. Focal areas of necrosis and hemorrhage are frequent: in US examination, they appear as anechoic areas (in case of recent hemorrhage) or hyperechoic areas (in case of organized necrosis or hemorrhage). The margins are mainly irregular and polylobulated [101]. CDUS commonly shows increased peripheral and internal chaotic vascularization, even if in a minority of cases they could be avascular if completely necrotic (Figure 11, Panel B).

SE: Embryonal carcinomas usually appear as hard lesions showing low/absent elastic strain [102] (Figure 11, Panel C).

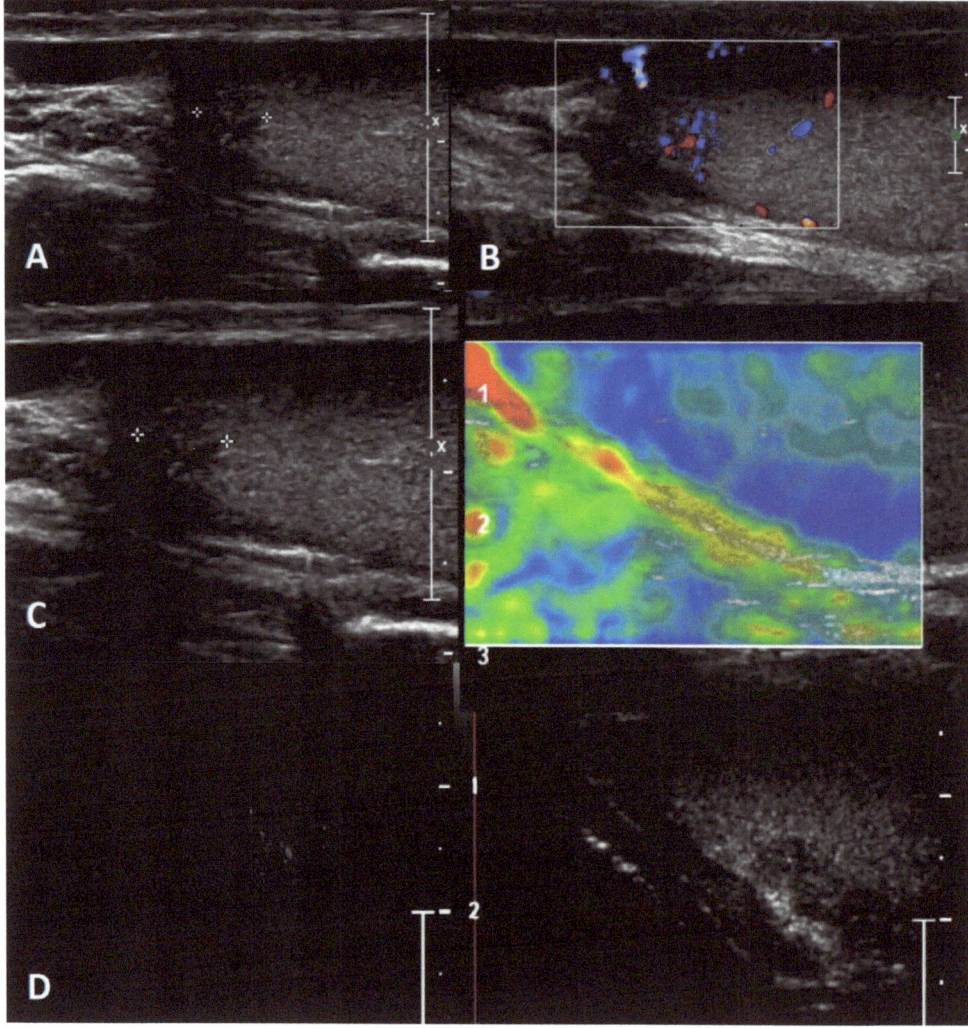

Figure 14. Sertoli cell tumor. GSUS demonstrated a mild hypoechoic lesion (panel **A**) with irregular margins in a 46-year-old patient referred for hypogonadism. CDUS showed markedly internal vascularization (panel **B**). In SE, the tumor showed absent elastic strain (panel **C**). CEUS confirmed the enhancement within the lesion (panel **D**).

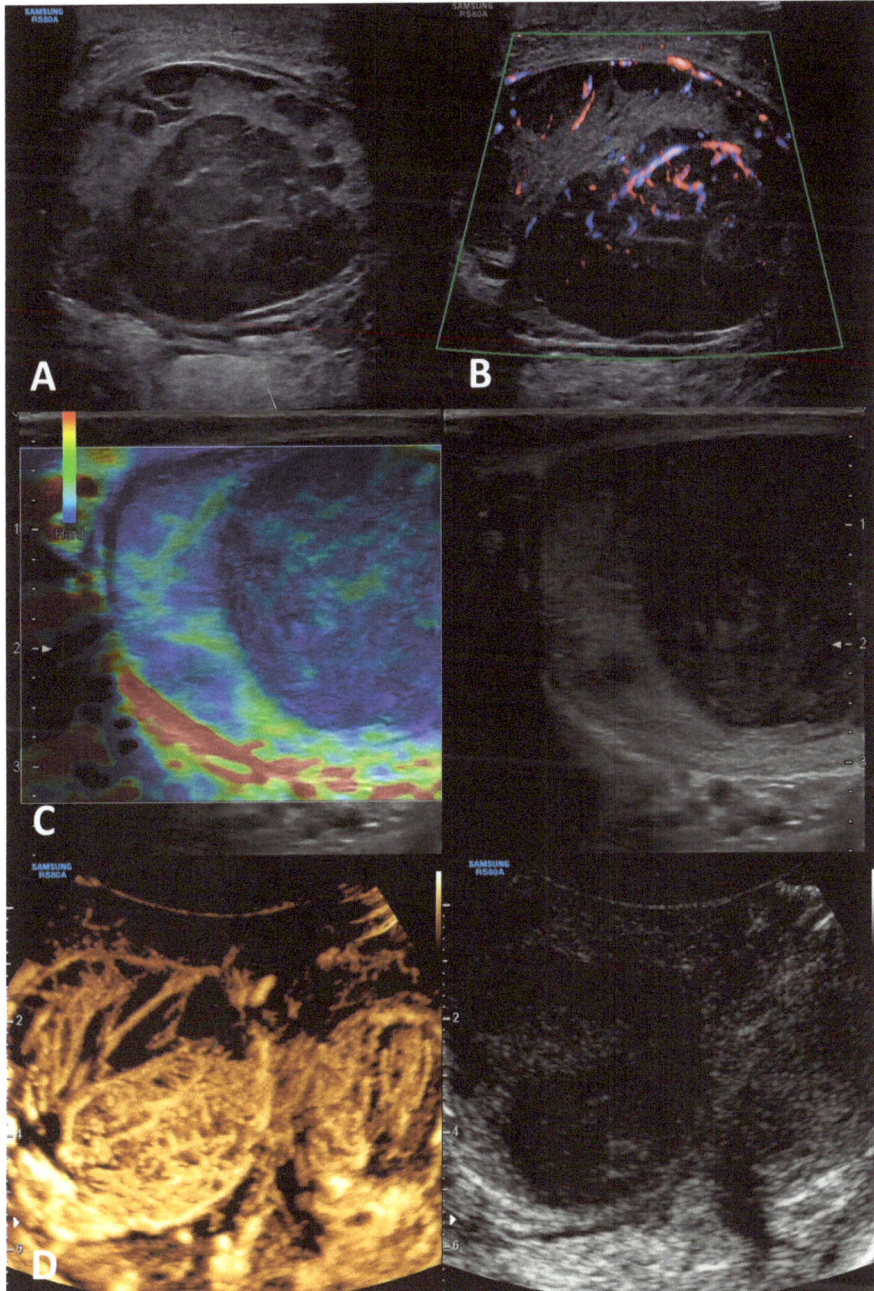

Figure 15. Lymphoma, nodular pattern. GSUS demonstrated a markedly hypoechoic lesion, with a multinodular aspect (panel **A**), with irregular margins, and interesting epididymis tail. CDUS showed markedly internal vascularization (panel **B**). In SE, the tumor showed an absent elastic strain (panel **C**). CEUS showed hyperenhancement of the lesions, with rapid wash-in and wash-out (panel **D**).

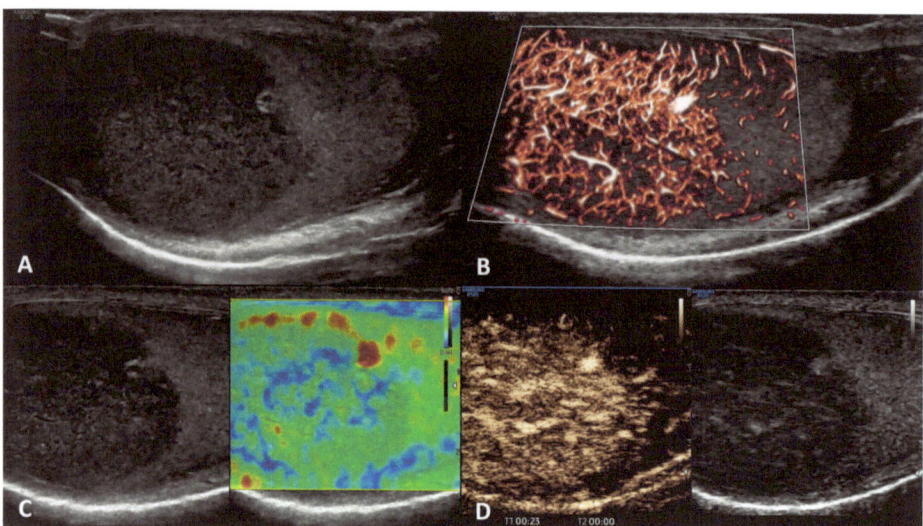

Figure 16. Leukemia. GSUS demonstrated a hypoechoic lesion (panel **A**) with regular margins. CDUS showed internal vascularization of the lesion (panel **B**). In SE, the lesion demonstrated an intermediate/soft elastic strain (panel **C**). In CEUS, the lesion appeared hyperenhanced due to its high vascularity (panel **D**).

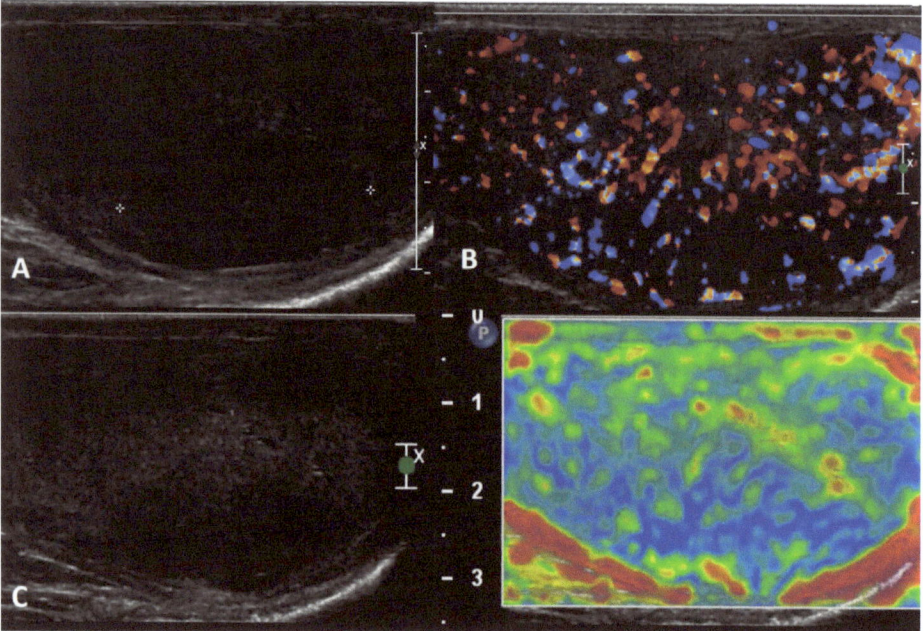

Figure 17. Plasmacytoma. GSUS demonstrated multiple, both mild and markedly hypoechoic lesions (panel **A**) with smooth margins in a 72 year-old-man referred for scrotal swelling, with a positive personal history of plasmacytoma. CDUS showed internal vascularization of the lesions and hypervascularization of the entire testis (panel **B**). In SE, the lesions demonstrated intermediate elastic strain (panel **C**).

CEUS: CEUS is usually not recommended for very large lesions with positive serum tumor markers, as embryonal carcinoma usually appears, but can be useful in smaller lesions. Embryonal carcinomas show an inhomogeneous hyperenhancement [103] of the lesion after CEUS administration with rapid wash-in and rapid wash-out (Figure 11, Panel D). However, in rare cases, the lesions may also fail to pick-up the contrast medium [40,103], making it more difficult to diagnose the differential diagnosis (i.e., with atypical epidermoid cyst).

Differential diagnosis: The differential diagnosis of embryonal carcinoma is usually with other ns-TGCTs, especially mixed ones due to large size, and is not always possible. Internal calcifications, if present, are usually hallmarks. Embryonal carcinoma with internal necrosis and calcified margins can be mistaken with an atypical epidermoid cyst (see above) [3]. Serum tumor markers can be helpful as well as the meticulous study of the margins, which are usually irregular in embryonal carcinoma and well-demarcated in epidermoid cyst.

5.2.2. Teratoma

Prevalence: Teratomas account for about 5–10% of TGCTs.

Clinical history and physical examination: See above (Section 5.2).

GSUS + CDUS: Teratoma is composed of different somatic tissues, derived from one or more germinal layers (endoderm, mesoderm, and ectoderm). They are usually divided into mature and immature tumors according to histology and in prepubertal and postpubertal according to the age of incidence. Prepubertal tumors are usually benign and have a conservative treatment [104], while postpubertal tumors (both mature and immature) can have malignant attitude and metastasize.

The US appearance varies according to the different histological features of the tumor [90]. They usually appear as well-defined lesions with regular margins. Echotexture can include cystic areas (cystic teratomas) with internal septa, with different content (serous, mucoid, keratinous) [91,105,106]. A differential diagnosis with simple, complex, or epidermoid cyst may sometimes be difficult. Focal calcifications are also common and are mainly due to the presence of cartilage and immature bone tissue [91]. CDUS commonly shows increased peripheral and internal vascularization in the solid portion of the lesion.

SE: As other TGCTs, teratomas usually appear as hard lesions showing low/absent elastic strain [102], but depending on the amount of liquid inside, they can also have higher elastic strain [95,102].

CEUS: Teratomas show hyperenhancement within the solid part of the lesions with rapid wash-in and rapid wash-out. Anechoic areas are usually non-enhanced.

Differential diagnosis: The differential diagnosis of teratoma is usually with other ns-TGCTs, especially mixed ones due to large size and is not always possible. Internal cysts, if present, different content, and internal septa are usually hallmarks.

5.2.3. Choriocarcinoma

Prevalence: Choriocarcinoma accounts for about 0.5–1% of TGCTs. They represent about 5–10% of mixed TGCTs.

Clinical history and physical examination: See above (Section 5.2). Specifically, choriocarcinomas have a more aggressive attitude compared to other ns-TGCTs, with a higher frequency of blood rather than lymphatic metastases [107]. β-hCG levels are usually very high and therefore they are frequently associated with gynecomastia [91].

GSUS + CDUS: Choriocarcinoma can appear as a large, solid inhomogeneous mass, with calcifications and areas with different echogenicity due to necrosis and/or hemorrhages [91,92,101]. However, the GS aspect is not specific and a differentiation from other non-seminomatous tumors is not always easy. In CDUS, peripheral and internal vascularization is highly represented.

SE: Choriocarcinomas usually appear as hard lesions showing low/absent elastic strain [102].

CEUS: Due to the aggressiveness of the tumor and the frequent positivity of serum testicular markers, the diagnosis can be conducted with GS- and CD-US and it is not necessary to perform CEUS. However, in CEUS, choriocarcinomas show hyperenhancement with rapid wash-in and rapid wash-out.

Differential diagnosis: The differential diagnosis of choriocarcinoma is usually with other ns-TGCTs and is not always possible. It could be difficult to distinguish pure forms from mixed ones.

5.2.4. Yolk Sac Tumor

Prevalence: Yolk sac tumor is very rare in adults (0–1%) in its pure form while it is the most common TGCT in children (60%). It represents 40% of mixed TGCTs.

Clinical history and physical examination: See above (Section 5.2). Of note, serum α-FP is usually high in these tumors [101].

GSUS + CDUS: Yolk sac tumors usually appear in CDUS as large, solid inhomogeneous masses, with multiple internal anechoic gaps [91,101]. In CDUS, peripheral and internal vascularization is highly represented.

SE: Yolk sac tumors usually appear as hard lesions showing low/absent elastic strain.

CEUS: Diagnosis is usually performed with GS and CDUS and it is not necessary to perform CEUS.

However, in CEUS, they show hyperenhancement with rapid wash-in and rapid wash-out.

Differential diagnosis: The differential diagnosis of yolk sac tumor is usually with other ns-TGCTs and is not always possible. It could be difficult to distinguish pure forms from mixed ones.

5.2.5. Mixed Germ Cell Tumor

Prevalence: Mixed germ cell tumors account for about 20–40% of TGCTs.

Clinical history and physical examination: See above (Section 5.2). Of note, mixed germ cell tumors are the most common of the ns-TGCTs and they include the various tumor types described above including the seminomatous and non- seminomatous components, with various percentages within the tumor lesion.

GSUS, CDUS, CEUS, and **SE** reflect the features of the different components and their representation within the lesion (Figure 12, Panel A–D).

5.3. Stromal Cell Tumors

Prevalence: Stromal cell tumors account for about 3–5% of testicular tumors in adults and 25% in children [104,108]. However, their prevalence is probably underestimated, and according to the recent scientific literature, they represent up to 22% of nonpalpable testicular nodules [109].

Clinical history and physical examination: In adults, stromal cell tumors are usually incidental findings detected in US performed for other reasons [110]. Specifically, according to many reports, stromal cell tumors, and in particular Leydig cell tumors (LCTs), are frequent incidental findings in infertile patients [108,111,112]. However, in the case of large tumors, enlargement of the scrotum is reported and can be the first reason for medical consultation.

In children and adolescents, LCTs can lead to precocious puberty due to the excessive androgen production, or gynecomastia, caused by excess estrogen due to androgen aromatization [113]. In adults, excessive androgen secretion is exceptional even in malignant LCTs and is usually not associated with peripheral effects [114]. Conversely, Sertoli cell tumors (SCTs) usually do not show any endocrine activity. In some cases, SCTs are a part of multiple neoplasia syndromes such as Carney complex and Peutz–Jegers [115,116]. Serum tumor markers are always negative in the case of stromal cell tumors and no specifical blood test marker exists for these tumors.

Unlike the TGCTs, the great majority of stromal cell tumors are benign, so testis-sparing surgery is now the standard of care in these tumors [117,118]. In selected patients, a strict radiological surveillance can also be performed [117].

5.3.1. Leydig Cell Tumor (LCT)

Prevalence: LCTs account for about 5% of all testicular tumors.

Clinical history and physical examination: See above (Section 5.3). Of note, malignancy is reported for 10–15% of LCTs [95]. Histological features of malignancy are cytologic atypia, necrosis, angiolymphatic invasion, increased mitotic activity, atypical mitotic figures, infiltrative margins, extension beyond testicular parenchyma, and DNA aneuploidy [95].

GSUS + CDUS: LCTs commonly appear in GSUS as round lesions with homogeneous hypoechoic echotexture and regular well-demarcated margins [40,119]. A hyperechoic halo surrounding the lesion can sometimes be found [120] (Figure 13, Panel A). Dimensions are usually small due to the slow cell growth, and they usually present as single lesions. LCTs are usually unilateral even if, in rare cases, they can involve both testicles [121]. CDUS can show peripheral and, sometimes, intralesional, blood flow [40,119] (Figure 13, Panel B).

SE: LCTs usually appear as hard lesions in SE, showing low/absent elastic strain [8,95,96] (Figure 13, Panel C).

CEUS: CEUS could be useful for differential diagnosis of LCTs with small seminomas (see below). After CEUS administration, LCT shows a homogeneous and intense hyperenhancement of the whole lesion [122]. A rapid wash-in and a slow wash-out are distinctive characteristics of LCTs [4,40,103] (Figure 13, Panel D). Leydig cells indeed strongly express an angiogenic mitogen, the endocrine gland–derived vascular endothelial growth factor (EG-VEGF) [123]. EG-VEGF may play a role in angiogenesis in LCT growth and therefore in an intense vascularization [122].

Differential diagnosis: Distinguishing LCT from small seminomas may sometimes not be straightforward. Nevertheless, differential diagnosis is imperative as the two tumors have a very different clinical course and therefore therapeutic direction [11]. The clinical context is not useful, as age of onset is similar, patients could be asymptomatic in both cases, and infertility could be a risk factor for both tumors. In the case of small lesions, they could be undetectable with clinical examination in both cases but, if palpable, both may have a firm consistency. Serum tumor markers can be negative in both cases. Microlithiasis of the surrounding parenchyma is more frequently identified in seminomas. In GS, both seminomas and LCTs appear as hypoechoic and homogeneous lesions, margins could be well-demarcated in both lesions, and CDUS usually shows internal vascularization in both lesions, even if it can appear more often as intralesional and arborized in seminomas and peripheral in LCTs. SE is similar in LCTs and seminomas as it shows hard lesions with low/absent elastic strain. Hence, CEUS can represent the decisive tool in the differential diagnosis between LCTs and seminomas since the contrast medium diffuses differently in the two lesions. Both seminomas and LCTs are homogeneously hyperenhanced compared to the surrounding parenchyma [20,40,122,124–126] with a rapid wash-in [40], while wash-out seems to be different, being slower in LCTs and faster in seminomas [4,40,103]. In addition, according to some reports, LCTs show a greater peak enhancement than seminomas in the wash-in phase [17,103]. These data may depend on the vascular architecture of LCTs, characterized by the high density of regular microvessels [104]. However, the literature does not fully agree on the results of the CEUS kinetics. This depends on very heterogeneous studies, which include different types of lesions and have small sample sizes [127].

Regarding the differential diagnosis between benign and malignant LCTs, no radiological feature can distinguish the nature of the lesion. Hence, although strict radiological surveillance can be performed if a LCT is suspected [98], testis-sparing surgery represents the standard of care in these tumors [117,118], and orchiectomy can be performed in the case of a malignancy in histology.

5.3.2. Sertoli Cell Tumor (SCT)

Prevalence: Sertoli cell tumors (SCTs) account for <1% of all testicular tumors, and can be found in men with a wide age range (18 to 80 years), although they are more frequent in young adults [128]. Rarely, SCTs are also reported in pediatric patients [129].

Clinical history and physical examination: See above (Section 5.3). Of note, malignancy is reported for 5% of SCTs [97].

GSUS + CDUS: SCTs can appear at GSUS as both hypoechoic and hyperechoic lesions, with possible intralesional calcifications (Figure 14, Panel A). Margins are well-demarcated. In some cases, there are large areas of calcification and inhomogeneous echotexture, identifying the so-called "calcifying Sertoli cell tumor": this specific subtype is usually associated with Carney complex or Peutz–Jegers syndrome [115,116]. CDUS shows a marked internal vascularization of these lesions (Figure 14, Panel B).

SE: SCTs usually appear as hard lesions showing low/absent elastic strain (Figure 14, Panel C) [8,95,96].

CEUS: SCTs show an homogeneous and intense hyperenhancement of the whole lesion with rapid wash-in and a wash-out similar to the parenchyma [40,103] (Figure 14, Panel D).

Differential diagnosis: Differential diagnosis includes LCTs and small seminomas and is sometimes difficult. The kinetic characteristics in CEUS can resemble both LCTs and seminomas, but the relative literature is very scarce as this histotype is rare.

5.4. Non-Primary Malignant Tumors

Among the neoplasms not deriving from testicular parenchyma, primary hematologic malignancies of the testes are the most frequent, namely non-Hodgkin lymphoma or primary testicular leukemia. In very rare cases, the testicle can also be the site of metastases [17].

5.4.1. Lymphoma

Prevalence: Testicular lymphomas represent 1–9% of all testicular tumors and are frequently B-cell type [130]. They usually affect men older than 50 years.

Clinical history and physical examination: Testicular lymphomas can appear as a primary or secondary localization of the disease, and they can be unilateral or bilateral. Patients are usually asymptomatic or paucisymptomatic. Symptoms include, as for other testicular tumors, firm testicular masses, testicular swelling, or testicular heaviness. Specific lymphoma symptoms could be present: fever, weight loss, sweating at night, itching.

GSUS + CDUS: In GSUS, lymphomas usually appear as hypoechoic lesions with infiltrating margins (Figure 15, Panel A). The vascular pattern is clearly visible within the lesion and consists of well-organized vessels arranged with a linear, non-branching pattern [17] (Figure 15, Panel B).

SE: SE reveals hard lesions showing low/absent elastic strain [17] (Figure 15, Panel C).

CEUS: Usually, CEUS shows hyperenhancement of the lesions, with rapid wash-in and wash-out [17], but qualitative and quantitative assessment do not add significant information to conventional CDUS (Figure 15, Panel D).

Differential diagnosis: The US differential diagnosis is usually with other testicular tumors that appear hypoechoic at GS (e.g., seminoma). The US hallmark of lymphomas are infiltrating margins and the vascular pattern, which besides the detection in men aged >50 years old can help in suggesting the diagnosis.

5.4.2. Primary Testicular Leukemia

Prevalence: Primary testicular leukemia is a rare presentation of leukemia, more frequent in children and young patients. Testicular involvement is found in 1% to 2.4% of boys with acute lymphoblastic leukemia, but is very rare in adult patients [131,132].

Clinical history and physical examination: Testicular localization may be simultaneous to the diagnosis of the primary disease or can occur after treatment/remission of the primary disease. Patients are usually asymptomatic. Physical examination can reveal testicular involvement by increased size, irregular swelling, and firm consistency of the testes [133].

GSUS + CDUS: GSUS appearance can include two patterns. On the one hand, an infiltrating pattern with irregular hypoechoic longitudinal striae radiating peripherally from the mediastinum to the entire testicle with CDUS showing increased vascularity of non-branching linear patterns has been described. On the other hand, a focal pattern with irregular hypoechoic nodules with smooth irregular margins with increased vascularity in CDUS can be found [17,102,134–136] (Figure 16, Panel A). The hypoechogenicity in US reflects the infiltration and aggregation of abnormal lymphoid lesions because the density of tumor cells and vessels is greater than that of normal testicular tissue [17,102,134] (Figure 16, Panel B).

SE: In SE, an increased testicular stiffness is reported [102,134] (Figure 16, Panel C).

CEUS: Regarding CEUS, lesions appear hyperenhanced due to their high vascularity [17] (Figure 16, Panel D).

Differential diagnosis: Primary testicular leukemia can mimic an inflammatory process of the testis such as orchitis. However, the lack of pain and normal appearance of the epididymis can guide the diagnosis [137].

5.4.3. Plasmacytoma

Prevalence: Patients with multiple myeloma can rarely present with an intratesticular plasmacytoma. So far, less than a hundred cases have been reported in the literature [138].

Clinical history and physical examination: In patients with a known diagnosis of multiple myeloma, intratesticular plasmacytoma should always be suspected. Diagnosis is usually due to a rapid testicular enlargement. The lesion can be hard and elastic at physical examination [139].

GSUS + CDUS: Plasmacytoma usually involves the whole testicle, which is enlarged and hypoechoic in GSUS (Figure 17, Panel A), with markedly increased vascularization in CDUS (Figure 17, Panel B).

SE: SE reveals a hard lesion showing low/absent elastic strain (Figure 17, Panel C).

CEUS: Regarding CEUS, lesions appear hyperenhanced due to their high vascularity [17].

Differential diagnosis: Differential diagnosis with orchitis may be difficult, even if the lack of pain and normal appearance of the epididymis can help [140].

5.4.4. Metastases

The testicle is a rare site for the metastatic localization of other tumors. Some literature reports include prostate [141], lung [142], gastrointestinal tumors [143,144], melanoma [145], pancreas [146], kidneys [147], bladder [148], thyroid [149], and neuroblastoma [150].

Clinical history and physical examination: In patients with a known diagnosis of extratesticular tumor and detection at palpation of a hard testicular nodule/mass, metastases should always be suspected.

GSUS + CDUS: In GSUS, metastases show variable patterns according to the site of the primary tumor. Usually, they present as irregular hypoechoic inhomogeneous lesions vascularized in CDUS [3].

SE: SE reveals a hard lesion showing low/absent elastic strain.

CEUS: Regarding CEUS, lesions appear hyperenhanced due to their high vascularity.

Differential diagnosis: US appearance is not specific; however, metastases are generally found in the setting of widespread disease and are rarely the first reason for presentation [3].

5.5. Burned-Out Tumor

Prevalence: 'Burned-out' testicular tumors are rare clinical entities that describe a spontaneously and completely regressed testicular tumor, which presents at the stage of metastases, in most cases in retroperitoneal lymph nodes, in the absence of clinical or US detection of a testicular nodule [151]. The cause of testicular mass regression is still unknown. Hypotheses of ischemia of the lesion or destruction by the immune system have been advocated [152]. Due to the rarity of burned-out tumors, no specific guidelines exist for diagnosis, clinical, and therapeutic management.

Clinical history and physical examination: Symptoms are often non-specific and include nausea, vomiting, and lower back pain due to retroperitoneal lymph-node enlargement, the most common site of metastasis. Retroperitoneal, supraclavicular, cervical, and axillary lymph nodes and, less often, lung and liver localization of metastases can be the first appearance of a 'burned-out' testicular tumor. A few patients complain of testicular symptoms [152]. Both seminomas and non-seminomas can have "burned-out" presentations. Commonly, serum tumor markers are very high [152].

GSUS + CDUS: No primary testicular lesion is identified, and the tumor is supposed to be reduced to a fibrotic scar, represented by a linear macrocalcification (>0.2–0.3 cm) with a rear shadow cone [153,154]. Histologically, it corresponds to psammoma bodies (smooth laminated intratubular calcifications) and hematoxyphilic bodies (non-laminated intratubular calcifications) [155–158]. Occasionally, signs of burned-out tumors are represented by hypoechoic irregular areas within the testicle with scarce vascularization [155–158]. Testicular atrophy and microlithiasis have also been reported in relation to burned-out tumors [155–157].

SE: In the parenchyma surrounding the scar/calcification, a focal area of increased stiffness can be observed in SE.

CEUS: The fibrotic scar and surrounding areas are usually not enhanced with CEUS [125].

Differential diagnosis: A burned-out tumor can be confused with a simple fibrotic scar or a linear macro-calcification. When the imaging is uncertain, serum tumor markers, which show high levels in burned-out tumors, must be performed to exclude distant spread of the disease.

6. Mp-US: Advantages, Limitations, and Future Perspectives

According to the aforementioned information, mp-US shows relevant advantages in relation to the investigation of testicular lesions. In fact, combining different US techniques, mp-US can provide a more detailed characterization of testicular lesions than a single US technique alone, helping in the differential diagnosis of benign or malignant lesions and in the effort to identify the type of lesion assessed [1–3]. However, mp-US also has some limitations. In some cases, even using mp-US, it can be difficult to discriminate the benign or malignant origin of a testicular lesion, and in the case of a "likely" malignant lesion, it is challenging to suggest a possible cancer type. Hence, to date, histology remains the only certain diagnostic tool to define the nature of a testicular lesion. In addition, while GS and CDUS are often sufficient to suggest the benign or malignant nature of a testicular lesion [1–3], and CEUS can help in better defining the nature of a lesion [7,29], SE added value in clinical practice remains to be proven [8,30,32] and, so far, its use in increasing the diagnostic accuracy of other US techniques is poor. Regardless, future perspectives of the imaging of testicular lesions are promising. Mp-US, eventually associated with other imaging techniques (e.g., magnetic resonance imaging), and the technical advancement of US devices will help to characterize testicular lesions more and more, with the aim to identify the nature of a testicular lesion with increasing accuracy. In addition, mp-US, eventually associated with other imaging techniques, will try to identify parameters suggesting an early tumor in men with testicular malignancy risk factors (e.g., cryptorchidism). In our opinion, in a few years, the new diagnostic paradigm will be "multiparametric imaging", combining more and more sophisticated US techniques and devices with other imaging techniques, in the attempt to increase the diagnostic accuracy of testicular lesions as much as possible.

7. Conclusions

Mp-US is a valuable diagnostic paradigm combining information derived from different US techniques (GSUS, CDUS, CEUS, and SE), which, along with clinical history and physical examination, can help in the differential diagnosis of testicular lesions. Mp-US can provide a more detailed characterization of testicular lesions than a single US technique alone. Although GS and CDUS are often sufficient to suggest the benign or malignant nature of testicular lesions, CEUS can be decisive in the differential diagnosis of unclear findings, and SE can help to strengthen the diagnosis. The knowledge of mp-US patterns of testicular lesions, summarized in this review, is useful to the physician in daily clinical practice to discriminate benign and malignant lesions, thus improving the management of critical patients by suggesting testicular salvage and US follow-up or orchiectomy.

Author Contributions: C.P. and F.L. conceived the study. All authors performed the literature search and collated the data. C.P., M.T., F.S., and F.L. wrote the manuscript with input from all the authors. P.S.S., D.Y.H., M.B., M.M., and A.M.I. provided critical feedback and helped shape the manuscript. C.P., A.M.I., and P.S.S. provided the multiparametric ultrasound pictures. All authors have read and agreed to the published version of the manuscript.

Funding: This research received no external funding.

Conflicts of Interest: The authors declare no conflict of interest.

References

1. Lotti, F.; Maggi, M. Ultrasound of the Male Genital Tract in Relation to Male Reproductive Health. *Hum. Reprod. Update* **2015**, *21*, 56–83. [CrossRef] [PubMed]
2. Lotti, F.; Bertolotto, M.; Maggi, M. Historical Trends for the Standards in Scrotal Ultrasonography: What Was, What Is and What Will Be Normal. *Andrology* **2021**, *9*, 1331–1355. [CrossRef] [PubMed]
3. Isidori, A.M.; Lenzi, A. *Ultrasound of the Testis for the Andrologist: Morphological and Functional Atlas*; Springer: Berlin/Heidelberg, Germany, 2018; ISBN 9783319518268.
4. Huang, D.Y.; Sidhu, P.S. Focal Testicular Lesions: Colour Doppler Ultrasound, Contrast-Enhanced Ultrasound and Tissue Elastography as Adjuvants to the Diagnosis. *Br. J. Radiol.* **2012**, *85*, S41–S53. [CrossRef] [PubMed]
5. Sidhu, P.S. Multiparametric Ultrasound (MPUS) Imaging: Terminology Describing the Many Aspects of Ultrasonography. *Ultraschall Med.* **2015**, *36*, 315–317. [CrossRef]
6. Shah, A.; Lung, P.F.; Clarke, J.L.; Sellars, M.E.; Sidhu, P.S. Re: New Ultrasound Techniques for Imaging of the Indeterminate Testicular Lesion May Avoid Surgery Completely. *Clin. Radiol.* **2010**, *65*, 496–497. [CrossRef] [PubMed]
7. Tenuta, M.; Sesti, F.; Bonaventura, I.; Mazzotta, P.; Pofi, R.; Gianfrilli, D.; Pozza, C. Use of Contrast Enhanced Ultrasound in Testicular Diseases: A Comprehensive Review. *Andrology* **2021**, *9*, 1369–1382. [CrossRef]
8. Pozza, C.; Gianfrilli, D.; Fattorini, G.; Giannetta, E.; Barbagallo, F.; Nicolai, E.; Cristini, C.; Di Pierro, G.B.; Franco, G.; Lenzi, A.; et al. Diagnostic Value of Qualitative and Strain Ratio Elastography in the Differential Diagnosis of Non-Palpable Testicular Lesions. *Andrology* **2016**, *4*, 1193–1203. [CrossRef]
9. Cantisani, V.; Di Leo, N.; Bertolotto, M.; Fresilli, D.; Granata, A.; Polti, G.; Polito, E.; Pacini, P.; Guiban, O.; Del Gaudio, G.; et al. Role of Multiparametric Ultrasound in Testicular Focal Lesions and Diffuse Pathology Evaluation, with Particular Regard to Elastography: Review of Literature. *Andrology* **2021**, *9*, 1356–1368. [CrossRef]
10. Dieckmann, K.-P.; Frey, U.; Lock, G. Contemporary Diagnostic Work-up of Testicular Germ Cell Tumours. *Nat. Rev. Urol.* **2013**, *10*, 703–712. [CrossRef]
11. Marko, J.; Wolfman, D.J.; Aubin, A.L.; Sesterhenn, I.A. Testicular Seminoma and Its Mimics: From the Radiologic Pathology Archives. *Radiographics* **2017**, *37*, 1085–1098. [CrossRef]
12. Song, G.; Xiong, G.-Y.; Fan, Y.; Huang, C.; Kang, Y.-M.; Ji, G.-J.; Chen, J.-C.; Xin, Z.-C.; Zhou, L.-Q. The Role of Tumor Size, Ultrasonographic Findings, and Serum Tumor Markers in Predicting the Likelihood of Malignant Testicular Histology. *Asian J. Androl.* **2019**, *21*, 196–200. [CrossRef] [PubMed]
13. Carmignani, L.; Gadda, F.; Gazzano, G.; Nerva, F.; Mancini, M.; Ferruti, M.; Bulfamante, G.; Bosari, S.; Coggi, G.; Rocco, F.; et al. High Incidence of Benign Testicular Neoplasms Diagnosed by Ultrasound. *J. Urol.* **2003**, *170*, 1783–1786. [CrossRef]
14. Rocher, L.; Ramchandani, P.; Belfield, J.; Bertolotto, M.; Derchi, L.E.; Correas, J.M.; Oyen, R.; Tsili, A.C.; Turgut, A.T.; Dogra, V.; et al. Incidentally Detected Non-Palpable Testicular Tumours in Adults at Scrotal Ultrasound: Impact of Radiological Findings on Management Radiologic Review and Recommendations of the ESUR Scrotal Imaging Subcommittee. *Eur. Radiol.* **2016**, *26*, 2268–2278. [CrossRef]
15. Yazici, S.; Del Biondo, D.; Napodano, G.; Grillo, M.; Calace, F.P.; Prezioso, D.; Crocetto, F.; Barone, B. Risk Factors for Testicular Cancer: Environment, Genes and Infections-Is It All? *Medicina* **2023**, *59*, 724. [CrossRef] [PubMed]

16. Schröder, C.; Lock, G.; Schmidt, C.; Löning, T.; Dieckmann, K.-P. Real-Time Elastography and Contrast-Enhanced Ultrasonography in the Evaluation of Testicular Masses: A Comparative Prospective Study. *Ultrasound Med. Biol.* **2016**, *42*, 1807–1815. [CrossRef]
17. Kachramanoglou, C.; Rafailidis, V.; Philippidou, M.; Bertolotto, M.; Huang, D.Y.; Deganello, A.; Sellars, M.E.; Sidhu, P.S. Multiparametric Sonography of Hematologic Malignancies of the Testis: Grayscale, Color Doppler, and Contrast-Enhanced Ultrasound and Strain Elastographic Appearances with Histologic Correlation. *J. Ultrasound Med.* **2017**, *36*, 409–420. [CrossRef]
18. Lock, G.; Schröder, C.; Schmidt, C.; Anheuser, P.; Loening, T.; Dieckmann, K.P. Contrast-Enhanced Ultrasound and Real-Time Elastography for the Diagnosis of Benign Leydig Cell Tumors of the Testis—A Single Center Report on 13 Cases. *Ultraschall Med.* **2014**, *35*, 534–539. [CrossRef]
19. Liu, H.; Dong, L.; Xiang, L.-H.; Xu, G.; Wan, J.; Fang, Y.; Ding, S.-S.; Jin, Y.; Sun, L.-P.; Xu, H.-X. Multiparametric Ultrasound for the Assessment of Testicular Lesions with Negative Tumoral Markers. *Asian J. Androl.* **2023**, *25*, 50–57. [CrossRef]
20. Auer, T.; De Zordo, T.; Dejaco, C.; Gruber, L.; Pichler, R.; Jaschke, W.; Dogra, V.S.; Aigner, F. Value of Multiparametric US in the Assessment of Intratesticular Lesions. *Radiology* **2017**, *285*, 640–649. [CrossRef] [PubMed]
21. Patrikidou, A.; Cazzaniga, W.; Berney, D.; Boormans, J.; de Angst, I.; Di Nardo, D.; Fankhauser, C.; Fischer, S.; Gravina, C.; Gremmels, H.; et al. European Association of Urology Guidelines on Testicular Cancer: 2023 Update. *Eur. Urol.* **2023**, *84*, 289–301. [CrossRef]
22. Bertolotto, M.; Muça, M.; Currò, F.; Bucci, S.; Rocher, L.; Cova, M.A. Multiparametric US for Scrotal Diseases. *Abdom. Radiol.* **2018**, *43*, 899–917. [CrossRef]
23. Lotti, F.; Frizza, F.; Balercia, G.; Barbonetti, A.; Behre, H.M.; Calogero, A.E.; Cremers, J.-F.; Francavilla, F.; Isidori, A.M.; Kliesch, S.; et al. The European Academy of Andrology (EAA) Ultrasound Study on Healthy, Fertile Men: An Overview on Male Genital Tract Ultrasound Reference Ranges. *Andrology* **2022**, *10* (Suppl. S2), 118–132. [CrossRef]
24. Lotti, F.; Frizza, F.; Balercia, G.; Barbonetti, A.; Behre, H.M.; Calogero, A.E.; Cremers, J.-F.; Francavilla, F.; Isidori, A.M.; Kliesch, S.; et al. The European Academy of Andrology (EAA) Ultrasound Study on Healthy, Fertile Men: Prostate-Vesicular Transrectal Ultrasound Reference Ranges and Associations with Clinical, Seminal and Biochemical Characteristics. *Andrology* **2022**, *10*, 1150–1171. [CrossRef]
25. Lotti, F.; Frizza, F.; Balercia, G.; Barbonetti, A.; Behre, H.M.; Calogero, A.E.; Cremers, J.-F.; Francavilla, F.; Isidori, A.M.; Kliesch, S.; et al. The European Academy of Andrology (EAA) Ultrasound Study on Healthy, Fertile Men: Scrotal Ultrasound Reference Ranges and Associations with Clinical, Seminal, and Biochemical Characteristics. *Andrology* **2021**, *9*, 559–576. [CrossRef] [PubMed]
26. Lotti, F.; Frizza, F.; Balercia, G.; Barbonetti, A.; Behre, H.M.; Calogero, A.E.; Cremers, J.-F.; Francavilla, F.; Isidori, A.M.; Kliesch, S.; et al. The European Academy of Andrology (EAA) Ultrasound Study on Healthy, Fertile Men: Clinical, Seminal and Biochemical Characteristics. *Andrology* **2020**, *8*, 1005–1020. [CrossRef]
27. Sidhu, P.S.; Cantisani, V.; Dietrich, C.F.; Gilja, O.H.; Saftoiu, A.; Bartels, E.; Bertolotto, M.; Calliada, F.; Clevert, D.-A.; Cosgrove, D.; et al. The EFSUMB Guidelines and Recommendations for the Clinical Practice of Contrast-Enhanced Ultrasound (CEUS) in Non-Hepatic Applications: Update 2017 (Long Version). *Ultraschall Med.* **2018**, *39*, e2–e44. [CrossRef] [PubMed]
28. Săftoiu, A.; Gilja, O.H.; Sidhu, P.S.; Dietrich, C.F.; Cantisani, V.; Amy, D.; Bachmann-Nielsen, M.; Bob, F.; Bojunga, J.; Brock, M.; et al. The EFSUMB Guidelines and Recommendations for the Clinical Practice of Elastography in Non-Hepatic Applications: Update 2018. *Ultraschall Med.* **2019**, *40*, 425–453. [CrossRef] [PubMed]
29. Bamber, J.; Cosgrove, D.; Dietrich, C.F.; Fromageau, J.; Bojunga, J.; Calliada, F.; Cantisani, V.; Correas, J.-M.; D'Onofrio, M.; Drakonaki, E.E.; et al. EFSUMB Guidelines and Recommendations on the Clinical Use of Ultrasound Elastography. Part 1: Basic Principles and Technology. *Ultraschall Med.* **2013**, *34*, 169–184. [CrossRef]
30. Correas, J.M.; Drakonakis, E.; Isidori, A.M.; Hélénon, O.; Pozza, C.; Cantisani, V.; Di Leo, N.; Maghella, F.; Rubini, A.; Drudi, F.M.; et al. Update on Ultrasound Elastography: Miscellanea. Prostate, Testicle, Musculo-Skeletal. *Eur. J. Radiol.* **2013**, *82*, 1904–1912. [CrossRef]
31. Hoag, N.A.; Afshar, K.; Youssef, D.; Masterson, J.S.T.; Murphy, J.; Macneily, A.E. Cystic Intratesticular Lesions in Pediatric Patients. *J. Pediatr. Surg.* **2013**, *48*, 1773–1777. [CrossRef]
32. Gooding, G.A.; Leonhardt, W.; Stein, R. Testicular Cysts: US Findings. *Radiology* **1987**, *163*, 537–538. [CrossRef] [PubMed]
33. Hamm, B.; Fobbe, F.; Loy, V. Testicular Cysts: Differentiation with US and Clinical Findings. *Radiology* **1988**, *168*, 19–23. [CrossRef] [PubMed]
34. Dogra, V.S.; Gottlieb, R.H.; Rubens, D.J.; Liao, L. Benign Intratesticular Cystic Lesions: US Features. *Radiographics* **2001**, *21*, S273–S281. [CrossRef] [PubMed]
35. Shah, K.H.; Maxted, W.C.; Chun, B. Epidermoid Cysts of the Testis: A Report of Three Cases and an Analysis of 141 Cases from the World Literature. *Cancer* **1981**, *47*, 577–582. [CrossRef]
36. Dogra, V.S.; Gottlieb, R.H.; Oka, M.; Rubens, D.J. Sonography of the Scrotum. *Radiology* **2003**, *227*, 18–36. [CrossRef]
37. Anheuser, P.; Kranz, J.; Stolle, E.; Höflmayer, D.; Büscheck, F.; Mühlstädt, S.; Lock, G.; Dieckmann, K.P. Testicular Epidermoid Cysts: A Reevaluation. *BMC Urol.* **2019**, *19*, 52. [CrossRef]
38. Patel, K.; Sellars, M.E.; Clarke, J.L.; Sidhu, P.S. Features of Testicular Epidermoid Cysts on Contrast-Enhanced Sonography and Real-Time Tissue Elastography. *J. Ultrasound Med.* **2012**, *31*, 115–122. [CrossRef]
39. Manning, M.A.; Woodward, P.J. Testicular Epidermoid Cysts: Sonographic Features with Clinicopathologic Correlation. *J. Ultrasound Med.* **2010**, *29*, 831–837. [CrossRef]

40. Isidori, A.M.; Pozza, C.; Gianfrilli, D.; Giannetta, E.; Lemma, A.; Pofi, R.; Barbagallo, F.; Manganaro, L.; Martino, G.; Lombardo, F.; et al. Differential Diagnosis of Nonpalpable Testicular Lesions: Qualitative and Quantitative Contrast-Enhanced US of Benign and Malignant Testicular Tumors. *Radiology* **2014**, *273*, 606–618. [CrossRef]
41. Engels, M.; Span, P.N.; van Herwaarden, A.E.; Sweep, F.C.G.J.; Stikkelbroeck, N.M.M.L.; Claahsen-van der Grinten, H.L. Testicular Adrenal Rest Tumors: Current Insights on Prevalence, Characteristics, Origin, and Treatment. *Endocr. Rev.* **2019**, *40*, 973–987. [CrossRef]
42. Jedrzejewski, G.; Ben-Skowronek, I.; Wozniak, M.M.; Brodzisz, A.; Budzynska, E.; Wieczorek, A.P. Testicular Adrenal Rest Tumors in Boys with Congenital Adrenal Hyperplasia: 3D US and Elastography—Do We Get More Information for Diagnosis and Monitoring? *J. Pediatr. Urol.* **2013**, *9*, 1032–1037. [CrossRef]
43. Corcioni, B.; Renzulli, M.; Marasco, G.; Baronio, F.; Gambineri, A.; Ricciardi, D.; Ortolano, R.; Farina, D.; Gaudiano, C.; Cassio, A.; et al. Prevalence and Ultrasound Patterns of Testicular Adrenal Rest Tumors in Adults with Congenital Adrenal Hyperplasia. *Transl. Androl. Urol.* **2021**, *10*, 562–573. [CrossRef] [PubMed]
44. Mansoor, N.M.; Huang, D.Y.; Sidhu, P.S. Multiparametric Ultrasound Imaging Characteristics of Multiple Testicular Adrenal Rest Tumours in Congenital Adrenal Hyperplasia. *Ultrasound* **2022**, *30*, 80–84. [CrossRef]
45. Tresoldi, A.S.; Betella, N.; Hasenmajer, V.; Pozza, C.; Vena, W.; Fiamengo, B.; Negri, L.; Cappa, M.; Lania, A.G.A.; Lenzi, A.; et al. Bilateral Testicular Masses and Adrenal Insufficiency: Is Congenital Adrenal Hyperplasia the Only Possible Diagnosis? First Two Cases of TARTS Described in Addison-Only X-Linked Adrenoleukodystrophy and a Brief Review of Literature. *J. Endocrinol. Investig.* **2021**, *44*, 391–402. [CrossRef] [PubMed]
46. Ricker, W.; Clark, M. Sarcoidosis: A Clinicopathologic Review of 300 Cases, Including 22 Autopsies. *Am. J. Clin. Pathol.* **1949**, *19*, 725–749. [CrossRef] [PubMed]
47. Bhatt, S.; Jafri, S.Z.H.; Wasserman, N.; Dogra, V.S. Imaging of Non-Neoplastic Intratesticular Masses. *Diagn. Interv. Radiol.* **2011**, *17*, 52–63. [CrossRef]
48. Stewart, V.R.; Sidhu, P.S. The Testis: The Unusual, the Rare and the Bizarre. *Clin. Radiol.* **2007**, *62*, 289–302. [CrossRef]
49. Rafailidis, V.; Robbie, H.; Konstantatou, E.; Huang, D.Y.; Deganello, A.; Sellars, M.E.; Cantisani, V.; Isidori, A.M.; Sidhu, P.S. Sonographic Imaging of Extra-Testicular Focal Lesions: Comparison of Grey-Scale, Colour Doppler and Contrast-Enhanced Ultrasound. *Ultrasound* **2016**, *24*, 23–33. [CrossRef]
50. Lung, P.F.C.; Fang, C.; Jaffer, O.S.; Deganello, A.; Shah, A.; Hedayati, V.; Obaro, A.; Yusuf, G.T.; Huang, D.Y.; Sellars, M.E.; et al. Vascularity of Intra-Testicular Lesions: Inter-Observer Variation in the Assessment of Non-Neoplastic Versus Neoplastic Abnormalities After Vascular Enhancement with Contrast-Enhanced Ultrasound. *Ultrasound Med. Biol.* **2020**, *46*, 2956–2964. [CrossRef]
51. De Cinque, A.; Corcioni, B.; Rossi, M.S.; Franceschelli, A.; Colombo, F.; Golfieri, R.; Renzulli, M.; Gaudiano, C. Case Report: Testicular Sarcoidosis: The Diagnostic Role of Contrast-Enhanced Ultrasound and Review of the Literature. *Front. Med.* **2020**, *7*, 610384. [CrossRef]
52. Gianfrilli, D.; Isidori, A.M.; Lenzi, A. Segmental Testicular Ischaemia: Presentation, Management and Follow-Up. *Int. J. Androl.* **2009**, *32*, 524–531. [CrossRef] [PubMed]
53. Patel, K.V.; Huang, D.Y.; Sidhu, P.S. Metachronous Bilateral Segmental Testicular Infarction: Multi-Parametric Ultrasound Imaging with Grey-Scale Ultrasound, Doppler Ultrasound, Contrast-Enhanced Ultrasound (CEUS) and Real-Time Tissue Elastography (RTE). *J. Ultrasound* **2014**, *17*, 233–238. [CrossRef] [PubMed]
54. Bilagi, P.; Sriprasad, S.; Clarke, J.L.; Sellars, M.E.; Muir, G.H.; Sidhu, P.S. Clinical and Ultrasound Features of Segmental Testicular Infarction: Six-Year Experience from a Single Centre. *Eur. Radiol.* **2007**, *17*, 2810–2818. [CrossRef] [PubMed]
55. Fernández-Pérez, G.C.; Tardáguila, F.M.; Velasco, M.; Rivas, C.; Dos Santos, J.; Cambronero, J.; Trinidad, C.; San Miguel, P. Radiologic Findings of Segmental Testicular Infarction. *AJR Am. J. Roentgenol.* **2005**, *184*, 1587–1593. [CrossRef]
56. Sweet, D.E.; Feldman, M.K.; Remer, E.M. Imaging of the Acute Scrotum: Keys to a Rapid Diagnosis of Acute Scrotal Disorders. *Abdom. Radiol.* **2020**, *45*, 2063–2081. [CrossRef]
57. Bertolotto, M.; Derchi, L.E.; Sidhu, P.S.; Serafini, G.; Valentino, M.; Grenier, N.; Cova, M.A. Acute Segmental Testicular Infarction at Contrast-Enhanced Ultrasound: Early Features and Changes during Follow-Up. *AJR Am. J. Roentgenol.* **2011**, *196*, 834–841. [CrossRef]
58. Yusuf, G.T.; Sidhu, P.S. A Review of Ultrasound Imaging in Scrotal Emergencies. *J. Ultrasound* **2013**, *16*, 171–178. [CrossRef]
59. Pavlica, P.; Barozzi, L. Imaging of the Acute Scrotum. *Eur. Radiol.* **2001**, *11*, 220–228. [CrossRef]
60. Valentino, M.; Bertolotto, M.; Derchi, L.; Bertaccini, A.; Pavlica, P.; Martorana, G.; Barozzi, L. Role of Contrast Enhanced Ultrasound in Acute Scrotal Diseases. *Eur. Radiol.* **2011**, *21*, 1831–1840. [CrossRef]
61. Lung, P.F.C.; Jaffer, O.S.; Sellars, M.E.; Sriprasad, S.; Kooiman, G.G.; Sidhu, P.S. Contrast-Enhanced Ultrasound in the Evaluation of Focal Testicular Complications Secondary to Epididymitis. *AJR Am. J. Roentgenol.* **2012**, *199*, W345–W354. [CrossRef]
62. Purushothaman, H.; Sellars, M.E.K.; Clarke, J.L.; Sidhu, P.S. Intratesticular Haematoma: Differentiation from Tumour on Clinical History and Ultrasound Appearances in Two Cases. *Br. J. Radiol.* **2007**, *80*, e184–e187. [CrossRef]
63. Ramanathan, S.; Bertolotto, M.; Freeman, S.; Belfield, J.; Derchi, L.E.; Huang, D.Y.; Lotti, F.; Markiet, K.; Nikolic, O.; Ramchandani, P.; et al. Imaging in Scrotal Trauma: A European Society of Urogenital Radiology Scrotal and Penile Imaging Working Group (ESUR-SPIWG) Position Statement. *Eur. Radiol.* **2021**, *31*, 4918–4928. [CrossRef]

64. Yusuf, G.; Konstantatou, E.; Sellars, M.E.; Huang, D.Y.; Sidhu, P.S. Multiparametric Sonography of Testicular Hematomas: Features on Grayscale, Color Doppler, and Contrast-Enhanced Sonography and Strain Elastography. *J. Ultrasound Med.* **2015**, *34*, 1319–1328. [CrossRef] [PubMed]
65. Öztürk, Ç.; Paşaoğlu, E.; Bölme Şavlı, T. A Lesion Mimicking Malignancy: Granulomatous Orchitis. *Bull. Uroonkol.* **2021**, *20*, 126–128. [CrossRef]
66. Civelli, V.F.; Heidari, A.; Valdez, M.C.; Narang, V.K.; Johnson, R.H. A Case of Testicular Granulomatous Inflammation Mistaken for Malignancy: Tuberculosis Identified Post Orchiectomy. *J. Investig. Med. High Impact Case Rep.* **2020**, *8*, 2324709620938947. [CrossRef]
67. Peyrí Rey, E.; Riverola Manzanilla, A.; Cañas Tello, M.A. Bilateral idiopathic granulomatous orchitis. *Actas Urol. Esp.* **2008**, *32*, 461–463. [CrossRef]
68. Wegner, H.E.; Loy, V.; Dieckmann, K.P. Granulomatous Orchitis—An Analysis of Clinical Presentation, Pathological Anatomic Features and Possible Etiologic Factors. *Eur. Urol.* **1994**, *26*, 56–60. [CrossRef]
69. Salmeron, I.; Ramirez-Escobar, M.A.; Puertas, F.; Marcos, R.; Garcia-Marcos, F.; Sanchez, R. Granulomatous Epidido-Orchitis: Sonographic Features and Clinical Outcome in Brucellosis, Tuberculosis and Idiopathic Granulomatous Epidido-Orchitis. *J. Urol.* **1998**, *159*, 1954–1957. [CrossRef] [PubMed]
70. Lung, P.F.C.; Sidhu, P.S. Role of Ultrasound in the Diagnosis of Testicular Lesions. *Imaging Med.* **2011**, *3*, 587–595. [CrossRef]
71. Nepal, P.; Ojili, V.; Songmen, S.; Kaur, N.; Olsavsky, T.; Nagar, A. "The Great Masquerader": Sonographic Pictorial Review of Testicular Tuberculosis and Its Mimics. *J. Clin. Imaging Sci.* **2019**, *9*, 27. [CrossRef]
72. Viswaroop, B.S.; Kekre, N.; Gopalakrishnan, G. Isolated Tuberculous Epididymitis: A Review of Forty Cases. *J. Postgrad. Med.* **2005**, *51*, 109–111. [PubMed]
73. Park, J.S.; Kim, J.; Elghiaty, A.; Ham, W.S. Recent Global Trends in Testicular Cancer Incidence and Mortality. *Medicine* **2018**, *97*, e12390. [CrossRef] [PubMed]
74. Gurney, J.K.; Florio, A.A.; Znaor, A.; Ferlay, J.; Laversanne, M.; Sarfati, D.; Bray, F.; McGlynn, K.A. International Trends in the Incidence of Testicular Cancer: Lessons from 35 Years and 41 Countries. *Eur. Urol.* **2019**, *76*, 615–623. [CrossRef]
75. Znaor, A.; Skakkebaek, N.E.; Rajpert-De Meyts, E.; Kuliš, T.; Laversanne, M.; Gurney, J.; Sarfati, D.; McGlynn, K.A.; Bray, F. Global Patterns in Testicular Cancer Incidence and Mortality in 2020. *Int. J. Cancer* **2022**, *151*, 692–698. [CrossRef] [PubMed]
76. Moch, H.; Amin, M.B.; Berney, D.M.; Compérat, E.M.; Gill, A.J.; Hartmann, A.; Menon, S.; Raspollini, M.R.; Rubin, M.A.; Srigley, J.R.; et al. The 2022 World Health Organization Classification of Tumours of the Urinary System and Male Genital Organs-Part A: Renal, Penile, and Testicular Tumours. *Eur. Urol.* **2022**, *82*, 458–468. [CrossRef]
77. Honecker, F.; Aparicio, J.; Berney, D.; Beyer, J.; Bokemeyer, C.; Cathomas, R.; Clarke, N.; Cohn-Cedermark, G.; Daugaard, G.; Dieckmann, K.-P.; et al. ESMO Consensus Conference on Testicular Germ Cell Cancer: Diagnosis, Treatment and Follow-Up. *Ann. Oncol.* **2018**, *29*, 1658–1686. [CrossRef]
78. Gilligan, T.D.; Seidenfeld, J.; Basch, E.M.; Einhorn, L.H.; Fancher, T.; Smith, D.C.; Stephenson, A.J.; Vaughn, D.J.; Cosby, R.; Hayes, D.F.; et al. American Society of Clinical Oncology Clinical Practice Guideline on Uses of Serum Tumor Markers in Adult Males with Germ Cell Tumors. *J. Clin. Oncol.* **2010**, *28*, 3388–3404. [CrossRef]
79. Barlow, L.J.; Badalato, G.M.; McKiernan, J.M. Serum Tumor Markers in the Evaluation of Male Germ Cell Tumors. *Nat. Rev. Urol.* **2010**, *7*, 610–617. [CrossRef]
80. Kanakis, G.A.; Nordkap, L.; Bang, A.K.; Calogero, A.E.; Bártfai, G.; Corona, G.; Forti, G.; Toppari, J.; Goulis, D.G.; Jørgensen, N. EAA Clinical Practice Guidelines-Gynecomastia Evaluation and Management. *Andrology* **2019**, *7*, 778–793. [CrossRef]
81. Hassan, H.C.; Cullen, I.M.; Casey, R.G.; Rogers, E. Gynaecomastia: An Endocrine Manifestation of Testicular Cancer. *Andrologia* **2008**, *40*, 152–157. [CrossRef]
82. Rajpert-De Meyts, E.; McGlynn, K.A.; Okamoto, K.; Jewett, M.A.S.; Bokemeyer, C. Testicular Germ Cell Tumours. *Lancet* **2016**, *387*, 1762–1774. [CrossRef]
83. Hanson, H.A.; Anderson, R.E.; Aston, K.I.; Carrell, D.T.; Smith, K.R.; Hotaling, J.M. Subfertility Increases Risk of Testicular Cancer: Evidence from Population-Based Semen Samples. *Fertil. Steril.* **2016**, *105*, 322–328. [CrossRef]
84. Skakkebaek, N.E.; Rajpert-De Meyts, E.; Buck Louis, G.M.; Toppari, J.; Andersson, A.-M.; Eisenberg, M.L.; Jensen, T.K.; Jørgensen, N.; Swan, S.H.; Sapra, K.J.; et al. Male Reproductive Disorders and Fertility Trends: Influences of Environment and Genetic Susceptibility. *Physiol. Rev.* **2016**, *96*, 55–97. [CrossRef] [PubMed]
85. Meyts, E.R.-D. Developmental Model for the Pathogenesis of Testicular Carcinoma in Situ: Genetic and Environmental Aspects. *Hum. Reprod. Update* **2006**, *12*, 303–323. [CrossRef] [PubMed]
86. Piltoft, J.S.; Larsen, S.B.; Dalton, S.O.; Johansen, C.; Baker, J.L.; Cederkvist, L.; Andersen, I. Early Life Risk Factors for Testicular Cancer: A Case-Cohort Study Based on the Copenhagen School Health Records Register. *Acta Oncol.* **2017**, *56*, 220–224. [CrossRef]
87. Pettersson, A.; Richiardi, L.; Nordenskjold, A.; Kaijser, M.; Akre, O. Age at Surgery for Undescended Testis and Risk of Testicular Cancer. *N. Engl. J. Med.* **2007**, *356*, 1835–1841. [CrossRef]
88. Williamson, S.R.; Delahunt, B.; Magi-Galluzzi, C.; Algaba, F.; Egevad, L.; Ulbright, T.M.; Tickoo, S.K.; Srigley, J.R.; Epstein, J.I.; Berney, D.M.; et al. The World Health Organization 2016 Classification of Testicular Germ Cell Tumours: A Review and Update from the International Society of Urological Pathology Testis Consultation Panel. *Histopathology* **2017**, *70*, 335–346. [CrossRef] [PubMed]

89. Kawamoto, A.; Hatano, T.; Saito, K.; Inoue, R.; Nagao, T.; Sanada, S. Sonographic Classification of Testicular Tumors by Tissue Harmonic Imaging: Experience of 58 Cases. *J. Med. Ultrason.* **2018**, *45*, 103–111. [CrossRef]
90. McDonald, M.W.; Reed, A.B.; Tran, P.T.; Evans, L.A. Testicular Tumor Ultrasound Characteristics and Association with Histopathology. *Urol. Int.* **2012**, *89*, 196–202. [CrossRef] [PubMed]
91. Woodward, P.J.; Sohaey, R.; O'Donoghue, M.J.; Green, D.E. From the Archives of the AFIP: Tumors and Tumorlike Lesions of the Testis: Radiologic-Pathologic Correlation. *Radiographics* **2002**, *22*, 189–216. [CrossRef]
92. Necas, M.; Muthupalaniappaan, M.; Barnard, C. Ultrasound Morphological Patterns of Testicular Tumours, Correlation with Histopathology. *J. Med. Radiat. Sci.* **2021**, *68*, 21–27. [CrossRef]
93. Barbonetti, A.; Martorella, A.; Minaldi, E.; D'Andrea, S.; Bardhi, D.; Castellini, C.; Francavilla, F.; Francavilla, S. Testicular Cancer in Infertile Men with and without Testicular Microlithiasis: A Systematic Review and Meta-Analysis of Case-Control Studies. *Front. Endocrinol.* **2019**, *10*, 164. [CrossRef]
94. Richenberg, J.; Belfield, J.; Ramchandani, P.; Rocher, L.; Freeman, S.; Tsili, A.C.; Cuthbert, F.; Studniarek, M.; Bertolotto, M.; Turgut, A.T.; et al. Testicular Microlithiasis Imaging and Follow-up: Guidelines of the ESUR Scrotal Imaging Subcommittee. *Eur. Radiol.* **2015**, *25*, 323–330. [CrossRef]
95. Goddi, A.; Sacchi, A.; Magistretti, G.; Almolla, J.; Salvadore, M. Real-Time Tissue Elastography for Testicular Lesion Assessment. *Eur. Radiol.* **2012**, *22*, 721–730. [CrossRef] [PubMed]
96. Aigner, F.; De Zordo, T.; Pallwein-Prettner, L.; Junker, D.; Schäfer, G.; Pichler, R.; Leonhartsberger, N.; Pinggera, G.; Dogra, V.S.; Frauscher, F. Real-Time Sonoelastography for the Evaluation of Testicular Lesions. *Radiology* **2012**, *263*, 584–589. [CrossRef] [PubMed]
97. Ishida, M.; Hasegawa, M.; Kanao, K.; Oyama, M.; Nakajima, Y. Non-Palpable Testicular Embryonal Carcinoma Diagnosed by Ultrasound: A Case Report. *Jpn. J. Clin. Oncol.* **2009**, *39*, 124–126. [CrossRef] [PubMed]
98. Scandura, G.; Verrill, C.; Protheroe, A.; Joseph, J.; Ansell, W.; Sahdev, A.; Shamash, J.; Berney, D.M. Incidentally Detected Testicular Lesions < 10 Mm in Diameter: Can Orchidectomy Be Avoided? *BJU Int.* **2018**, *121*, 575–582. [CrossRef]
99. Stepanas, A.V.; Samaan, N.A.; Schultz, P.N.; Holoye, P.Y. Endocrine Studies in Testicular Tumor Patients with and without Gynecomastia: A Report of 45 Cases. *Cancer* **1978**, *41*, 369–376. [CrossRef]
100. Gerber, D.; Wright, H.C.; Sussman, R.D.; Stamatakis, L. Embryonal Carcinoma Presenting as a Calcified Solitary Testicular Mass on Ultrasound. *BMJ Case Rep.* **2017**, *2017*, bcr-2017. [CrossRef]
101. Katabathina, V.S.; Vargas-Zapata, D.; Monge, R.A.; Nazarullah, A.; Ganeshan, D.; Tammisetti, V.; Prasad, S.R. Testicular Germ Cell Tumors: Classification, Pathologic Features, Imaging Findings, and Management. *Radiographics* **2021**, *41*, 1698–1716. [CrossRef]
102. Fang, C.; Huang, D.Y.; Sidhu, P.S. Elastography of Focal Testicular Lesions: Current Concepts and Utility. *Ultrasonography* **2019**, *38*, 302–310. [CrossRef]
103. Xue, N.; Zhang, S.; Wang, G. The Value of Contrast-Enhanced Ultrasonography in the Diagnosis of Primary Testicular Non-Neoplastic and Neoplastic Lesions in Adults. *BMC Urol.* **2022**, *22*, 210. [CrossRef] [PubMed]
104. Anderson, K.H.; Romao, R.L.P. Testicular Tumors in Children and Adolescents: Long-Term Endocrine and Fertility Issues. *Transl. Androl. Urol.* **2020**, *9*, 2393–2399. [CrossRef]
105. Liu, P.; Phillips, M.J.; Edwards, V.D.; Ein, S.; Daneman, A. Sonographic Findings of Testicular Teratoma with Pathologic Correlation. *Pediatr. Radiol.* **1992**, *22*, 99–101. [CrossRef]
106. Epifanio, M.; Baldissera, M.; Esteban, F.G.; Baldisserotto, M. Mature Testicular Teratoma in Children: Multifaceted Tumors on Ultrasound. *Urology* **2014**, *83*, 195–197. [CrossRef] [PubMed]
107. Pagliaro, L.C. Role of High-Dose Chemotherapy with Autologous Stem-Cell Rescue in Men with Previously Treated Germ Cell Tumors. *J. Clin. Oncol.* **2017**, *35*, 1036–1040. [CrossRef] [PubMed]
108. Lagabrielle, S.; Durand, X.; Droupy, S.; Izard, V.; Marcelli, F.; Huyghe, E.; Ferriere, J.-M.; Ferretti, L. Testicular Tumours Discovered during Infertility Workup Are Predominantly Benign and Could Initially Be Managed by Sparing Surgery. *J. Surg. Oncol.* **2018**, *118*, 630–635. [CrossRef]
109. Maxwell, F.; Savignac, A.; Bekdache, O.; Calvez, S.; Lebacle, C.; Arama, E.; Garrouche, N.; Rocher, L. Leydig Cell Tumors of the Testis: An Update of the Imaging Characteristics of a Not So Rare Lesion. *Cancers* **2022**, *14*, 3652. [CrossRef]
110. Leonhartsberger, N.; Ramoner, R.; Aigner, F.; Stoehr, B.; Pichler, R.; Zangerl, F.; Fritzer, A.; Steiner, H. Increased Incidence of Leydig Cell Tumours of the Testis in the Era of Improved Imaging Techniques. *BJU Int.* **2011**, *108*, 1603–1607. [CrossRef]
111. Pozza, C.; Pofi, R.; Tenuta, M.; Tarsitano, M.G.; Sbardella, E.; Fattorini, G.; Cantisani, V.; Lenzi, A.; Isidori, A.M.; Gianfrilli, D.; et al. Clinical Presentation, Management and Follow-up of 83 Patients with Leydig Cell Tumors of the Testis: A Prospective Case-Cohort Study. *Hum. Reprod.* **2019**, *34*, 1389–1403. [CrossRef]
112. Holm, M.; Rajpert-De Meyts, E.; Andersson, A.-M.; Skakkebaek, N.E. Leydig Cell Micronodules Are a Common Finding in Testicular Biopsies from Men with Impaired Spermatogenesis and Are Associated with Decreased testosterone/LH Ratio. *J. Pathol.* **2003**, *199*, 378–386. [CrossRef] [PubMed]
113. Rajpert-De Meyts, E.; Aksglaede, L.; Bandak, M.; Toppari, J.; Jørgensen, N. Testicular Cancer: Pathogenesis, Diagnosis and Management with Focus on Endocrine Aspects. In *Endotext*; Feingold, K.R., Anawalt, B., Blackman, M.R., Boyce, A., Chrousos, G., Corpas, E., de Herder, W.W., Dhatariya, K., Dungan, K., Hofland, J., et al., Eds.; MDText.com, Inc.: South Dartmouth, MA, USA, 2023.

114. Cheville, J.C.; Sebo, T.J.; Lager, D.J.; Bostwick, D.G.; Farrow, G.M. Leydig Cell Tumor of the Testis: A Clinicopathologic, DNA Content, and MIB-1 Comparison of Nonmetastasizing and Metastasizing Tumors. *Am. J. Surg. Pathol.* **1998**, *22*, 1361–1367. [CrossRef]
115. Washecka, R.; Dresner, M.I.; Honda, S.A.A. Testicular Tumors in Carney's Complex. *J. Urol.* **2002**, *167*, 1299–1302. [CrossRef]
116. Grogg, J.; Schneider, K.; Bode, P.K.; Kranzbühler, B.; Eberli, D.; Sulser, T.; Lorch, A.; Beyer, J.; Hermanns, T.; Fankhauser, C.D. Sertoli Cell Tumors of the Testes: Systematic Literature Review and Meta-Analysis of Outcomes in 435 Patients. *Oncologist* **2020**, *25*, 585–590. [CrossRef] [PubMed]
117. Connolly, S.S.; D'Arcy, F.T.; Gough, N.; McCarthy, P.; Bredin, H.C.; Corcoran, M.O. Carefully Selected Intratesticular Lesions Can Be Safely Managed with Serial Ultrasonography. *BJU Int.* **2006**, *98*, 1005–1007. [CrossRef] [PubMed]
118. Paffenholz, P.; Held, L.; Loosen, S.H.; Pfister, D.; Heidenreich, A. Testis Sparing Surgery for Benign Testicular Masses: Diagnostics and Therapeutic Approaches. *J. Urol.* **2018**, *200*, 353–360. [CrossRef]
119. Maizlin, Z.V.; Belenky, A.; Kunichezky, M.; Sandbank, J.; Strauss, S. Leydig Cell Tumors of the Testis: Gray Scale and Color Doppler Sonographic Appearance. *J. Ultrasound Med.* **2004**, *23*, 959–964. [CrossRef]
120. Grand, T.; Hermann, A.-L.; Gérard, M.; Arama, E.; Ouerd, L.; Garrouche, N.; Rocher, L. Precocious Puberty Related to Leydig Cell Testicular Tumor: The Diagnostic Imaging Keys. *Eur. J. Med. Res.* **2022**, *27*, 67. [CrossRef]
121. Akman, H.; Ege, G.; Yildiz, S.; Cakiroglu, G. Incidental Bilateral Leydig Cell Tumor of the Testes. *Urol. Int.* **2003**, *71*, 316–318. [CrossRef]
122. Drudi, F.M.; Valentino, M.; Bertolotto, M.; Malpassini, F.; Maghella, F.; Cantisani, V.; Liberatore, M.; De Felice, C.; D'Ambrosio, F. CEUS Time Intensity Curves in the Differentiation Between Leydig Cell Carcinoma and Seminoma: A Multicenter Study. *Ultraschall Med.* **2016**, *37*, 201–205. [CrossRef]
123. Samson, M.; Peale, F.V., Jr.; Frantz, G.; Rioux-Leclercq, N.; Rajpert-De Meyts, E.; Ferrara, N. Human Endocrine Gland-Derived Vascular Endothelial Growth Factor: Expression Early in Development and in Leydig Cell Tumors Suggests Roles in Normal and Pathological Testis Angiogenesis. *J. Clin. Endocrinol. Metab.* **2004**, *89*, 4078–4088. [CrossRef] [PubMed]
124. Lock, G.; Schmidt, C.; Helmich, F.; Stolle, E.; Dieckmann, K.-P. Early Experience with Contrast-Enhanced Ultrasound in the Diagnosis of Testicular Masses: A Feasibility Study. *Urology* **2011**, *77*, 1049–1053. [CrossRef]
125. Luzurier, A.; Maxwell, F.; Correas, J.M.; Benoit, G.; Izard, V.; Ferlicot, S.; Teglas, J.P.; Bellin, M.F.; Rocher, L. Qualitative and Quantitative Contrast-Enhanced Ultrasonography for the Characterisation of Non-Palpable Testicular Tumours. *Clin. Radiol.* **2018**, *73*, 322.e1–322.e9. [CrossRef]
126. Lerchbaumer, M.H.; Auer, T.A.; Marticorena, G.S.; Stephan, C.; Hamm, B.; Jung, E.-M.; Fischer, T. Diagnostic Performance of Contrast-Enhanced Ultrasound (CEUS) in Testicular Pathologies: Single-Center Results. *Clin. Hemorheol. Microcirc.* **2019**, *73*, 347–357. [CrossRef]
127. Pinto, S.P.S.; Huang, D.Y.; Dinesh, A.A.; Sidhu, P.S.; Ahmed, K. A Systematic Review on the Use of Qualitative and Quantitative Contrast-Enhanced Ultrasound in Diagnosing Testicular Abnormalities. *Urology* **2021**, *154*, 16–23. [CrossRef]
128. Young, R.H.; Koelliker, D.D.; Scully, R.E. Sertoli Cell Tumors of the Testis, Not Otherwise Specified: A Clinicopathologic Analysis of 60 Cases. *Am. J. Surg. Pathol.* **1998**, *22*, 709–721. [CrossRef]
129. Harms, D.; Kock, L.R. Testicular Juvenile Granulosa Cell and Sertoli Cell Tumours: A Clinicopathological Study of 29 Cases from the Kiel Paediatric Tumour Registry. *Virchows Arch.* **1997**, *430*, 301–309. [CrossRef]
130. Vitolo, U.; Ferreri, A.J.M.; Zucca, E. Primary Testicular Lymphoma. *Crit. Rev. Oncol. Hematol.* **2008**, *65*, 183–189. [CrossRef] [PubMed]
131. Nguyen, H.T.K.; Terao, M.A.; Green, D.M.; Pui, C.-H.; Inaba, H. Testicular Involvement of Acute Lymphoblastic Leukemia in Children and Adolescents: Diagnosis, Biology, and Management. *Cancer* **2021**, *127*, 3067–3081. [CrossRef] [PubMed]
132. Gutjahr, P.; Humpl, T. Testicular Lymphoblastic Leukemia/lymphoma. *World J. Urol.* **1995**, *13*, 230–232. [CrossRef] [PubMed]
133. de Jesus, L.E.; Dekermacher, S.; Resende, G.C.; Justiniano, R.R. Testicular Involvement in Pediatric Acute Lymphocytic Leukemia: What to Do about It? *Int. Braz. J. Urol* **2022**, *48*, 981–987. [CrossRef] [PubMed]
134. Koh, S.Y.; Lee, S.; Lee, S.B.; Cho, Y.J.; Choi, Y.H.; Cheon, J.-E.; Kim, W.S. Shear-Wave Elastography for the Assessment of Testicular Involvement of Hematologic Malignancies in Children and Young Adults: A Feasibility Study. *Ultrasonography* **2022**, *41*, 325–334. [CrossRef]
135. Mazzu, D.; Jeffrey, R.B., Jr.; Ralls, P.W. Lymphoma and Leukemia Involving the Testicles: Findings on Gray-Scale and Color Doppler Sonography. *AJR Am. J. Roentgenol.* **1995**, *164*, 645–647. [CrossRef] [PubMed]
136. Arrigan, M.; Smyth, L.; Harmon, M.; Flynn, C.; Sheehy, N. Imaging Findings in Recurrent Extramedullary Leukaemias. *Cancer Imaging* **2013**, *13*, 26–35. [CrossRef] [PubMed]
137. Hermann, A.-L.; L'Herminé-Coulomb, A.; Irtan, S.; Audry, G.; Cardoen, L.; Brisse, H.J.; Vande Perre, S.; Pointe, H.D.L. Imaging of Pediatric Testicular and Para-Testicular Tumors: A Pictural Review. *Cancers* **2022**, *14*, 3180. [CrossRef]
138. Khan, M.; Rajarubendra, N.; Azer, S.; Skene, A.; Harrison, S.J.; Campbell, B.; Lawrentschuk, N. Plasmacytoma of the Testis in a Patient with Relapsed and Refractory Multiple Myeloma: Case Report and Review of the Literature. *Urol. Ann.* **2015**, *7*, 530–533. [CrossRef]
139. Shimokihara, K.; Kawahara, T.; Chiba, S.; Takamoto, D.; Yao, M.; Uemura, H. Extramedullary Plasmacytoma of the Testis: A Case Report. *Urol. Case Rep.* **2018**, *16*, 101–103. [CrossRef] [PubMed]

140. Schiavo, C.; Mann, S.A.; Mer, J.; Suvannasankha, A. Testicular Plasmacytoma Misdiagnosed as Orchitis. *BMJ Case Rep.* **2018**, *2018*, bcr-2017. [CrossRef]
141. McCann, C.; Doherty, A.; Flynn, C.; Mulholland, C. Prostate Cancer Metastasis to the Testis: An Unexpected Presentation of a Solitary Recurrence. *BMJ Case Rep.* **2021**, *14*, e237853. [CrossRef]
142. Birker, I.L.; van der Zee, J.A.; Keizer, K.M. Uncommon Testicular Metastasis of a Primary Neuroendocrine Tumour of the Lung. *Can. Urol. Assoc. J.* **2013**, *7*, E614–E617. [CrossRef]
143. Hatoum, H.A.; Abi Saad, G.S.; Otrock, Z.K.; Barada, K.A.; Shamseddine, A.I. Metastasis of Colorectal Carcinoma to the Testes: Clinical Presentation and Possible Pathways. *Int. J. Clin. Oncol.* **2011**, *16*, 203–209. [CrossRef] [PubMed]
144. Qazi, H.A.R.; Manikandan, R.; Foster, C.S.; Fordham, M.V. Testicular Metastasis from Gastric Carcinoma. *Urology* **2006**, *68*, 890.e7–890.e8. [CrossRef] [PubMed]
145. Dusaud, M.; Adjadj, L.; Debelmas, A.; Souraud, J.B.; Durand, X. Malignant Melanoma Revealed by Testicular Metastasi. *Int. J. Surg. Case Rep.* **2015**, *12*, 102–105. [CrossRef] [PubMed]
146. Hou, G.; Jiang, Y.; Cheng, X. Testicular Metastasis of Pancreatic Carcinoma on FDG-PET/CT. *Clin. Nucl. Med.* **2020**, *45*, 85–86. [CrossRef]
147. Rouvinov, K.; Neulander, E.Z.; Kan, E.; Asali, M.; Ariad, S.; Mermershtain, W. Testicular Metastasis from Renal Cell Carcinoma: A Case Report and Review of the Literature. *Case Rep. Oncol.* **2017**, *10*, 388–391. [CrossRef] [PubMed]
148. Turo, R.; Smolski, M.; Hatimy, U.; Bromage, S.J.; Brown, S.C.W.; Brough, R.; Collins, G.N. A Rare Case of Testicular Metastasis of Bladder Transitional Cell Carcinoma. *Can. Urol. Assoc. J.* **2014**, *8*, E181–E183. [CrossRef]
149. Appetecchia, M.; Barnabei, A.; Pompeo, V.; Sentinelli, S.; Baldelli, R.; Corsello, S.M.; Torino, F. Testicular and Inguinal Lymph Node Metastases of Medullary Thyroid Cancer: A Case Report and Review of the Literature. *BMC Endocr. Disord.* **2014**, *14*, 84. [CrossRef]
150. Simon, T.; Hero, B.; Berthold, F. Testicular and Paratesticular Involvement by Metastatic Neuroblastoma. *Cancer* **2000**, *88*, 2636–2641. [CrossRef]
151. Sidhu, P.S.; Sriprasad, S.; Bushby, L.H.; Sellars, M.E.; Muir, G.H. Impalpable Testis Cancer. *BJU Int.* **2004**, *93*, 888. [CrossRef]
152. Iannantuono, G.M.; Strigari, L.; Roselli, M.; Torino, F. A Scoping Review on the "Burned out" or "Burnt out" Testicular Cancer: When a Rare Phenomenon Deserves More Attention. *Crit. Rev. Oncol. Hematol.* **2021**, *165*, 103452. [CrossRef]
153. Sidhu, P.S.; Muir, G.H. Extragonadal Tumor and Testicular Microlithiasis: "Burned-out" Tumors Are Represented by Macrocalcification. *J. Ultrasound Med.* **2011**, *30*, 1604–1605. [CrossRef] [PubMed]
154. Pedersen, M.R.; Bartlett, E.C.; Brown, C.; Rafaelsen, S.R.; Sellars, M.E.; Sidhu, P.S. Is Testicular Macrocalcification a Risk for Malignancy?: Tumor Development on Ultrasonographic Follow-up of Preexisting Intratesticular Macrocalcification. *J. Ultrasound Med.* **2018**, *37*, 2949–2953. [CrossRef] [PubMed]
155. Rocher, L.; Glas, L.; Bellin, M.F.; Ferlicot, S.; Izard, V.; Benoit, G.; Albiges, L.; Fizazi, K.; Correas, J.-M. Burned-Out Testis Tumors in Asymptomatic Infertile Men: Multiparametric Sonography and MRI Findings. *J. Ultrasound Med.* **2017**, *36*, 821–831. [CrossRef]
156. Comiter, C.V.; Renshaw, A.A.; Benson, C.B.; Loughlin, K.R. Burned-out Primary Testicular Cancer: Sonographic and Pathological Characteristics. *J. Urol.* **1996**, *156*, 85–88. [CrossRef] [PubMed]
157. Tasu, J.-P.; Faye, N.; Eschwege, P.; Rocher, L.; Bléry, M. Imaging of Burned-out Testis Tumor: Five New Cases and Review of the Literature. *J. Ultrasound Med.* **2003**, *22*, 515–521. [CrossRef]
158. Fabre, E.; Jira, H.; Izard, V.; Ferlicot, S.; Hammoudi, Y.; Theodore, C.; Di Palma, M.; Benoit, G.; Droupy, S. "Burned-out" Primary Testicular Cancer. *BJU Int.* **2004**, *94*, 74–78. [CrossRef]

Disclaimer/Publisher's Note: The statements, opinions and data contained in all publications are solely those of the individual author(s) and contributor(s) and not of MDPI and/or the editor(s). MDPI and/or the editor(s) disclaim responsibility for any injury to people or property resulting from any ideas, methods, instructions or products referred to in the content.

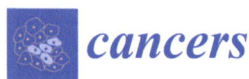

Review

Imaging of Peritoneal Carcinomatosis in Advanced Ovarian Cancer: CT, MRI, Radiomic Features and Resectability Criteria

Valentina Miceli [1,†], Marco Gennarini [1,†], Federica Tomao [2], Angelica Cupertino [1], Dario Lombardo [1], Innocenza Palaia [2], Federica Curti [1], Sandrine Riccardi [1], Roberta Ninkova [1], Francesca Maccioni [1], Paolo Ricci [1], Carlo Catalano [1], Stefania Maria Rita Rizzo [3,4], and Lucia Manganaro [1,*]

1. Department of Radiological, Oncology and Patological Sciences, "Sapienza" University of Rome, 00185 Rome, Italy; valentina.miceli@uniroma1.it (V.M.); marco.gennarini@uniroma1.it (M.G.); angelica.cupertino@uniroma1.it (A.C.); dario.lombardo@uniroma1.it (D.L.); federica.curti@uniroma1.it (F.C.); sandrine.riccardi@uniroma1.it (S.R.); robertavalerieva.ninkova@uniroma1.it (R.N.); francesca.maccioni@uniroma1.it (F.M.); paolo.ricci@uniroma1.it (P.R.); carlo.catalano@uniroma1.it (C.C.)
2. Department of Gynecological, Obstetrical and Urological Sciences, "Sapienza" University of Rome, 00185 Rome, Italy; federica.tomao@uniroma1.it (F.T.); innocenza.palaia@uniroma1.it (I.P.)
3. Clinica di Radiologia EOC, Istituto Imaging della Svizzera Italiana (IIMSI), 6900 Lugano, Switzerland; stefania.maria.rita.rizzo@usi.ch
4. Facoltà di Scienze Biomediche, Università della Svizzera Italiana (USI), 6900 Lugano, Switzerland
* Correspondence: lucia.manganaro@uniroma1.it
† These authors contributed equally to this work.

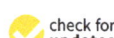

Citation: Miceli, V.; Gennarini, M.; Tomao, F.; Cupertino, A.; Lombardo, D.; Palaia, I.; Curti, F.; Riccardi, S.; Ninkova, R.; Maccioni, F.; et al. Imaging of Peritoneal Carcinomatosis in Advanced Ovarian Cancer: CT, MRI, Radiomic Features and Resectability Criteria. *Cancers* 2023, *15*, 5827. https://doi.org/10.3390/cancers 15245827

Academic Editor: Athina C Tsili

Received: 27 October 2023
Revised: 4 December 2023
Accepted: 6 December 2023
Published: 13 December 2023

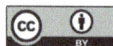

Copyright: © 2023 by the authors. Licensee MDPI, Basel, Switzerland. This article is an open access article distributed under the terms and conditions of the Creative Commons Attribution (CC BY) license (https:// creativecommons.org/licenses/by/ 4.0/).

Simple Summary: Ovarian cancer is the second most frequent gynecological cancer in Western countries and the most common cause of death due to gynecological malignancies with an estimated five-year survival rate of 39%. The high aggressiveness and mortality are mainly related to the speed of abdominal spread: 70% of patients are diagnosed at an advanced stage of disease (stage III–IV FIGO) or in the presence of peritoneal carcinomatosis (PC), and about 60% of women will develop a recurrence. In this context, imaging plays an essential role for proper staging and follow-up and in selecting patients eligible for complete cytoreduction (CCR), the most important treatment and prognostic factor for patients.

Abstract: PC represents the most striking picture of the loco-regional spread of ovarian cancer, configuring stage III. In the last few years, many papers have evaluated the role of imaging and therapeutic management in patients with ovarian cancer and PC. This paper summed up the literature on traditional approaches to the imaging of peritoneal carcinomatosis in advanced ovarian cancer, presenting classification systems, most frequent patterns, routes of spread and sites that are difficult to identify. The role of imaging in diagnosis was investigated, with particular attention to the reported sensitivity and specificity data—computed tomography (CT), magnetic resonance imaging (MRI), positron emission tomography-CT (PET-CT)—and to the peritoneal cancer index (PCI). In addition, we explored the therapeutic possibilities and radiomics applications that can impact management of patients with ovarian cancer. Careful staging is mandatory, and patient selection is one of the most important factors influencing complete cytoreduction (CCR) outcome: an accurate pre-operative imaging may allow selection of patients that may benefit most from primary cytoreductive surgery.

Keywords: ovarian cancer; peritoneal disease; radiomic; imaging; cytoreduction

1. Introduction

Ovarian cancer (OC) is the most common cause of death due to gynecologic malignancies, with an estimated five-year survival rate of 39% [1], which varies according to stage of presentation (75% in stage I, 17–20% in stage IV) [2].

OC tends to spread and grow early within the peritoneal cavity and generally occurs at an advanced stage (stages III–IV at time of diagnosis: 70% of patients with OC at the time of diagnosis already have peritoneal disease) [3] (Table 1).

Table 1. Figo staging of ovarian cancer.

Stage	Description
I	Tumor confined to the ovaries or fallopian tube(s) IA: Limited to one ovary (capsule intact) or fallopian tube IB: Limited to both ovaries (capsule intact) or fallopian tubes IC: Limited to one or both ovaries or fallopian tubes, with any of the following: IC1: Surgical spill intraoperatively IC2: Capsule ruptured before surgery, or tumor on ovarian or fallopian tube surface IC3: Malignant cells present in the ascites or peritoneal washing
II	Tumor involves one or both ovaries or fallopian tubes or is primary peritoneal cancer and involves other pelvic organs IIA: Extension and/or implants on the uterus and/or fallopian tubes and/or ovaries IIB: Extension to the other pelvic intraperitoneal tissue
III	Tumor involves one or both ovaries or fallopian tubes or primary peritoneal cancer and spreads beyond the pelvis but not outside the abdominal cavity IIIA: Cancer involves the pelvic structures and the retroperitoneal lymph nodes, without macroscopic visible tumor outside of the pelvis IIIB: Cancer involves structures outside of the pelvis (<2 cm) IIIC: Cancer involves structures outside of the pelvis (>2 cm). This included surface implants along abdominal solid organs, without parenchymal involvement.
IV	Distant metastasis excluding peritoneal metastases IVA: Metastatic pleural effusion IVB: Parenchymal metastatic lesion and/or metastases to extra-abdominal organs (including inguinal and thoracic lymph nodes)

PC is defined as the implantation of neoplastic cells in the peritoneal cavity and is a relatively frequent condition in the advanced stages of many neoplasms of the digestive system (colon, stomach, pancreas) [4].

The onset of carcinomatosis represents the most striking picture of the loco-regional spread of the disease, configuring stage III, associated with progression of disease and poor prognosis, causing more than 80% of deaths.

Because of this spread, often the most common symptom is neoplastic ascites, the result of fluid production by peritoneal cells and production of serum and mucin by cancer cells [5].

The treatment plan for patients with OC varies depending on the stage of presentation, and the clinical course is usually characterized by surgery and multiple chemotherapy strategies combined [6].

In patients diagnosed with early or advanced-stage OC, the established treatment protocol involves optimal cytoreductive surgery (CRS) aiming to achieve minimal residual tumor size (less than 1 cm) and subsequent platinum-based chemotherapy. This combination represents the standard of care and is the foremost factor influencing clinical outcomes.

CRS embodies the principle of surgical thoroughness, striving for the complete elimination of macroscopically visible disease or any minute millimeter-sized residue [7].

After initial management for late-stage disease, most patients will achieve remission. However, the risk of recurrence remains high (>70–80%), often occurs within 18 months of treatment and is linked to post-surgical residues of the disease and to the chemosensitivity of the tumor; the main site of recurrent disease is the peritoneal cavity [8].

An accurate staging is mandatory to assess the spread of disease and to select patients with resectable peritoneal disease for whom a complete cytoreduction can be achieved.

The peritoneal cancer index (PCI) is a preoperative score system that considers the size and distribution of implants on the peritoneal surface and is the most widespread and comparable carcinomatosis staging system [9].

Despite imaging advancement, diagnostic laparoscopy is still the gold standard for quantifying peritoneal disease [10] by allowing an estimate of tumor extent by PCI.

Multidetector computed tomography (MDCT) is the pillar for the initial staging of patients with OC: it allows the evaluation of the primary tumor, the identification of peritoneal implants and the evaluation of distant metastases both in lymph nodes and in solid organs [11–13].

MRI, due to its high contrast resolution, has an accuracy similar to that of CT in staging and even higher than CT in the identification of small peritoneal implants (even without ascites) or in the evaluation of the local extent of the disease. Its usefulness remains, however, limited to selected cases, due to lower spatial resolution, long duration, lower availability, and higher costs of the investigation. 18F-fluorodeoxyglucose positron emission tomography-computed tomography (18FDG PET-CT) is not usually recommended for staging purposes. Its use may be helpful during follow-up in case of suspected recurrence, if CT and MRI results are negative and tumor markers are increased [14].

The optimal treatment in patients with OC is represented by surgical cytoreduction and adjuvant platinum-based chemotherapy, with potential subsequent maintenance strategies established on the basis of two different biomarkers (BRCA status and homologous recombination deficiency status) [15].

The purpose of this review is, therefore, to provide an overview of peritoneal carcinosis in patients with OC, and critically evaluate the most frequent patterns, the routes of diffusion and the sites that are difficult to identify for the radiologist, with particular attention to the role of imaging (CT, MRI, PET-CT) for correct staging. Additionally, the increasing role of radiomic analysis in the staging of patients with advanced OC will be investigated, as a predictive factor in surgical resectability and in the prognosis.

2. Materials and Methods

As of September 2023, a structured search was performed using the PubMed database that included all relevant original articles about peritoneal carcinomatosis in OC. No start date limits or language restrictions were used; the research was expanded by also checking the references of the recovered articles for further potentially eligible studies. The search terms consisted of (ovarian cancer) AND (peritoneal carcinomatosis) AND (survival) OR (peritoneal carcinomatosis index) OR (radiomics) OR (treatment). Data mining was performed independently by two reviewers, and any disagreement was discussed with a third auditor.

From the set of articles selected during our literature search, we specifically chose to include studies that offered insights into pathology and imaging techniques. Any editorial comments, conference abstracts and short communications were omitted.

After conducting an initial assessment based on factors such as title, topic, and methodology, articles that were not in line with the objective of our review were excluded. Subsequently, those containing subjective opinions, personal perspectives or anecdotal content were also eliminated.

Our initial literature search yielded 150 articles. Following the application of our predefined criteria, 65 articles were excluded from the review. Ultimately, 87 published articles met the requirements for inclusion in this review [1–87] (Figure 1).

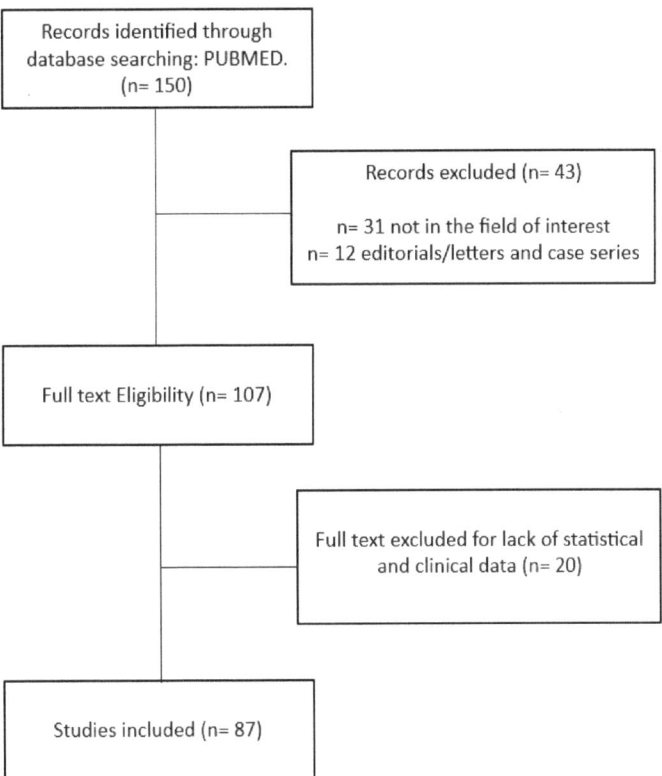

Figure 1. Study selection flow chart.

3. Surgical Staging and Treatment

The primary objective of cytoreductive surgery is to resect all macroscopic tumors or at least to reduce the largest tumor residuals to less than a centimeter.

When obtaining a complete cytoreduction is technically not feasible due to the spread of disease, or when a patient is unable to tolerate an extensive surgery, then interval debulking surgery (IDS) could be an alternative. IDS implies three cycles of neoadjuvant chemotherapy (NACT) followed by cytoreductive surgery and a further three cycles of adjuvant chemotherapy eventually followed by maintenance treatment based on the molecular characteristics of the tumor. Residual disease at the end of surgery is still considered as the most important prognostic factor impacting survival of patients affected by advanced OC [16,17].

The benefit to survival obtained by a neoadjuvant chemotherapeutic approach followed by cytoreductive surgery compared to primary debulking surgery is still debated.

The EORTC55971 trial [18] and the CHORUS trial [19] reported analogous values in both similar progression-free survival (PFS; 12 months) and over-all survival (OS; 29 vs. 24 months) for patients affected by advanced OC receiving neoadjuvant chemotherapy and interval debulking surgery compared with upfront debulking surgery. However, in both of these studies, the percentage of patients with complete upfront debulking surgery was very low (<20%). For this reason, a Trial on Radical Upfront Surgical Therapy (TRUST), requiring a qualification process for participating centers in order to reduce an eventual variability of the surgical outcomes, is currently ongoing and expected to conclude in 2024.

In this scenario, identifying those criteria leading to an optimal cytoreduction is a very important issue.

According to the most recent ESGO guidelines [14], patients affected by advanced OC are not candidates for primary surgery if the following spread of disease is present:

- Diffuse deep infiltration of the root of small bowel mesentery
- Diffuse carcinomatosis of the small bowel involving such large parts that resection would lead to a short bowel syndrome (remaining bowel < 1.5 m)
- Diffuse involvement/deep infiltration of:
    - stomach/duodenum;
    - head or middle part of pancreas
- Involvement of coeliac trunk, hepatic arteries, left gastric artery, Hepatic hilum infiltration or hepatic metastases
- Multiple parenchymal lung metastases (preferably histologically proven)
- Non-resectable lymph nodes
- Brain metastases

Evidence-based standardized evaluation of the disease extent and of patient condition are essential to predict the possibility of residual macroscopic disease after upfront debulking surgery. Particularly, specific clinical factors (e.g., comorbidities, age, World Health Organization performance status WHO—PS) should also be considered in the pre-operative assessment of operability.

Regarding the spread of the disease, imaging strategies, serum markers and staging, surgical approaches have all been investigated for the prediction of cytoreduction both at primary debulking surgery and at interval debulking surgery, with variable results.

Diagnostic laparoscopy can provide a definitive histopathological diagnosis and detailed information about the intra-abdominal disease burden [20,21].

In a prospective study involving 113 patients with advanced OC, Fagotti et al. [21] investigated by laparoscopy the presence of omental cake, peritoneal and diaphragmatic extensive carcinosis, bowel and stomach infiltration, mesenteric retraction, and spleen and/or liver superficial metastasis. For each patient, a laparoscopic evaluation was conducted, and the total predictive index value (PIV) was computed by aggregating the scores associated with all parameters.

The overall accuracy rate of the laparoscopic procedure to predict an optimal debulking ranged between 77.3 and 100%. The authors observed that when the PIV was greater than or equal to 8, the probability of optimally resecting the disease by laparotomy was equal to 0, and the rate of futile exploratory laparotomy was 40.5%. Vizzielli et al. [22] stratified patients into three groups based on the volume of the disease: high tumor load (HTL) for PIV ≥ 8, intermediate tumor load (ITL) for PIV equal to 6 and 4, and low tumor load (LTL) for PIV < 4, showing that tumor spread according to PIV was an independent prognostic factor impacting either PFS and OS, together with residual tumor (RT) and performance status.

Some other trials investigated the role of diagnostic laparoscopy, with the Fagotti score being still the most adopted in clinical practice [23,24].

In summary, diagnostic laparoscopy is an accurate tool for staging in patients with advanced OC. Some limitations have been noted, including the inability to palpate the liver surface and diaphragm, challenges in visualizing certain anatomical sites due to adhesions in the upper abdomen [25] or in detecting implants of carcinomatosis beyond the gastrosplenic ligament, in the lesser sac, mesenteric root and in the retroperitoneum [23].

Moreover, the presence of huge, fixed masses in the Douglas pouch can reduce the performance of diagnostic laparoscopy. Despite its overall safety, minor complications have been reported. In a study including a series of 145 patients, only one patient showed a serosal injury that was immediately treated [26].

4. Imaging

Pre-operative imaging strategies, including CT, MRI, and 18FDG PET-CT, have been largely tested to assess the extent of disease.

However, the best option technique for staging OC and for detecting all of the implants of PC to assess the non-resectability of the disease does not exist yet.

Among all of the imaging strategies, CT is the most used for preoperative workup and to predict the likelihood of suboptimal cytoreduction.

With the aim of predicting surgical outcome, some promising imaging models with their related scoring systems have been proposed, however, not yet reproduced for external validation. Several authors have evaluated the use of preoperative CT in assessing tumor resectability with different prediction models. A number of researchers created novel scoring systems that yielded AUC values between 0.67 and 0.97 [27,28], whereas others conducted validation studies on preexisting scoring systems, like the peritoneal cancer index, which produced AUC values in the range of 0.55 to 0.76 [29–31].

If identified on CT scan, disease localizations such as diffuse peritoneal thickening, mesenteric disease, suprarenal lymph nodes, ascites, and diaphragmatic or hepatic site disease could be included in potential scoring systems along with clinical features such as age, performance status, and serum tumor markers such as CA 125 value, as they are frequently associated with residual disease.

In recent years, dual energy CT (DECT), a recently introduced technological advancement, has been playing an innovative role by enabling the simultaneous capture of a series of images at different radiant energies during a single CT acquisition [32].

This technique leverages the variations in low-energy and high-energy attenuation of different tissues. In the field of oncology, it enhances the precision and accuracy of identifying neoplasia, allowing for a more targeted approach. Moreover, it offers the possibility of reducing the radiation dose administered to the patient without compromising image quality [32].

Through the utilization of post-processing techniques on DECT data, it becomes feasible to obtain monochromatic images at a specific energy level ranging from 40 to 140 keV.

In the context of advanced OC, this technology could serve as a diagnostic tool for identifying subdiaphragmatic, hepatic, and perisplenic carcinoma implants that may not have been explored surgically [33].

Peritoneal carcinomatosis implants exhibit variable attenuation values, with densitometric characteristics such as those of soft tissue, calcium, and fluid. These characteristics are best visualized through low-kilovolt monochrome images, which highlight contrast differences between tissues at various energy levels. Particularly, DECT excels in detecting implants smaller than 1 cm, proving to be a valuable asset in enhancing the effectiveness of staging for advanced OC, thereby contributing positively to surgical outcomes [33].

However, some of the models reporting good performance for predicting residual disease failed in the external validation phase.

In this context, the external validation of a radiological scoring system appliable for evaluating the spread of the disease, and its diagnostic performance before integration into diagnostic algorithms, is essential.

Finally, recent evidence showed that post-operative imaging-based evaluations of the residual disease differ depending on the intraoperative judgment of the surgeons [34,35].

Particularly, Lorusso et al. [34], analyzed 64 patients with FIGO stage III–IV OC who underwent optimal primary cytoreduction in the same institution with a CT scan performed within 30 days of the surgery. The authors observed that surgeons reported a residual tumor (RT) = 0, 0.1 < RT < 0.5 cm, and 0.6 < RT < 1 cm in 53 (82.8%), 9 (14.1%) and 2 (3.1%) cases, respectively, with postoperative CT scan disagreeing in 13 out of 64 (20.3%) cases. Progression-free survival (PFS) of patients with a positive and negative postoperative CT scan for RT was 5 months (95% confidence interval (CI) 1–15 months) and 28 months (95% CI 2–46 months), respectively ($p < 0.0001$). Evidence of the disease using postoperative CT was an independent prognostic factor in multivariate analysis (hazard ratio (HR) = 8.87, 95% CI = 3.23–24.31, $p < 0.0001$).

Furthermore, in the study by Heitz et al. [35], the authors hypothesized that an early tumor regrowth might be a contributor to the discordance between surgical assessment and radiologic assessment/integrated assessment. The risk of losing the prognostic factor of complete resection, if chemotherapy is started later than 31 days after primary surgery, was greater than 15%. These data stressed the importance of the timing of chemotherapy initiation (Table 2).

Table 2. Imaging study results.

	Modality	Authors	Title	Patients	Aim of Study	Sensitivity (%)	Specificity (%)
1	CT	Choi H.J. et al., 2010 [44]	Region-based diagnostic performance of multidetector CT for detecting peritoneal seeding in OC patients	57	To determine the accuracy of CT compared with the surgical findings (peritoneal seeding, metastatic lymph nodes) in OC patients	45	72
2	CT MRI	Tempany C.M.C. et al., 2000 [39]	Staging of advanced OC: comparison of imaging modalities-report from the radiological diagnostic oncology group	118	To compare multiple imaging modalities for diagnosing and staging advanced OC	92 95	82 80
3	CT	Mazzei M.A. et al., 2013 [43]	Accuracy of MDCT in the preoperative definition of peritoneal cancer index (PCI) in patients with advanced OC who underwent peritonectomy and hyperthermic intraperitoneal chemotherapy	43	To assess MDCT accuracy in preoperatively defining the peritoneal cancer index (PCI) in individuals with advanced ovarian cancer	100	40
4	CT MRI	Qayyuma A. et al., 2004 [41]	Role of CT and MR imaging in predicting optimal cytoreduction of newly diagnosed primary epithelial OC	137	To ascertain the comparative precision of CT and MR imaging in identifying non-surgically manageable tumor sites before cytoreductive surgery in patients with primary ovarian cancer	79 71	99 100
5	MRI	Ricke J. et al., 2002 [51]	Prospective evaluation of contrast-enhanced MRI in the depiction of peritoneal spread in primary or recurrent OC	57	To evaluate MRI accuracy in the staging of intra-abdominal tumor dissemination in ovarian cancer	90.9	57.1
6	PET/CT CT	Kim H.W. et al., 2013 [58]	Peritoneal carcinomatosis in Patients with OC—Enhanced CT Versus 18F-FDG PET/CT	46	To conduct a comparative analysis of the diagnostic accuracy between FDG PET/CT and enhanced abdominal CT	96.2 88.5	90 65
7	WB-DWI/MRI	Michielsen K. et al., 2014 [53]	Whole-body MRI with diffusion-weighted sequence for staging of patients with suspected ovarian cancer: a clinical feasibility study in comparison to CT and FDG-PET/CT	32	To evaluate whole-body DWI/MRI diagnostic effectiveness in staging and determining operability, in contrast to CT and FDG-PET/CT, for individuals with suspected ovarian cancer	91	91
8	CT F-FDG PET/CT	Lopez-Lopez V. et al., 2016 [59]	Use of (18)F-FDG PET/CT in the preoperative evaluation of patients diagnosed with peritoneal carcinomatosis of ovarian origin, candidates to cytoreduction and hipec. A pending issue	59	To evaluate the clinical usefulness of the results obtained with 18F-FDG PET/CT in relation to CT in the preoperative staging of patients with peritoneal carcinomatosis secondary to primary or recurrent OC	35 24	98 93

4.1. Computed Tomography

According to the international guidelines, CT represents the imaging modality of choice for OC staging, showing a high accuracy (up to 94%) [11,36].

CT allows evaluation of the extent of the primary tumor, the identification of any peritoneal implants of carcinomatosis and lymph node involvement, and the investigation of the presence of distant metastases (Figure 2).

Strengths of the procedure include wide availability, low cost, high spatial resolution, short scanning time and the possibility of multiplanar image reconstructions (MPRs) [37].

The correct protocol for acquiring CT images to highlight carcinomatosis implants involves the use of intravenous iodine contrast medium (CM) and image acquisition in the portal venous phase (70–90 s) and MPR with a layer thickness of 1–3 mm in multiple planes (axial, coronal and sagittal). Sagittal and coronal reconstructions allow a better evaluation of the subphrenic space and abdominal recesses. Oral CM can be administered to differentiate digestive structures from serous and mesenteric implants [11,38], although it is not currently recommended because it may obscure the presence of calcified peritoneal deposits.

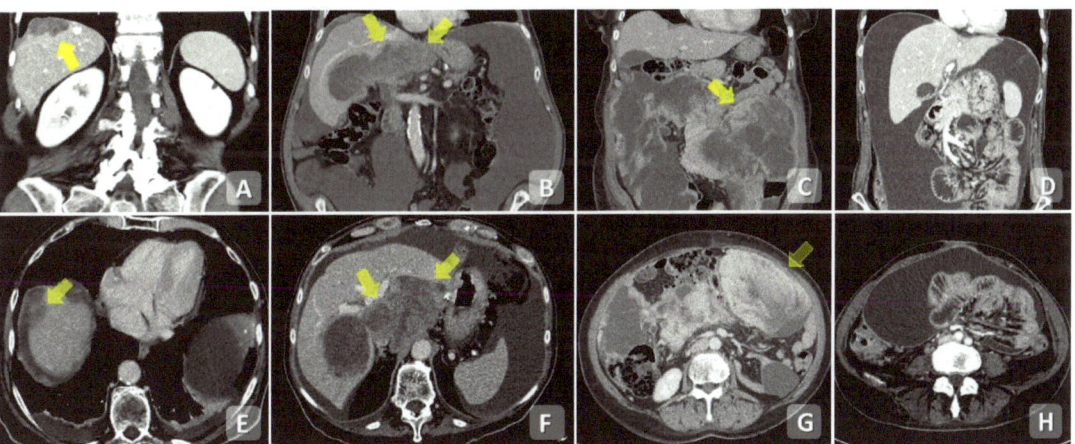

Figure 2. Contrast-enhanced CT scan, axial planes (**E–H**) and MPRs (**A–D**). Extensive infiltration of the diaphragmatic dome (**A,E**) and hepatic hilum (**B,F**). Diffuse mesenteric infiltration (**C,G,D,H**). Note the presence of free peritoneal fluid and pleural effusion.

The diagnostic accuracy of CT examination to identify peritoneal carcinomatosis implants is reported to be between 70–90% at all stages of the disease [39].

Considering the heterogeneity of size, morphology, and location of carcinomatosis implants, sensitivity was reported with a wide gap, ranging from 25 to 90% [40,41].

Indeed, CT has several disadvantages, such as low soft-tissue resolution, which limits the ability to characterize primary tumors. CT also has limitations in detecting small volume carcinomatosis (<1 cm), especially on the surface of the small bowel or on mesentery root.

In addition, other limitative factors in the detection of carcinosis implants can be the absence of ascites, localization in "challenging" sites such as small bowel, shortage of intra-abdominal adipose tissue and inadequacy of intestinal opacification [38].

Coakley et al. achieved an overall sensitivity of 85–93%, with 25–50% sensitivity in metastases < 1 cm [12], whereas De Bree et al. reported a sensitivity of 9–24% in similarly sized implants [42,43].

Choi HJ et al. showed a lower sensitivity (35.1%) and specificity (68%) for the detection of peritoneal carcinomatosis < 1 cm compared to implants > 1 cm (52.4 and 75%, respectively; $p = 0.037$) [44].

4.2. Magnetic Resonance Imaging

MRI is performed in cases where CT examination is contraindicated (pregnant patients or allergies to iodized CM), if the CT findings are inadequate/doubtful for the presence of metastases or if the implants are in sites where CT proves inadequate, such as subphrenic spaces, lesser omentum, serosal, and mesenteric deposits [45].

The MRI study protocol includes T1- and T2-weighted image sequences on multiple planes (axial, sagittal and coronal) with and without adipose tissue signal suppression, DWI on axial plane at least using two b factor (0, 1000 s/mm^2), over the entire abdomen and pelvis, and dynamic contrast-enhanced MRI after injection of paramagnetic CM.

T2-weighted images and DWI, including apparent diffusion coefficient (ADC) maps, are pivotal to improve the identification of even small peritoneal carcinomatous implants, especially on the mesentery, bowel serosa and peritoneal reflections, due to the significant contrast between the lesion and surrounding peritoneal tissues [45] (Figure 3).

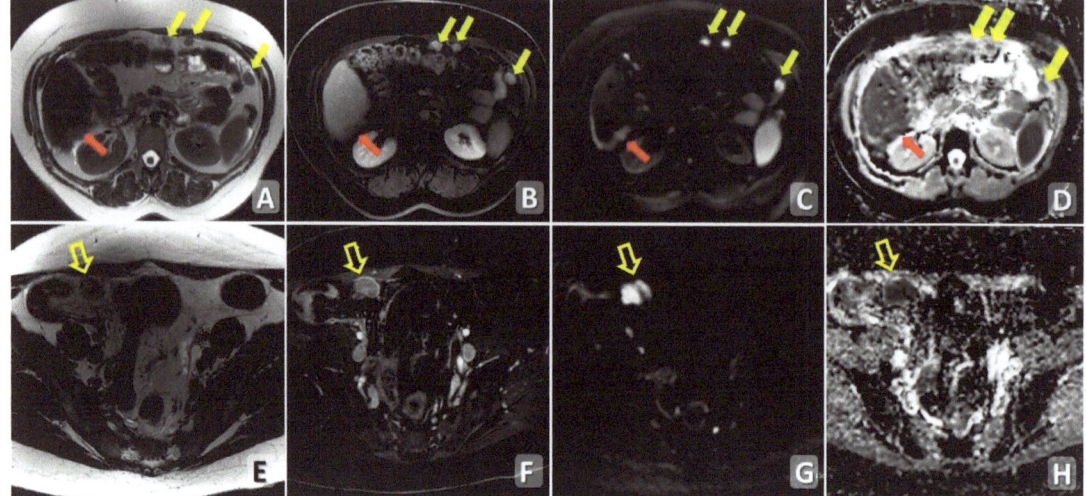

Figure 3. MRI axial T2WI (**A,E**), post-contrast fat-suppressed T1WI (**B,F**), DWI (**C,G**) and ADC map (**D,H**) showing multiple centimetric nodules of peritoneal carcinosis. Upper row: multiple nodules of PC (yellow arrows) showing post-contrast enhancement (**B**) and signal restriction in DWI/ADC (**C,D**). Additionally, a plaque of PC is localized on the Glissonian surface well recognizable in DWI (red arrow) at high b value (**C,D**). Lower row: macronodule of PC in the right iliac fossa (empty arrows) showing post-contrast enhancement (**F**) and signal restriction in DWI/ADC (**G,H**).

Moreover, involved peritoneal lining may be shown by dynamic contrast-enhanced MRI as a delayed enhancement.

Nevertheless, the usefulness of MRI remains limited by potential artifacts (e.g., motion or magnetic susceptibility artifacts), long duration of the investigation, lower availability, higher costs, long interpretation times and simultaneous analysis of the abdomen and pelvis.

Concerning the sensitivity and specificity of the MRI in detecting peritoneal carcinomatosis implants, Fujii et al. found values of 90% and 95.5%, respectively, with the use of DWI sequences [46].

Yu et al. found that the sensitivity and specificity of MRI for detecting peritoneal deposits in ovarian neoplasm were 88% and 99%, respectively [47].

Compared to CT, MRI demonstrated a superior sensitivity and accuracy (MRI: 95% and 88% vs. CT: 55% and 63%, respectively) thanks to the use of DWI at high b values and the administration of paramagnetic CM [48,49].

Concerning sizes, MRI was shown to have better sensitivity (85–90%) than CT in the detection of implants < 1 cm [50], but little difference was seen in one of the largest series in which the majority of patients (88%) had implants > 2 cm and presence of ascites (sensitivities of MR and CT, respectively, 95% and 92%) [39,51].

In recent years, the development of new techniques, such as whole-body diffusion-weighted imaging (WB-DWI/MRI) improved the diagnostic accuracy.

Rizzo et al., in a cohort of 92 patients evaluated by CT and WB-DWI/MRI, showed significantly higher accuracy of WB-DWI/MRI specifically for involvement of mesentery, lumbo-aortic lymph nodes, pelvis, large bowel, and sigmoid-rectum [52].

Findings by Michielsen et al. [53] indicated that WB-DWI/MRI outperformed CT in terms of sensitivity (94% vs. 66%), specificity (98% vs. 77%), and accuracy (96% vs. 71%) for detecting disease sites that suggested non-resectability.

Conversely, when applying the ESMO-ESGO criteria for non-resectability, Fischerova et al. found no statistically significant variations in the outcomes between WB-DWI/MRI, pelvic and abdominal ultrasound, and contrast-enhanced CT when predicting residual disease upon completion of the surgery [54].

4.3. PET-CT

According to the European Society for Medical Oncology (ESMO), PET-CT is not recommended as an imaging technique for initial management of epithelial ovarian carcinoma [55].

The main disadvantage of 18F FDG PET-CT is the limited spatial resolution (5–6 mm) in detection of small-volume carcinomatosis, especially on the small bowel/colon serosa or their mesenteries; moreover, the results may be misinterpreted due to the uptake of 18F FDG caused by physiological movements (e.g., of the digestive tract) or non-malignant and inflammatory lesions, giving rise to false-positive results [56–58].

Michielsen et al. found a lower sensitivity of PET-CT in PC detection in small bowel mesentery (33%), colon serosa (27%) and colon mesentery (25%) compared to CT (63%, 45% and 50%, respectively). Specificity was, however, overlapping [53].

Lopez-Lopez et al. compared the 18F FDG PET-CT with CT in 59 patients, showing a sensitivity of 35% and 24%, respectively, whereas CT had higher specificity (98% vs. 93%) [59].

18F FDGPET-CT may still be used for staging as a problem-solving tool if unclear CT findings are detected (such as indeterminate lymph node involvement in the retroperitoneum or mediastinum), providing in a single test, anatomical and functional information of carcinosis implants.

4.4. PET-MRI

PET-MRI is an emerging fusion technique that, despite the few studies carried out, has shown important results in the OC characterization thanks to high soft tissue contrast of MRI along with functional imaging of FDG uptake. In a pilot study, compared to DW-MRI, PET-MRI turned out to have higher sensitivity for detection of carcinomatosis in 31 patients with OC, especially in "challenging sites" (three out of four in small bowel regions) [60].

Combined PET-MRI has proven to be helpful in the characterization of ovarian tumors with a sensitivity and specificity of 94% and 100%, respectively, compared to PET-CT (74–80%) and MRI (84–60%) [61].

Although this promising hybrid imaging technique could soon be included for a better evaluation of OC peritoneal carcinomatosis, further investigations are needed for clarification of its role.

5. Diffusion Pathways

Peritoneal extension of OC is considered a negative prognostic factor associated with higher risk of recurrence and high mortality compared to cancers diagnosed at an early stage (I or II) [62].

Spread of ovarian carcinoma to the abdominal cavity usually occurs through the peritoneal circulation [63]. In order to understand how the tumor spreads within the peritoneum, it is necessary to know its anatomy and function. The peritoneum is a serous membrane composed of two layers continuous with each other: the outer parietal layer, lining the abdominal cavity and pelvis, and the inner visceral layer, lining the intraperitoneal visceral organs; the latter reflects and folds to line the visceral organs and keep them suspended in the cavity, thus forming mesenteries, omenta and ligaments that divide the abdomen into several compartments. The space between the parietal and visceral layers of the peritoneum is the peritoneal cavity and is filled with a slight amount of fluid, which allows frictionless movement of the visceral organs.

Such spaces and supporting structures can serve as gateways for intraperitoneal tumor spread and the establishment of carcinomatosis implants [37,64].

Peritoneal fluid is not stationary; rather, it follows a dynamic circulation related to diaphragmatic respiratory movements: in the upright position, peritoneal fluid accumulates in most of the declivous portions of the abdomen, such as the recto-uterine and paravesical recesses. Fluid flows from the pelvis to the paracolic gutter, and then to the subdiaphragmatic regions during the expiratory phase whereby the diaphragm moves upward and generates negative intraabdominal pressure, drawing back the fluid in a cranial direction.

On the right side, fluid moves from the paracolic gutter to the anterior subhepatic space and into the right hepatic spaces. On the left side, fluid ascending toward the paracolic gutter is arrested by the left phrenicocolic ligament, so its progression into the perisplenic spaces is confined. In addition, the falciform ligament is an anatomical barrier to fluid progression from the right subdiaphragmatic spaces to the left perisplenic spaces.

The kinetics of intraperitoneal fluid explain why implants of peritoneal carcinomatosis are more often located in the paracolic gutters and right subdiaphragmatic spaces, rather than in the left ones, and on higher constriction sites such as Douglas' pouch and the right lower quadrant [63,65].

6. Disease Patterns

Implants of peritoneal carcinomatosis should be characterized by different morphological and dimensional features since they are extremely important for an ideal presurgical and pretreatment evaluation.

Number (solitary or multiple) and density or intensity with and without intravenous injection of contrast are other parameters to evaluate.

Nodules of peritoneal carcinomatosis could be morphologically divided into solid, cystic and mixed implants with either a solid component or a cystic component, although rarely, mixed solid and cystic or purely cystic lesions are found [4,62] (Figure 4).

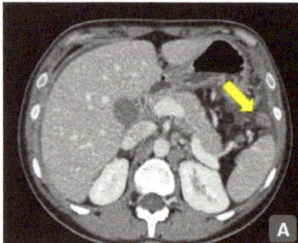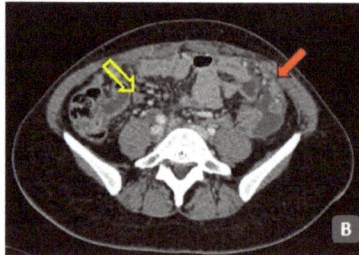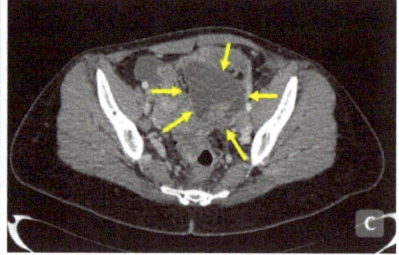

Figure 4. Axial contrast-enhanced CT of the abdomen. (**A**) Upper abdomen. Perisplenic carcinosis with micro and macronodular pattern (solid arrow). (**B**) Close to the ileocecal junction (empty arrow) an inhomogeneous density of adipose tissue is present with nodules and septa as reticular-nodular pattern of PC. Omental cake is present in the left side (arrow). (**C**) Ovarian mass with mixed solid/cystic components (small arrows). Diffuse infiltration of the sigmoid colon is present.

Moreover, serous cystadenocarcinoma, an OC subtype, can produce calcified peritoneal metastatic deposits [66].

Some cystic implants are low in attenuation and mimic loculated fluid [67].

Micronodular pattern refers to milky spots of peritoneal implants smaller than 5 mm involving the parietal or visceral peritoneum and mesenteric fat; on the contrary, nodular pattern is characterized instead by oval shape implants or coalescing small lesions (>5 mm) diffusely involving the tunica serosa and mesenteric, sometimes presenting spiculated margins.

Micronodular patterns observed in the mesentery can appear as thickening of the root with a stellate pattern [67].

Nodular lesions coalescing in irregular soft-tissue thickenings of variable extension that coat the viscera refer to plaque-like patterns. This type of lesion is typically found in the subdiaphragmatic spaces involving liver and spleen surfaces and presenting lower attenuation than the parenchyma on contrast-enhanced scans [68].

Large plaques involving omental fat and surrounded by reactive fibrotic tissue are referred to as "omental cakes" (Figure 5).

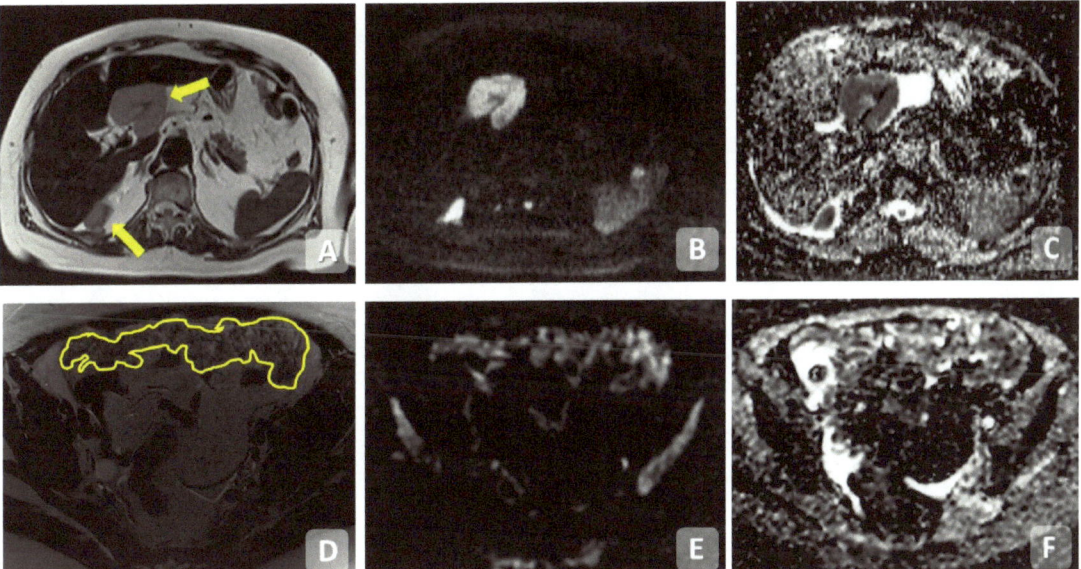

Figure 5. MRI images of peritoneal carcinomatosis. Upper row: (**A**) Axial T2WI, (**B**) DWI, (**C**) ADC—carcinomatosis nodule in perihilar and posterior pericapsular hepatic area (arrows); lower row, (**D**) T2WI, (**E**) DWI, (**F**) ADC—carcinomatosis with omental cake pattern (underlined).

Implants of several centimeters, resulting from the confluence of smaller nodules, can lead to soft-tissue masses (mass-like pattern), usually found in the pelvis; Masses measuring 10 cm or larger are called "bulky tumor" [4].

Subcutaneous nodules in the anterior abdominal wall may sometimes be the first clinical manifestation of OC (Sister Mary Josef's nodules). They are typically found in the periumbilical zone and can be direct extensions of omental disease [69].

Diffusely infiltrating tumor or focal soft-tissue masses on the bowel surface and mesentery can tether the loops and straighten the mesenteric vasculature, eventually causing bowel obstruction and dilatation of proximal loops (ileal freezing) [4,68].

7. Scoring System in Diagnostic Imaging
7.1. Peritoneal Cancer Index (PCI)

The peritoneal cancer index, adapted for imaging, is the only externally validated system. With the aim of creating a peritoneal evaluation system useful in the concise, clinically relevant, and statistically assessable preoperative and follow-up setting, Sugarbaker devised the PCI, a scoring system determined by the distribution and size of the tumor within the abdominopelvic cavity found on direct examination or through CT.

Tracing two sagittal lines and two transverse lines divides the abdomen into nine abdominopelvic regions that are numbered from 0 to 8, starting from the umbilical region and proceeding clockwise. The small intestine, unlike the large intestine that is evaluated in the respective abdominal regions 0–9, is evaluated separately and is divided into four further regions called 9 to 12 (9: upper jejunum; 10: lower jejunum; 11: superior ileum; 12: inferior ileum). For each of these regions, the volume of the tumor that occupies it is then indicated: V0 indicates the absence of tumor localization in the abdominopelvic region described; V1 indicates the presence of nodules with a diameter < 0.5 cm; V2 indicates nodules with a diameter between 0.5 and 5 cm; V3 indicates nodules with a diameter > 5 cm [70] (Figure 6).

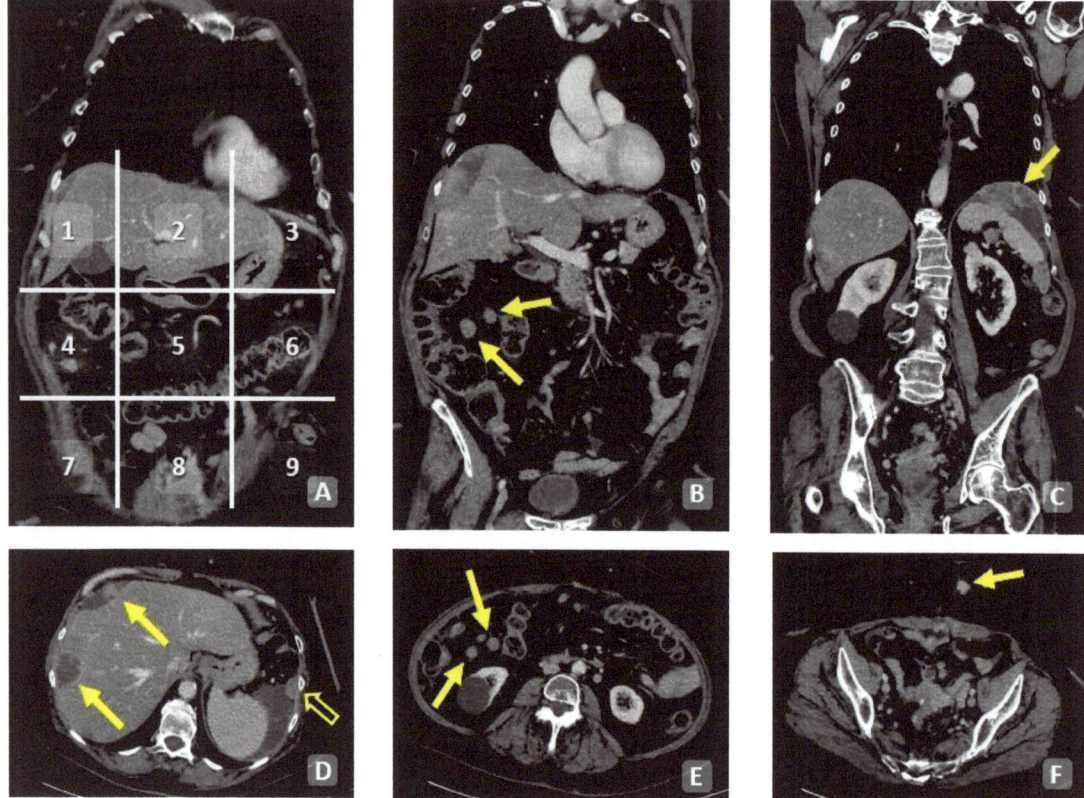

Figure 6. A 73-year-old patient. Coronal (**A–C**) and axial (**D–F**) contrast-enhanced CT scan of the abdomen. Division into quadrants of the abdomen with PCI numbering (**A**). Macronodules of peritoneal carcinomatosis in the context of the mesentery (arrows, (**B,E**)). Left subphrenic plaque of peritoneal carcinomatosis (**C**). Multifocal extensive infiltration of the hepatic surface (**D**). Subcutaneous implantation of peritoneal carcinomatosis (**E**).

Evaluation of the correlation between preoperative CT-PCI and surgical outcome and overall survival in patients with epithelial OC demonstrated that preoperative CT-PCI correlates with the probability of post-operative residual disease in patients undergoing primary cytoreduction. In addition, it showed that the serous histotype is significantly associated with higher CT-PCI scores and that it has higher prevalence in the upper abdominal and intestinal regions than in the other histotypes [31].

PCI is considered a prognostic indicator of survival in OC. Patients with PCI < 10 show better survival than those with PCI > 10, and even excluding stage IV patients from the analysis, PCI remains a significant survival index. Patients with PCI > 10 do not have prolonged survival and are, therefore, considered a high-risk group even if they have performed complete or near complete cytoreduction and standard treatment with systemic chemotherapy [71]. In patients with advanced epithelial OC, it has been proposed to evaluate PCI only in the regions corresponding to the small intestine and the hepatoduodenal ligament (9–12 + 2), as it has been demonstrated that they are more predictive for a complete resection and for survival based on the sum of the total PCI [72].

Evaluation of the prognostic value of small bowel PCI in patients with advanced epithelial OC undergoing cytoreduction and hyperthermic intraperitoneal chemotherapy (HIPEC) shows that both small bowel PCI and cytoreduction completeness are independent prognostic factors of overall survival, while age and timing of HIPEC have not been identified as independent prognostic factors [73].

Currently a clinical trial, "Imaging Study in Advanced ovArian Cancer (ISAAC)", is investigating the diagnostic performance of the peritoneal cancer index using ultrasound, WB-DWI/MRI and CT [29].

On the basis of previous results comparing imaging methods with the surgical approach for PCI, CT-PCI showed lower accuracy than surgical PCI in both high- and low-volume patients of disease. The difference in CT-PCI compared to surgical PCI is significant both in patients with OC and in patients treated with neoadjuvant chemotherapy for peritoneal disease [74]. Mikkelsen et al. [75] compared the efficacy of DW-MRI, CT and FDG PET/CT in PCI vs. surgical assessment. The mean surgical PCI was 18 (range 3–32), and all three imaging modalities often underestimated surgical PCI with a mean difference from surgical PCI of 4.2 (95% CI: 2.6–5.8) for CT, 4.4 for DW-MRI (95% CI: 2.9–5.8) and 5.3 for FDG PET/CT (95% CI: 3.6–7.0) in the absence of statistically significant differences between the three different imaging modalities.

A PCI > 20 evaluated by laparotomy and an albumin concentration < 33 g/L can predict the onset of high-grade complications after OC surgery. The main high-grade complication (28/62 patients—45.2%) in these patients was pleural effusion [76] (Table 3).

Table 3. PCI study results.

	Author	Title	Patients	Results
1	Rosendahl M, et al. (2018) [72]	Specific regions, rather than the entire Peritoneal Carcinosis Index, are predictive of complete resection and survival in advanced epithelial ovarian cancer	673	The predictive value of complete resection and survival is higher when specific PCI regions related to the small intestine and hepatoduodenal ligament are chosen compared to considering the entire PCI.
2	Tentes A.-A. K, et al. (2003) [71]	Peritoneal Cancer Index: a prognostic indicator of survival in advanced ovarian cancer	60	The extent of peritoneal spread in advanced ovarian cancer can be thoroughly evaluated through the peritoneal cancer index. This index plays a crucial role as a prognostic factor for survival and proves valuable in identifying distinct subgroups.
3	Avesani G, et al. (2020) [31]	Radiological assessment of Peritoneal Cancer Index on preoperative CT in ovarian cancer is related to surgical outcome and survival	297	The evaluation of preoperative CT-assessed PCI is linked to the likelihood of residual disease following cytoreductive surgery. Nevertheless, its effectiveness as a primary screening test to consistently pinpoint patients suitable for complete cytoreductive surgery is limited. CT-PCI exhibits a positive correlation with both disease-free survival and overall survival, thus serving as a potentially valuable independent prognostic factor.
4	Lomnytska M, et al. (2021) [76]	Peritoneal Cancer Index predicts severe complications after ovarian cancer surgery	256	Peritoneal cancer index ≥ 21 was an independent predictor of high-grade complications after ovarian cancer surgery. Increased peritoneal cancer index also impacted overall survival negatively, but high-grade complications did not influence overall survival.
5	Iavazzo C, et al. (2021) [73]	Small Bowel PCI Score as a prognostic factor of ovarian cancer patients undergoing cytoreductive surgery (CRS) with hyperthermic intraperitoneal chemotherapy (HIPEC), a retrospective analysis of 130 patients	130	A statistically significant correlation between small bowel-PCI score and overall survival of patients with advanced ovarian cancer was revealed.
6	Mikkelsen MS, et al. (2021) [75]	Assessment of peritoneal metastases with DW-MRI, CT, and FDG PET/CT before cytoreductive surgery for advanced stage epithelial ovarian cancer	50	None of the imaging modalities, including DW-MRI, CT, and FDG PET/CT, demonstrated superiority in the preoperative evaluation of surgical PCI in patients scheduled for upfront CRS for advanced stage EOC.
7	Goswami G, et al. (2019) [74]	Accuracy of CT scan in predicting the surgical PCI in patients undergoing cytoreductive surgery with/without HIPEC-a prospective single institution study	50	CT-PCI shows lower accuracy than surgical PCI in both high- and low-volume patients of disease. The difference in CT-PCI compared to surgical PCI is significant both in patients with ovarian cancer and in patients treated with neoadjuvant chemotherapy for peritoneal disease.

7.2. Bowel, Upper Abdomen, Mesentery in Peritoneal Metastasis (BUMPY)

Recently, another score has been proposed by Nougaret et al. [7] on the basis of radiological criteria to assess resectability in OC. Nougaret collected such planting sites under the acronym BUMPy (Bowel, Upper abdomen, Mesentery in Peritoneal metastasis). It is well known that some sites of carcinomatosis correlate with a suboptimal cytoreduction or require particular attention on the surgical level. Regarding localizations, peritoneal implants are divided into resectable and unresectable. Resectable implants are classified into implants with limited involvement of the small bowel (few nodules with serous involvement and nodules on the antimesenteric side) and of the mesentery (scattered nodules). Unresectable implants are classified into implants with diffuse involvement of the mesentery (many nodules, retractile and infiltrative pattern) and of the small bowel (tumor-like pattern, and both serosa and adjacent mesentery involved in multiple segments). The author suggests analyzing the images following the direction of peritoneal flow. The analysis is carried out on the coronal plane starting from the pelvis describing the involvement of the Douglas cord and then moving up right towards the paracolic gutter, the serous membrane of the ascending colon and the Morrison pouch. It continues with the evaluation of the hepatic capsule and the right hemidiaphragm. This is followed by the evaluation of the gastrohepatic ligament, the serous of the transverse mesocolon and the gastric ligament, then the left hemidiaphragm, the gastrosplenic ligament, the spleen, the descending colon and the left paracolic gutter. Finally, the mesentery is evaluated. At the end of the analysis on the coronal plane, it is suggested to repeat the evaluation on the axial plane (Figure 7).

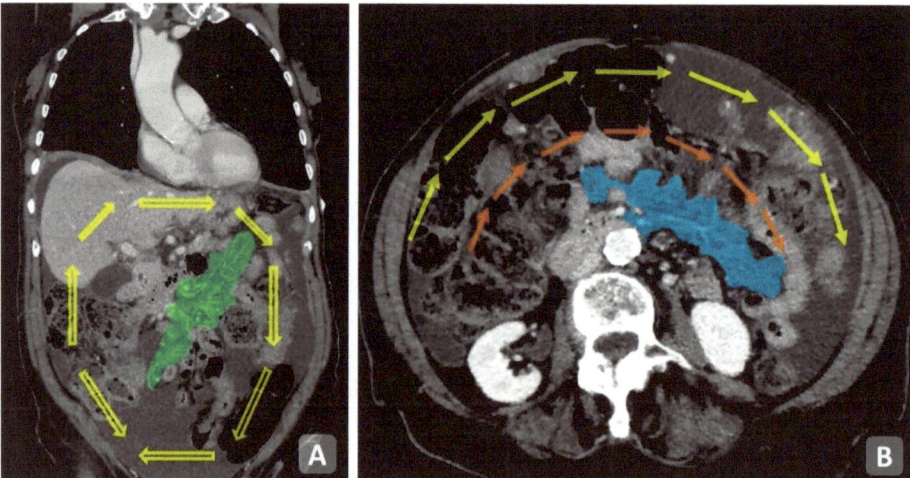

Figure 7. Coronal plane showing peritoneal fluid flow direction (arrows) and mesentery (green area) (**A**). Axial plane showing suggested evaluation direction (double wagon wheel-like) and mesentery (blue area) (**B**).

8. Radiomics

The process of radiomics analysis is based on established steps, each one in continuous evolution over time thanks to technological and mathematical advances, and they are the same for all radiomics studies, independently from the anatomy, pathology, and outcomes under examination [77–79]. The main steps are image acquisition and segmentation, feature extraction, feature selection and model construction [80].

Although some studies have so far evaluated radiomics and radiogenomics of OC, only a few of them have evaluated the possibility to predict the cytoreduction.

Thanks to advancements in The Cancer Genome Atlas (TCGA), a prognostic algorithm for high-grade serous OC has been defined with four different subtypes: differentiated, immunoreactive, mesenchymal, and proliferative. Vargas et al. explored the relationships between subjective qualitative CT features and the different subtypes of OC, showing that the mesenchymal subtype was significantly associated with higher risk of peritoneal involvement and the presence of mesenteric infiltration on CT [81], which is considered one of the reasons for failure of cytoreduction. In a different study including 38 patients, 12 quantitative metrics were selected to represent the inter-site imaging heterogeneity, and these metrics were associated with incomplete surgical resection (similarity-level cluster shade, inter-site similarity-level cluster prominence, and inter-site cluster variance) [82].

Rizzo et al. evaluated CT radiomics features in 101 patients, extracted from the primary tumor alone and combined with clinical data, showing that radiomic features related to mass size, randomness and homogeneity were associated with residual tumor at surgery [83], which still represents the most important feature for a complete cytoreduction and for prognosis.

Meier et al. assessed associations between inter site texture heterogeneity parameters derived from CT, survival, and BRCA mutation status in 88 OC patients. They showed that high values of the three metrics used for the model were significantly associated with lower complete surgical resection status in BRCA-negative patients, but not in BRCA-positive patients, although the model was not able to distinguish the presence or absence of BRCA mutation [84].

More recently, studies based on MRI are underway in evaluating radiomic features in OC. To this end, Yu et al. assessed MR radiomic features in 86 patients with OC with the aim of predicting the peritoneal carcinomatosis. The authors showed that the radiomics nomogram constructed by combining radiomics characteristics and clinicopathological risk factors showed a better diagnostic effect than the clinical model and the radiomics model alone [85]. Likewise, in a recent study, Song et al. generated a radiomic signature based on MRI features to predict the presence of peritoneal carcinomatosis before surgery in 89 patients. The nomogram, comprising the radiomics signature (based on six features), pelvic fluid, and CA-125 level, showed the best discrimination with an AUC of 0.969 in the training cohort and 0.944 in the validation cohort [86].

Although there is strong interest in radiomics for the prediction of peritoneal carcinomatosis and prognosis in OC patients, there are currently many tools based on artificial intelligence that do not include imaging data, thus showing the gap that still exists in this field. In the future, more precise descriptions of the methods and integration of multi-omics models may lead to an out-performance of single-omic datasets [87], offering adjunctive help for prognostication and treatment planning for OC patients (Table 4).

Table 4. Radiomics study results.

	Author	Title	Patients	Results
1	Vargas HA, et al. (2018) [81]	Radiogenomics of High-Grade Serous Ovarian Cancer: Multireader Multi-Institutional Study from the Cancer Genome Atlas Ovarian Cancer Imaging Research Group	92	Combinations of imaging features contained predictive signal for time to progression and CLOVAR profile. Interobserver agreement was strong for some features, but could be improved for others.
2	Vargas HA, et al. (2017) [82]	A novel representation of inter-site tumour heterogeneity from pre-treatment computed tomography textures classifies ovarian cancers by clinical outcome	38	Of the 12 inter-site texture heterogeneity metrics evaluated, those capturing the differences in texture similarities across sites were associated with shorter overall survival and incomplete surgical resection.
3	Rizzo S et al. (2018) [77]	Radiomics of high-grade serous ovarian cancer: association between quantitative CT features, residual tumour and disease progression within 12 months.	101	This study found significant associations between radiomic features and prognostic factors, such as residual tumour and progressive disease at 12 months

Table 4. Cont.

	Author	Title	Patients	Results
4	Meier A et al. (2019) [84]	Association between CT-texture-derived tumor heterogeneity, outcomes, and BRCA mutation status in patients with high-grade serous ovarian cancer.	88	Higher inter-site cluster variance was associated with lower PFS ($p = 0.006$) and OS ($p = 0.003$). Higher inter-site cluster prominence was associated with lower PFS ($p = 0.02$) and higher inter-site cluster entropy (SE) correlated with lower OS ($p = 0.01$). High values of the three metrics were significantly associated with lower complete surgical resection status in BRCA-negative patients
5	Yu XY et al. (2021) [85]	Multiparameter MRI Radiomics Model Predicts Preoperative Peritoneal Carcinomatosis in Ovarian Cancer	88	The radiomics model from the multiparametric-MRI combined sequence showed a higher area under the curve than the model from FS-T2WI, DWI, and DCE-MRI alone. A radiomics nomogram constructed by combining radiomics features and clinicopathological risk factors showed a better diagnostic effect than the clinical model and the radiomics model.
6	Song XL et al. (2021) [86]	Radiomics based on multisequence magnetic resonance imaging for the preoperative prediction of peritoneal metastasis in ovarian cancer.	89	The radiomics signature generated by 6 selected features showed a favorable discriminatory ability to predict peritoneal metastases. The nomogram, comprising the radiomics signature, pelvic fluid, and CA-125 level, showed more favorable discrimination.

9. Conclusions

The high aggressiveness of OC leads to frequent peritoneal dissemination. Utilizing various imaging techniques, including CT, MRI, and PET-CT, plays a crucial role in guiding the diagnostic workflow for patients due to their sensitivity and specificity in identifying various morphological patterns and disease spread pathways. Disease staging systems like PCI and its derivatives establish a threshold for directing treatment decisions and assessing prognosis in patients. Radiomics may serve a significant role in identifying suitable candidates for surgical treatment and predicting optimal cytoreduction. Moreover, it has the potential to aid in prospective risk stratification for PC, showing promise as a valuable addition, though further research in this area is currently required.

Author Contributions: Conceptualization: S.M.R.R., F.M. and P.R.; Methodology: I.P. and F.T.; Writing—Original draft: V.M., M.G., A.C. and D.L.; Resources: F.C., S.R. and R.N.; Writing—Review and Editing: L.M. and F.T.; Supervision: L.M. and C.C. All authors have read and agreed to the published version of the manuscript.

Funding: This research received no external funding.

Conflicts of Interest: The authors declare no conflict of interest.

Abbreviations

CI: confidence interval; CCR: complete cytoreduction; CM: Contrast medium; CRS: cytoreductive surgery; CT: Computed tomography; HR: hazard ratio; HTL: high tumor load; IDS: interval debulking surgery; ITL: intermediate tumor load; LTL: low tumor load; MDCT: Multi Detector Computed Tomography; MPR: multiplanar image reconstructions; MRI: Magnetic resonance imaging, NACT: neoadjuvant chemotherapy; OC: ovarian cancer OS: overall survival; PC: peritoneal carcinomatosis, PCI: Peritoneal Cancer Index; PET-CT: Positron emission tomography-Computed tomography; PFS: progression-free survival; PIV: predictive index value; RT: residual tumor; WB-DW-MRI: whole-body diffusion-weighted MRI.

References

1. Jemal, A.; Tiwari, R.; Murray, T.; Ghafoor, A.; Samuels, A.; Ward, E.; Feuer, E.; Feuer, M. Cancer statistics, 2004. *CA Cancer J. Clin.* **2004**, *54*, 8–29. [CrossRef] [PubMed]
2. Munkarah, A.R.; Coleman, R.L. Critical evaluation of secondary cytoreduction in recurrent ovarian cancer. *Gynecol. Oncol.* **2004**, *95*, 273–280. [CrossRef] [PubMed]
3. Lheureux, S.; Braunstein, M.; Oza, A. Epithelial ovarian cancer: Evolution of management in the era of precision medicine. *CA Cancer J. Clin.* **2019**, *69*, 280–304. [CrossRef]
4. Iafrate, F.; Ciolina, M.; Sammartino, P.; Baldassari, P.; Rengo, M.; Lucchesi, P.; Sibio, S.; Accarpio, F.; Di Giorgio, A.; Laghi, A. Peritoneal carcinomatosis: Imaging with 64-MDCT and 3T MRI with diffusion-weighted imaging. *Abdom. Imaging* **2012**, *37*, 616–627. [CrossRef] [PubMed]
5. Fagotti, A.; Gallotta, V.; Romano, F.; Fanfani, F.; Rossitto, C.; Naldini, A.; Vigliotta, M.; Scambia, G. Peritoneal carcinosis of ovarian origin. *World J. Gastrointest. Oncol.* **2010**, *2*, 102–108. [CrossRef] [PubMed]
6. Winter, W.E.; Maxwell, G.L.; Tian, C.; Carlson, J.W.; Ozols, R.F.; Rose, P.G.; Markman, M.; Armstrong, D.K.; Muggia, F. Gynecologic Oncology Group Study. Prognostic factors for stage III epithelial ovarian cancer: A Gynecologic Oncology Group Study. *J. Clin. Oncol. Off. J. Am. Soc. Clin. Oncol.* **2007**, *25*, 3621–3627. [CrossRef] [PubMed]
7. Nougaret, S.; Sadowski, E.; Lakhman, Y.; Rousset, P.; Lahaye, M.; Worley, M.; Sgarbura, O.; Shinagare, A.B. The BUMPy road of peritoneal metastases in ovarian cancer. *Diagn. Interv. Imaging* **2022**, *103*, 448–459. [CrossRef] [PubMed]
8. Armstrong, D.K.; Bundy, B.; Wenzel, L.; Huang, H.Q.; Baergen, R.; Lele, S.; Copeland, L.J.; Walker, J.L.; Burger, R.A.; Gynecologic Oncology Group. Intraperitoneal cisplatin and paclitaxel in ovarian cancer. *N. Engl. J. Med.* **2006**, *354*, 34–43. [CrossRef]
9. Reginelli, A.; Giacobbe, G.; Del Canto, M.T.; Alessandrella, M.; Balestrucci, G.; Urraro, F.; Russo, G.M.; Gallo, L.; Danti, G.; Miele, V. Peritoneal Carcinosis: What the Radiologist Needs to Know. *Diagnostics* **2023**, *13*, 1974. [CrossRef]
10. Rodolfino, E.; Devicienti, E.; Miccò, M.; Del Ciello, A.; Di Giovanni, S.E.; Giuliani, M.; Conte, C.; Gui, B.; Valentini, A.L.; Bonomo, L. Diagnostic accuracy of MDCT in the evaluation of patients with peritoneal carcinomatosis from ovarian cancer: Is delayed enhanced phase really effective? *Eur. Rev. Med. Pharmacol. Sci.* **2016**, *20*, 4426–4434.
11. Forstner, R.; Hricak, H.; Occhipinti, K.A.; Powell, C.B.; Frankel, S.D.; Stern, J.L. Ovarian cancer: Staging with CT and MR imaging. *Radiology* **1995**, *197*, 619–626. [CrossRef] [PubMed]
12. Coakley, F.V.; Choi, P.H.; Gougoutas, C.A.; Pothuri, B.; Venkatraman, E.; Chi, D.; Bergman, A.; Hricak, H. Peritoneal metastases: Detection with spiral CT in patients with ovarian cancer. *Radiology* **2002**, *223*, 495–499. [CrossRef] [PubMed]
13. Funicelli, L.; Travaini, L.L.; Landoni, F.; Trifirò, G.; Bonello, L.; Bellomi, M. Peritoneal carcinomatosis from ovarian cancer: The role of CT and [^{18}F]FDG-PET/CT. *Abdom. Imaging* **2010**, *35*, 701–707. [CrossRef] [PubMed]
14. Colombo, N.; Sessa, C.; du Bois, A.; Ledermann, J.; McCluggage, W.G.; McNeish, I.; Morice, P.; Pignata, S.; Ray-Coquard, I.; ESMO-ESGO Ovarian Cancer Consensus Conference Working Group. ESMO-ESGO consensus conference recommendations on ovarian cancer: Pathology and molecular biology, early and advanced stages, borderline tumours and recurrent disease†. *Ann. Oncol. Off. J. Eur. Soc. Med. Oncol.* **2019**, *30*, 672–705. [CrossRef]
15. Shashikant, L.; Kesterson Joshua, P. In Pursuit of Optimal Cytoreduction in Ovarian Cancer Patients: The Role of Surgery and Surgeon. *J. Obstet. Gynaecol. India* **2009**, *59*, 209–216.
16. du Bois, A.; Reuss, A.; Pujade-Lauraine, E.; Harter, P.; Ray-Coquard, I.; Pfisterer, J. Role of surgical outcome as prognostic factor in advanced epithelial ovarian cancer: A combined exploratory analysis of 3 prospectively randomized phase 3 multicenter trials: By the Arbeitsgemeinschaft Gynaekologische Onkologie Studiengruppe Ovarialkarzinom (AGO-OVAR) and the Groupe d'Investigateurs Nationaux Pour les Etudes des Cancers de l'Ovaire (GINECO). *Cancer* **2009**, *115*, 1234–1244. [CrossRef]
17. Bristow, R.; Tomacruz, R.; Armstrong, D.; Trimble, E.; Montz, F. Survival Effect of Maximal Cytoreductive Surgery for Advanced Ovarian Carcinoma During the Platinum Era: A Meta-Analysis. *J. Clin. Oncol. Off. J. Am. Soc. Clin. Oncol.* **2023**, *41*, 4065–4076. [CrossRef]
18. Vergote, I.; Tropé, C.G.; Amant, F.; Kristensen, G.B.; Ehlen, T.; Johnson, N.; Verheijen, R.H.M.; Burg, M.E.L.; van der Lacave, A.J.; NCIC Clinical Trials Group. Neoadjuvant chemotherapy or primary surgery in stage IIIC or IV ovarian cancer. *N. Engl. J. Med.* **2010**, *363*, 943–953. [CrossRef]
19. Kehoe, S.; Hook, J.; Nankivell, M.; Jayson, G.C.; Kitchener, H.; Lopes, T.; Luesley, D.; Perren, T.; Bannoo, S.; Swart, A.M. Primary chemotherapy versus primary surgery for newly diagnosed advanced ovarian cancer (CHORUS): An open-label, randomised, controlled, non-inferiority trial. *Lancet* **2015**, *386*, 249–257. [CrossRef]
20. Fagotti, A.; Ferrandina, G.; Fanfani, F.; Ercoli, A.; Lorusso, D.; Rossi, M.; Scambia, G. A laparoscopy-based score to predict surgical outcome in patients with advanced ovarian carcinoma: A pilot study. *Ann. Surg. Oncol.* **2006**, *13*, 1156–1161. [CrossRef]
21. Fagotti, A.; Ferrandina, G.; Fanfani, F.; Garganese, G.; Vizzielli, G.; Carone, V.; Salerno, M.G.; Scambia, G. Prospective validation of a laparoscopic predictive model for optimal cytoreduction in advanced ovarian carcinoma. *Am. J. Obstet. Gynecol.* **2008**, *199*, e1–e6. [CrossRef] [PubMed]
22. Vizzielli, G.; Costantini, B.; Tortorella, L.; Petrillo, M.; Fanfani, F.; Chiantera, V.; Ercoli, A.; Iodice, R.; Scambia, G.; Fagotti, A. Influence of intraperitoneal dissemination assessed by laparoscopy on prognosis of advanced ovarian cancer: An exploratory analysis of a single-institution experience. *Ann. Surg. Oncol.* **2014**, *21*, 3970–3977. [CrossRef] [PubMed]

23. Fagotti, A.; Vizzielli, G.; De Iaco, P.; Surico, D.; Buda, A.; Mandato, V.D.; Petruzzelli, F.; Ghezzi, F.; Garzarelli, S.; Scambia, G. A multicentric trial (Olympia-MITO 13) on the accuracy of laparoscopy to assess peritoneal spread in ovarian cancer. *Am. J. Obstet. Gynecol.* **2013**, *209*, 462.e1–462.e11. [CrossRef] [PubMed]
24. Fagotti, A.; Ferrandina, G.; Vizzielli, G.; Fanfani, F.; Gallotta, V.; Chiantera, V.; Costantini, B.; Margariti, P.A.; Gueli Alletti, S.; Scambia, G. Phase III randomised clinical trial comparing primary surgery versus neoadjuvant chemotherapy in advanced epithelial ovarian cancer with high tumour load (SCORPION trial): Final analysis of peri-operative outcome. *Eur. J. Cancer* **2016**, *59*, 22–33. [CrossRef] [PubMed]
25. El-Agwany, A.S. Laparoscopy and Computed Tomography Imaging in Advanced Ovarian Tumors: A Roadmap for Prediction of Optimal Cytoreductive Surgery. *Gynecol. Minim. Invasive Ther.* **2018**, *7*, 66–69. [CrossRef] [PubMed]
26. Hanna, D.N.; Ghani, M.O.; Hermina, A.; Mina, A.; Bailey, C.E.; Idrees, K.; Magge, D. Diagnostic Laparoscopy in Patients with Peritoneal Carcinomatosis Is Safe and Does Not Delay Cytoreductive Surgery with Hyperthermic Intraperitoneal Chemotherapy. *Am. Surg.* **2022**, *88*, 698–703. [CrossRef]
27. Bristow, R.E.; Duska, L.R.; Lambrou, N.C.; Fishman, E.K.; O'Neill, M.J.; Trimble, E.L.; Montz, F.J. A model for predicting surgical outcome in patients with advanced ovarian carcinoma using computed tomography. *Cancer* **2000**, *89*, 1532–1540. [CrossRef]
28. Gerestein, C.G.; Eijkemans, M.J.; Bakker, J.; Elgersma, O.E.; Burg, M.E.L.V.D.; Kooi, G.S.; Burger, C.W. Nomogram for Suboptimal Cytoreduction at Primary Surgery for Advanced Stage Ovarian Cancer. *Anticancer Res.* **2011**, *31*, 4043–4049.
29. Pinto, P.; Burgetova, A.; Cibula, D.; Haldorsen, I.S.; Indrielle-Kelly, T.; Fischerova, D. Prediction of Surgical Outcome in Advanced Ovarian Cancer by Imaging and Laparoscopy: A Narrative Review. *Cancers* **2023**, *15*, 1904. [CrossRef]
30. Feng, Z.; Wen, H.; Jiang, Z.; Liu, S.; Ju, X.; Chen, X.; Xia, L.; Xu, J.; Bi, R.; Wu, X. A triage strategy in advanced ovarian cancer management based on multiple predictive models for R0 resection: A prospective cohort study. *J. Gynecol. Oncol.* **2018**, *29*, e65. [CrossRef]
31. Avesani Arshad, M.; Lu, H.; Fotopoulou, C.; Cannone, F.; Melotti, R.; Aboagye, E.; Rockall, A. Radiological assessment of Peritoneal Cancer Index on preoperative CT in ovarian cancer is related to surgical outcome and survival. *La Radiol. Med.* **2020**, *125*, 770–776. [CrossRef] [PubMed]
32. Elsherif, S.B.; Zheng, S.; Ganeshan, D.; Iyer, R.; Wei, W.; Bhosale, P.R. Does dual-energy CT differentiate benign and malignant ovarian tumours? *Clin. Radiol.* **2020**, *75*, 606–614. [CrossRef] [PubMed]
33. Benveniste, A.P.; de Castro Faria, S.; Broering, G.; Ganeshan, D.M.; Tamm, E.P.; Iyer, R.B.; Bhosale, P. Potential Application of Dual-Energy CT in Gynecologic Cancer: Initial Experience. *Am. J. Roentgenol.* **2017**, *208*, 695–705. [CrossRef] [PubMed]
34. Lorusso, D.; Sarno, I.; Di Donato, V.; Palazzo, A.; Torrisi, E.; Pala, L.; Marchiano, A.; Raspagliesi, F. Is postoperative computed tomography evaluation a prognostic indicator in patients with optimally debulked advanced ovarian cancer? *Oncology* **2014**, *87*, 293–299. [CrossRef]
35. Heitz, F.; Harter, P.; Åvall-Lundqvist, E.; Reuss, A.; Pautier, P.; Cormio, G.; Colombo, N.; Reinthaller, A.; Vergote, I.; de Bois, A. Early tumor regrowth is a contributor to impaired survival in patients with completely resected advanced ovarian cancer. An exploratory analysis of the Intergroup trial AGO-OVAR 12. *Gynecol. Oncol.* **2019**, *152*, 235–242. [CrossRef]
36. Kang, S.; Reinhold, C.; Atri, M.; Benson, C.; Bhosale, P.; Jhingran, A.; Lakhman, Y.; Maturen, K.; Nicola, R.P.G. ACR Appropriateness Criteria®Staging and Follow-Up of Ovarian Cancer. *J. Am. Coll. Radiol. JACR* **2018**, *15*, S198–S207. [CrossRef]
37. Kose, S. Role of Computed Tomography in the Evaluation of Peritoneal Carcinomatosis. *J. Belg. Soc. Radiol.* **2023**, *107*, 1–27. [CrossRef] [PubMed]
38. Nougaret, S.; Addley, H.; Colombo, P.; Fujii, S.; Ss, S.; Tirumani, S.; Jardon, K.; Sala, E.; Reinhold, R. Ovarian carcinomatosis: How the radiologist can help plan the surgical approach. *Radiogr. A Rev. Publ. Radiol. Soc. N. Am. Inc.* **2012**, *32*, 775–800. [CrossRef]
39. Tempany, C.; Zou, K.; Silverman, S.; Brown, D.; Kurtz, A.; McNeil, B. Staging of advanced ovarian cancer: Comparison of imaging modalities--report from the Radiological Diagnostic Oncology Group. *Radiology* **2000**, *215*, 761–767. [CrossRef]
40. Pfannenberg, C.; Königsrainer, I.; Aschoff, P.; Oksüz, M.; Zieker, D.; Beckert, S.; Symons, S.; Nieselt, K.; Glatzle, J.; Königsrainer, A. (18)F-FDG-PET/CT to select patients with peritoneal carcinomatosis for cytoreductive surgery and hyperthermic intraperitoneal chemotherapy. *Ann. Surg. Oncol.* **2009**, *16*, 1295–1303. [CrossRef]
41. Qayyum, A.; Coakley, F.V.; Westphalen, A.C.; Hricak, H.; Okuno, W.T.; Powell, B. Role of CT and MR imaging in predicting optimal cytoreduction of newly diagnosed primary epithelial ovarian cancer. *Gynecol. Oncol.* **2005**, *96*, 301–306. [CrossRef] [PubMed]
42. de Bree, E.; Koops, W.; Kröger, R.; van Ruth, S.; Witkamp, A.J.; Zoetmulder, F. Peritoneal carcinomatosis from colorectal or appendiceal origin: Correlation of preoperative CT with intraoperative findings and evaluation of interobserver agreement. *J. Surg. Oncol.* **2004**, *86*, 64–73. [CrossRef] [PubMed]
43. Mazzei, M.A.; Khader, L.; Cirigliano, A.; Cioffi Squitieri, N.; Guerrini, S.; Forzoni, B.; Marrelli, D.; Roviello, F.; Mazzei, F.G.; Volterrani, L. Accuracy of MDCT in the preoperative definition of Peritoneal Cancer Index (PCI) in patients with advanced ovarian cancer who underwent peritonectomy and hyperthermic intraperitoneal chemotherapy (HIPEC). *Abdom. Imaging* **2013**, *38*, 1422–1430. [CrossRef] [PubMed]
44. Choi, H.J.; Lim, M.C.; Bae, J.; Cho, K.S.; Jung, D.C.; Kang, S.; Yoo, C.W.; Seo, S.S.; Park, S.Y. Region-based diagnostic performance of multidetector CT for detecting peritoneal seeding in ovarian cancer patients. *Arch. Gynecol. Obstet.* **2011**, *283*, 353–360. [CrossRef]

45. Low, R.N. Diffusion-Weighted MR Imaging for Whole Body Metastatic Disease and Lymphadenopathy. *Magn. Reson. Imaging Clin. N. Am.* **2009**, *17*, 245–261. [CrossRef] [PubMed]
46. Fujii, S.; Matsusue, E.; Kanasaki, Y.; Kanamori, Y.; Nakanishi, J.; Sugihara, S.; Kigawa, J.; Terakawa, N.; Ogawa, T. Detection of peritoneal dissemination in gynecological malignancy: Evaluation by diffusion-weighted MR imaging. *Eur. Radiol.* **2008**, *18*, 18–23. [CrossRef]
47. Yu, X.; Lee, E.Y.P.; Lai, V.; Chan, Q. Correlation between tissue metabolism and cellularity assessed by standardized uptake value and apparent diffusion coefficient in peritoneal metastasis. *J. Magn. Reson. Imaging JMRI* **2014**, *40*, 99–105. [CrossRef]
48. Low, R.N.; Barone, R.M.; Lucero, J. Comparison of MRI and CT for predicting the Peritoneal Cancer Index (PCI) preoperatively in patients being considered for cytoreductive surgical procedures. *Ann. Surg. Oncol.* **2015**, *22*, 1708–1715. [CrossRef]
49. Bozkurt, M.; Doganay, S.; Kantarci, M.; Yalcin, A.; Eren, S.; Atamanalp, S.S.; Yuce, I.; Yildirgan, M.I. Comparison of peritoneal tumor imaging using conventional MR imaging and diffusion-weighted MR imaging with different b values. *Eur. J. Radiol.* **2011**, *80*, 224–228. [CrossRef]
50. Low, R.N.; Barone, R.M.; Lacey, C.; Sigeti, J.S.; Alzate, G.D.; Sebrechts, C.P. Peritoneal tumor: MR imaging with dilute oral barium and intravenous gadolinium-containing contrast agents compared with unenhanced MR imaging and CT. *Radiology* **1997**, *204*, 513–520. [CrossRef]
51. Ricke, J.; Sehouli, J.; Hach, C.; Hänninen, E.L.; Lichtenegger, W.; Felix, R. Prospective evaluation of contrast-enhanced MRI in the depiction of peritoneal spread in primary or recurrent ovarian cancer. *Eur. Radiol.* **2003**, *13*, 943–949. [CrossRef]
52. Rizzo, S.; De Piano, F.; Buscarino, V.; Pagan, E.; Bagnardi, V.; Zanagnolo, V.; Colombo, N.; Maggioni, A.; Del Grande, M.; Aletti, G. Pre-operative evaluation of epithelial ovarian cancer patients: Role of whole body diffusion weighted imaging MR and CT scans in the selection of patients suitable for primary debulking surgery. A single-centre study. *Eur. J. Radiol.* **2020**, *123*, 108786. [CrossRef] [PubMed]
53. Michielsen, K.; Vergote, I.; Op de Beeck, K.; Amant, F.; Leunen, K.; Moerman, P.; Deroose, C.; Souverijns, G.; Dymarkowski, S.; Vandecaveye, V. Whole-body MRI with diffusion-weighted sequence for staging of patients with suspected ovarian cancer: A clinical feasibility study in comparison to CT and FDG-PET/CT. *Eur. Radiol.* **2014**, *24*, 889–901. [CrossRef] [PubMed]
54. Fischerova, D.; Pinto, P.; Burgetova, A.; Masek, M.; Slama, J.; Kocian, R.; Frühauf, F.; Zikan, M.; Dusek, L.; Cibula, D. Preoperative staging of ovarian cancer: Comparison between ultrasound, CT and whole-body diffusion-weighted MRI (ISAAC study). *Ultrasound Obstet. Gynecol.* **2022**, *59*, 248–262. [CrossRef] [PubMed]
55. Ledermann, J.A.; Raja, F.A.; Fotopoulou, C.; Gonzalez-Martin, A.; Colombo, N.; Sessa, C. ESMO Guidelines Working Group. Newly diagnosed and relapsed epithelial ovarian carcinoma: ESMO Clinical Practice Guidelines for diagnosis, treatment and follow-up. *Ann. Oncol. Off. J. Eur. Soc. Med. Oncol.* **2013**, *24* (Suppl. S6), vi24–vi32. [CrossRef]
56. Pannu, H.K.; Bristow, R.E.; Cohade, C.; Fishman, E.K.; Wahl, R.L. PET-CT in recurrent ovarian cancer: Initial observations. *Radiogr. A Rev. Publ. Radiol. Soc. N. Am. Inc* **2004**, *24*, 209–223. [CrossRef] [PubMed]
57. Anthony, M.P.; Khong, P.L.; Zhang, J. Spectrum of (18)F-FDG PET/CT appearances in peritoneal disease. *AJR. Am. J. Roentgenol.* **2009**, *193*, W523–W529. [CrossRef]
58. Kim, H.W.; Won, K.S.; Zeon, S.K.; Ahn, B.C.; Gayed, I.W. Peritoneal carcinomatosis in patients with ovarian cancer: Enhanced CT versus 18F-FDG PET/CT. *Clin. Nucl. Med.* **2013**, *38*, 93–97. [CrossRef]
59. Lopez-Lopez, V.; Cascales-Campos, P.A.; Gil, J.; Frutos, L.; Andrade, R.J.; Fuster-Quiñonero, M.; Feliciangeli, E.; Gil, E.; Parrilla, P. Use of (18)F-FDG PET/CT in the preoperative evaluation of patients diagnosed with peritoneal carcinomatosis of ovarian origin, candidates to cytoreduction and hipec. A pending issue. *Eur. J. Radiol.* **2016**, *85*, 1824–1828. [CrossRef]
60. Jónsdóttir, B.; Ripoll, M.A.; Bergman, A.; Silins, I.; Poromaa, I.S.; Ahlström, H.; Stålberg, K. Validation of 18F-FDG PET/MRI and diffusion-weighted MRI for estimating the extent of peritoneal carcinomatosis in ovarian and endometrial cancer -a pilot study. *Cancer Imaging Off. Publ. Int. Cancer Imaging Soc.* **2021**, *21*, 34. [CrossRef]
61. Fiaschetti, V.; Calabria, F.; Crusco, S.; Meschini, A.; Nucera, F.; Schillaci, O.; Simonetti, G. MR-PET fusion imaging in evaluating adnexal lesions: A preliminary study. *La Radiol. Med.* **2011**, *116*, 1288–1302. [CrossRef] [PubMed]
62. Forstner, R. Radiological staging of ovarian cancer: Imaging findings and contribution of CT and MRI. *Eur. Radiol.* **2007**, *17*, 3223–3235. [CrossRef] [PubMed]
63. Purbadi, S.; Anggraeni, T.; Vitria, A. Early stage epithelial ovarian cancer metastasis through peritoneal fluid circulation. *J. Ovarian Res.* **2021**, *14*, 1–5. [CrossRef] [PubMed]
64. Le, O. Patterns of peritoneal spread of tumor in the abdomen and pelvis. *World J. Radiol.* **2013**, *5*, 106–112. [CrossRef] [PubMed]
65. Bailly, C.; Bailly-Glatre, A.; Alfidja, A.; Vincent, C.; Dauplat, J.; Pomel, C. Peritoneal carcinosis in ovarian cancer: Conventional imaging (CT-scan and MRI. *Bull. Du Cancer* **2009**, *96*, 1155–1162. [CrossRef]
66. Agarwal, A.; Yeh, B.; Breiman, R.; Qayyum, A.; Coakley, F. Peritoneal calcification: Causes and distinguishing features on CT. *AJR. Am. J. Roentgenol.* **2004**, *182*, 441–445. [CrossRef]
67. Kawamoto, S.; Urban, B.; Fishman, E. CT of epithelial ovarian tumors. *Radiogr. A Rev. Publ. Radiol. Soc. N. Am. Inc* **1999**, *19*, S85–S102. [CrossRef] [PubMed]
68. Pannu, H.K.; Bristow, R.E.; Montz, F.J.; Fishman, E.K. Multidetector CT of peritoneal carcinomatosis from ovarian cancer. *Radiogr. A Rev. Publ. Radiol. Soc. N. Am. Inc.* **2003**, *23*, 687–701. [CrossRef]

69. Brasanac, D.; Boricic, I.; Todorovic, V.; Basta-Jovanovic, G. Umbilical metastasis (Sister Joseph's nodule) as a first sign of a disseminated ovarian carcinoma: Comparative immunohistochemical analysis of primary tumor and its metastases. *Int. J. Gynecol. Cancer Off. J. Int. Gynecol. Cancer Soc.* **2005**, *15*, 377–381. [CrossRef]
70. Jacquet, P.; Sugarbaker, P. Clinical research methodologies in diagnosis and staging of patients with peritoneal carcinomatosis. *Cancer Treat. Res.* **1996**, *82*, 359–374. [CrossRef]
71. Tentes, A.A.K.; Tripsiannis, G.; Markakidis, S.K.; Karanikiotis, C.N.; Tzegas, G.; Georgiadis, G.; Avgidou, K. Peritoneal cancer index: A prognostic indicator of survival in advanced ovarian cancer. *Eur. J. Surg. Oncol. J. Eur. Soc. Surg. Oncol. Br. Assoc. Surg. Oncol.* **2003**, *29*, 69–73. [CrossRef] [PubMed]
72. Rosendahl, M.; Harter, P.; Bjørn, S.F.; Høgdall, C. Specific Regions, Rather than the Entire Peritoneal Carcinosis Index, are Predictive of Complete Resection and Survival in Advanced Epithelial Ovarian Cancer. *Int. J. Gynecol. Cancer Off. J. Int. Gynecol. Cancer Soc.* **2018**, *28*, 316–322. [CrossRef] [PubMed]
73. Iavazzo, C.; Fotiou, A.; Psomiadou, V.; Lekka, S.; Katsanos, D.; Spiliotis, J. Small Bowel PCI Score as a Prognostic Factor of Ovarian Cancer Patients Undergoing Cytoreductive Surgery (CRS) with Hyperthermic Intraperitoneal Chemotherapy (HIPEC), a Retrospective Analysis of 130 Patients. *Indian J. Surg. Oncol.* **2021**, *12*, 258–265. [CrossRef] [PubMed]
74. Goswami, G.; Kammar, P.; Mangal, R.; Shaikh, S.; Patel, M.D.; Bhatt, A. Accuracy of CT Scan in Predicting the Surgical PCI in Patients Undergoing Cytoreductive Surgery with/without HIPEC-a Prospective Single Institution Study. *Indian J. Surg. Oncol.* **2019**, *10*, 296–302. [CrossRef] [PubMed]
75. Mikkelsen, M.S.; Petersen, L.K.; Blaakaer, J.; Marinovskij, E.; Rosenkilde, M.; Andersen, G.; Bouchelouche, K.; Iversen, L.H. Assessment of peritoneal metastases with DW-MRI, CT, and FDG PET/CT before cytoreductive surgery for advanced stage epithelial ovarian cancer. *Eur. J. Surg. Oncol. J. Eur. Soc. Surg. Oncol. Br. Assoc. Surg. Oncol.* **2021**, *47*, 2134–2141. [CrossRef] [PubMed]
76. Lomnytska, M.; Karlsson, E.; Jonsdottir, B.; Lejon, A.M.; Stålberg, K.; Poromaa, I.S.; Silins, I.; Graf, W. Peritoneal cancer index predicts severe complications after ovarian cancer surgery. *Eur. J. Surg. Oncol. J. Eur. Soc. Surg. Oncol. Br. Assoc. Surg. Oncol.* **2021**, *47*, 2915–2924. [CrossRef] [PubMed]
77. Rizzo, S.; Botta, F.; Raimondi, S.; Origgi, D.; Fanciullo, C.; Morganti, A.G.; Bellomi, M. Radiomics: The facts and the challenges of image analysis. *Eur. Radiol. Exp.* **2018**, *2*, 36. [CrossRef] [PubMed]
78. Jong, E.E.C.; de Elmpt, W.; van Rizzo, S.; Colarieti, A.; Spitaleri, G.; Leijenaar, R.T.H.; Jochems, A.; Hendriks, L.E.L.; Troost, E.G.C.; Lambin, P. Applicability of a prognostic CT-based radiomic signature model trained on stage I-III non-small cell lung cancer in stage IV non-small cell lung cancer. *Lung Cancer* **2018**, *124*, 6–11. [CrossRef]
79. Chianca, V.; Albano, D.; Messina, C.; Vincenzo, G.; Rizzo, S.; Del Grande, F.; Sconfienza, L.M. An update in musculoskeletal tumors: From quantitative imaging to radiomics. *La Radiol. Med.* **2021**, *126*, 1095–1105. [CrossRef]
80. Nougaret, S.; McCague, C.; Tibermacine, H.; Vargas, H.A.; Rizzo, S.; Sala, E. Radiomics and radiogenomics in ovarian cancer: A literature review. *Abdom. Radiol.* **2021**, *46*, 2308–2322. [CrossRef]
81. Vargas, H.A.; Huang, E.P.; Lakhman, Y.; Ippolito, J.E.; Bhosale, P.; Mellnick, V.; Shinagare, A.B.; Anello, M.; Kirby, J.; Sala, E. Radiogenomics of High-Grade Serous Ovarian Cancer: Multireader Multi-Institutional Study from the Cancer Genome Atlas Ovarian Cancer Imaging Research Group. *Radiology* **2017**, *285*, 482–492. [CrossRef] [PubMed]
82. Vargas, H.A.; Veeraraghavan, H.; Micco, M.; Nougaret, S.; Lakhman, Y.; Meier, A.A.; Sosa, R.; Soslow, R.A.; Levine, D.A.; Sala, E. A novel representation of inter-site tumour heterogeneity from pre-treatment computed tomography textures classifies ovarian cancers by clinical outcome. *Eur. Radiol.* **2017**, *27*, 3991–4001. [CrossRef] [PubMed]
83. Rizzo, S.; Botta, F.; Raimondi, S.; Origgi, D.; Buscarino, V.; Colarieti, A.; Tomao, F.; Aletti, G.; Zanagnolo, V.; Bellomi, M. Radiomics of high-grade serous ovarian cancer: Association between quantitative CT features, residual tumour and disease progression within 12 months. *Eur. Radiol.* **2018**, *28*, 4849–4859. [CrossRef] [PubMed]
84. Meier, A.; Veeraraghavan, H.; Nougaret, S.; Lakhman, Y.; Sosa, R.; Soslow, R.A.; Sutton, E.J.; Hricak, H.; Sala, E.; Vargas, H.A. Association between CT-texture-derived tumor heterogeneity, outcomes, and BRCA mutation status in patients with high-grade serous ovarian cancer. *Abdom. Radiol.* **2019**, *44*, 2040–2047. [CrossRef] [PubMed]
85. Yu, X.Y.; Ren, J.; Jia, Y.; Wu, H.; Niu, G.; Liu, A.; Gao, Y.; Hao, F.; Xie, L. Multiparameter MRI Radiomics Model Predicts Preoperative Peritoneal Carcinomatosis in Ovarian Cancer. *Front. Oncol.* **2021**, *11*, 765652. [CrossRef]
86. Song, X.L.; Ren, J.L.; Yao, T.Y.; Zhao, D.; Niu, J. Radiomics based on multisequence magnetic resonance imaging for the preoperative prediction of peritoneal metastasis in ovarian cancer. *Eur. Radiol.* **2021**, *31*, 8438–8446. [CrossRef]
87. Hatamikia, S.; Nougaret, S.; Panico, C.; Avesani, G.; Nero, C.; Boldrini, L.; Sala, E.; Woitek, R. Ovarian cancer beyond imaging: Integration of AI and multiomics biomarkers. *Eur. Radiol. Exp.* **2023**, *7*, 50. [CrossRef]

Disclaimer/Publisher's Note: The statements, opinions and data contained in all publications are solely those of the individual author(s) and contributor(s) and not of MDPI and/or the editor(s). MDPI and/or the editor(s) disclaim responsibility for any injury to people or property resulting from any ideas, methods, instructions or products referred to in the content.

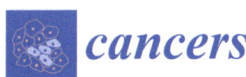

Article

Performance of MRI for Detection of ≥pT1b Disease in Local Staging of Endometrial Cancer

Leonie Van Vynckt [1], Philippe Tummers [2], Hannelore Denys [3], Menekse Göker [2], Sigi Hendrickx [4], Eline Naert [3], Rawand Salihi [2], Koen Van de Vijver [5], Gabriëlle H. van Ramshorst [6], Donatienne Van Weehaeghe [4], Katrien Vandecasteele [7], Geert M. Villeirs [4] and Pieter J. L. De Visschere [4,*]

1. Faculty of Medicine and Health Sciences, Ghent University, 9000 Ghent, Belgium
2. Department of Obstetrics and Gynecology, Ghent University Hospital, 9000 Ghent, Belgium
3. Department of Medical Oncology, Ghent University Hospital, 9000 Ghent, Belgium
4. Department of Radiology and Nuclear Medicine, Ghent University Hospital, Corneel Heymanslaan 10, 9000 Ghent, Belgium
5. Department of Pathology, Ghent University Hospital, 9000 Ghent, Belgium
6. Department of Gastrointestinal Surgery, Ghent University Hospital, 9000 Ghent, Belgium
7. Department of Radiation Oncology, Ghent University Hospital, 9000 Ghent, Belgium
* Correspondence: pieter.devisschere@ugent.be; Tel.: +32-93322925

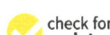

Citation: Van Vynckt, L.; Tummers, P.; Denys, H.; Göker, M.; Hendrickx, S.; Naert, E.; Salihi, R.; Van de Vijver, K.; van Ramshorst, G.H.; Van Weehaeghe, D.; et al. Performance of MRI for Detection of ≥pT1b Disease in Local Staging of Endometrial Cancer. Cancers 2024, 16, 1142. https://doi.org/10.3390/cancers16061142

Academic Editor: Athina C Tsili

Received: 19 January 2024
Revised: 11 March 2024
Accepted: 12 March 2024
Published: 13 March 2024

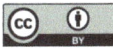

Copyright: © 2024 by the authors. Licensee MDPI, Basel, Switzerland. This article is an open access article distributed under the terms and conditions of the Creative Commons Attribution (CC BY) license (https://creativecommons.org/licenses/by/4.0/).

Simple Summary: Magnetic resonance imaging (MRI) can be used for the preoperative local staging of endometrial cancer (EC). The purpose of this study was to assess the performance of MRI for the detection of ≥pT1b disease (i.e., tumor invasion in ≥50% of the myometrium, into the cervical stroma or spread outside the uterus) and to evaluate whether tumor size measured via MRI was predictive for ≥pT1b disease, independent of imaging signs of invasion. We found that MRI had good performance for the detection of ≥pT1b disease and that a tumor diameter of ≥40 mm and a tumor volume of ≥20 mL were highly predictive for the presence of ≥pT1b disease. Our results support the use of MRI in the preoperative staging of EC and suggest including size criteria in EC staging guidelines.

Abstract: Magnetic resonance imaging (MRI) can be used for the preoperative local staging of endometrial cancer (EC). The presence of ≥pT1b disease (i.e., tumor invasion in ≥50% of the myometrium, into the cervical stroma or spread outside the uterus) has important prognostic value and implications for the decision to perform lymphadenectomy. The purpose of this study was to assess the performance of MRI for the detection of ≥pT1b disease and to evaluate whether tumor size measured via MRI was predictive for ≥pT1b disease, independent of imaging signs of deep invasion. MRI T-staging and tumor diameter and volume were correlated with histopathology of the hysterectomy specimen in 126 patients. MRI had a sensitivity, specificity, positive predictive value, negative predictive value and accuracy of 70.0%, 83.3%, 79.2%, 75.3% and 77.0%, respectively, for the detection of ≥pT1b disease. A tumor diameter of ≥40 mm and volume of ≥20 mL measured via MRI were predictive for ≥pT1b disease at rates of 78.3% and 87.1%, respectively. An EC size of at least 5 mm upon MRI was predictive for ≥pT1b disease in more than 50% of cases. Our results support the use of MRI in the preoperative staging of EC and suggest including size criteria in EC staging guidelines.

Keywords: endometrial cancer; magnetic resonance imaging; MRI; staging

1. Introduction

Endometrial cancer (EC) is the most common gynecological cancer in developed countries and the sixth most common cancer among women worldwide [1–3]. The incidence is increasing, presumably due to the rising prevalence of risk factors such as obesity and aging of the population [2–4]. There are many genetic factors associated with an increased risk for EC of which the most important is Lynch Syndrome [5,6]. Most patients with EC are postmenopausal women presenting with abnormal vaginal bleeding [3–5,7]. The first examination performed in the diagnostic work-up is a transvaginal ultrasound (TVU). Endometrial thickness greater than 4 mm in a postmenopausal woman is suspicious and warrants histopathological sampling to confirm the diagnosis of EC [8,9]. Historically, two types of EC were defined. Type I included the most common endometroid adenocarcinomas (80–85%), further divided into three grades (well, moderately and poorly differentiated). Type II (10–15%) included non-endometrioid types such as serous, clear cell and undifferentiated tumors with a relatively worse prognosis [1,3–7]. Based on new developments, a molecular classification has now replaced this traditional morphological classification. The International Federation of Gynaecology and Obstetrics (FIGO) guidelines were updated in 2023 and have increased focus on these newer molecular aspects [10]. In parallel, the TNM classification (UICC 8th edition of 2017) is used for the staging of EC, in which pT1a indicates EC limited to the endometrium or <50% of the myometrium, pT1b indicates EC invasion in $\geq$50% of the myometrium, pT2 indicates EC invasion into the cervical stroma and pT3 or higher indicates spread outside the uterus.

The standard treatment for localized EC includes hysterectomy with bilateral salpingo-oophorectomy and bilateral sentinel lymph node (SLN) procedure for both treatment and staging purposes. When the SLN is not found or an SLN procedure is not possible, a lymphadenectomy may be performed additionally, depending on the size of the tumor or its histological type. Lymph node metastasis is the strongest predictor of recurrence and is related with aggressive histological types and $\geq$pT1b disease. It has been shown that $\geq$pT1b disease is associated with a 6-fold higher prevalence of pelvic and para-aortic lymph node metastases as compared to <50% myometrial invasion, and therefore lymph node surgery is generally recommended in these cases in addition to hysterectomy [2,7,10–16].

Preoperative imaging, particularly assessing the extent of myometrial invasion, cervical invasion, lymph node metastasis and distant metastasis, is used to optimize treatment decision and to tailor surgery [2,8,15,17,18]. In addition to TVU, magnetic resonance imaging (MRI), computed tomography (CT) and positron emission tomography (PET)-CT may be used for local staging and for the assessment of lymph nodes and distant metastasis [7,8,18]. MRI is the preferred imaging modality for local staging of EC [12,19]. MRI may be useful for surgical planning because when $\geq$pT1b disease is preoperatively visualized, the recommended lymphadenectomy can then be performed immediately with the hysterectomy, avoiding a second operation. Moreover, EC tumor size can be measured relatively easily via preoperative MRI and may be a useful biomarker in the management of EC. EC tumor size has been suggested to be an independent prognostic factor and may even predict distant failure more accurately as compared to the depth of myometrial invasion [20–24].

There is still some controversy about the value of routine preoperative MRI in the local staging of EC. The European Society of Urogenital Radiology (ESUR) recommends the use of MRI for the preoperative assessment of the depth of myometrial invasion [12,19], but in the current 2023 FIGO staging guidelines, MRI is not mentioned [10].

Therefore, the purpose of this study was to assess the performance of MRI for the local staging of EC, especially in the assessment of $\geq$pT1b disease and to evaluate whether tumor size measured via MRI was predictive for the presence of $\geq$pT1b disease, independent of imaging signs of invasion.

2. Materials and Methods

This is a retrospective analysis of all patients diagnosed with EC at our institution who underwent MRI for local staging before surgery between February 2009 and September 2022. The scans were performed according to the routine diagnostic MRI scanning protocol used at the time of the referral. For each patient, the MRI scanning protocol and imaging findings were registered. All the MRIs were reviewed by an expert urogenital radiologist with 14 years of experience, blinded for the histopathological staging. The following parameters were assessed: TNM-stage (UICC 8th edition of 2017) on MRI, invasion of the tumor into the myometrium, visualization of enlarged lymph nodes (>10 mm axis in case of a round lymph node and 8 mm short axis in case of an oval lymph node) and presence of myomas. The size of the EC was measured in latero-lateral diameter (LL), anterior–posterior diameter (AP) and cranio-caudal diameter (CC) in mm. The volume of the tumors was estimated based on three-dimensional measurements using the ellipsoid formula AP × LL × CC × 0.52. The imaging findings were correlated with the pathological TNM-stage of the hysterectomy specimen and lymphadenectomy when applicable.

For statistical analysis, IIBM SPSS Statistics version 29 was used. We grouped the staging in a binary manner with threshold $\geq$pT1b disease (i.e., tumor invasion in $\geq$50% of the myometrium, into the cervical stroma or spread outside the uterus) versus $\leq$pT1a disease (i.e., tumor limited to the endometrium or invasion in <50% of the myometrium). Sensitivity, specificity, positive predictive value (PPV), negative predictive value (NPV) and accuracy were calculated using a cross-table between pathological staging ($\geq$pT1b/<pT1a, considered as the gold standard) and MRI-based staging ($\geq$iT1b/$\leq$iT1a).

The largest EC diameters measured via MRI were translated into binary variables with threshold values of 5, 10, 20, 30, 40 and 50 mm. The EC volumes measured via MRI were converted into binary variables with threshold values of 3, 5, 10, 20 and 30 mL. The area under the curve (AUC) of the receiver operating characteristic (ROC) was analyzed for EC diameter and volume. The McNemar test was used to analyze the relationship between binary pathological staging ($\geq$pT1b/$\leq$pT1a) and binary MRI-based staging ($\geq$iT1b/$\leq$iT1a). The Wilcoxon signed-rank test was used to analyze the relationship between pathological staging (pT1a, pT1b, pT2, pT3a, pT3b and pT4) and MRI-based staging (iT0, iT1a, iT1b, iT2, iT3a, iT3b and iT4). Subsequently, pathological staging ($\geq$pT1b/$\leq$pT1a) were correlated with tumor diameters and tumor volumes by using the Wilcoxon signed-rank test. This study was approved by our institution's ethics committee (ONZ-2022-0167).

3. Results

A total of 126 patients were included (Table 1). In 86.5% (109/126), the scan protocol consisted of axial, coronal and sagittal T2-weighted images (T2-WI), sagittal dynamic contrast enhanced T1-weighted images (T1-WI) and axial T1-WI. In 8.7% (11/126), triplanar T2-WI and axial non-enhanced T1-WI were scanned. In 4.8% (6/126), triplanar T2-WI and axial non-enhanced T1-WI were supplemented with axial diffusion-weighted images (DWI). Further, 66.7% (84/126) of the scans were performed on a 1.5 Tesla scanner and 33.3% (42/126) were performed on a 3.0 Tesla system.

On MRI, the EC was considered to be limited to the inner half of the myometrium in 37.3% (47/126) and suspected to invade more than half of the myometrium in 62.7% (79/126) of the patients. In 7.1% (9/126), cervical stroma invasion was suspected. In 7.2% (9/126), enlarged lymph nodes were visualized through MRI, of which 55.5% (5/9) were limited to the pelvis and 44.4% (4/9) to the pelvic and para-aortic lymph nodes. In 48.4% (61/126) of the patients, concomitant uterine myomas were present.

The mean LL diameter of the EC measured via MRI was 26.0 mm (SD 20.1 mm), the mean AP diameter was 20.4 mm (SD 17.7 mm), and the mean CC diameter was 30.4 mm (SD 23.3 mm). The mean largest diameter measured by MRI was 32.9 mm (SD 24.2 mm). The mean estimated tumor volume was 24.5 mL with a maximum of 752.1 mL. The tumor was invisible on MRI in 11.1% (14/126) (recorded as T0). According to MRI, the tumor was considered iT1a in 46.8% (59/126), iT1b in 28.6% (36/126), iT2 in 6.3% (8/126), iT3a in 4.8% (6/126), iT3b in 1.6% (2/126) and iT4 in 0.8% (1/126).

The histological type of EC was endometrioid adenocarcinoma in 90.5% (114/126) of cases, of which 56.1% (64/114) were grade 1, 28.9% (33/114) were grade 2 and 14.9% (17/114) were grade 3. Other histological types were serous carcinomas in 4.8% (6/126), carcinosarcoma in 1.6% (2/126), clear cell carcinoma in 0.8% (1/126) or a mixed type in 2.4% (3/126). The pathological T-stage was pT1a in 52.4% (66/126), pT1b in 31% (39/126), pT2 in 5.6% (7/126), pT3a in 4.0% (5/126), pT3b in 6.3% (8/126) and pT4 in 0.8% (1/126).

Regarding the hysterectomy specimen, no residual tumoral tissue was found in 4% (5/126) of the patients, although the cancer was detected on prior diagnostic pipelle or curettage. They were included in the pT1a stage group.

Table 1. Patients included in the study.

		Age at Diagnosis	Mean 67 Year [SD 10]
Histological type		Endometrioid carcinoma	90.5% (N = 114)
		Grade 1	56.1% (N = 64)
		Grade 2	28.9% (N = 33)
		Grade 3	14.9% (N = 17)
		Clear cell carcinoma	0.8% (N = 1)
		Serous cell carcinoma	4.8% (N = 6)
		Carcinosarcoma	1.6% (N = 2)
		Mixed	2.4% (N = 3)
Pathological T-stage		pT1a	52.3% (N = 66)
		pT1b	31.0% (N = 39)
		pT2	5.6% (N = 7)
		pT3a	4.0% (N = 5)
		pT3b	6.3% (N = 8)
		pT4	0.8% (N = 1)
Pathological N-stage		pN0	9.4% (N = 119)
		pN1	5.6% (N = 7)
		pN2	0.0% (N = 0)
MRI technical features	Scan protocol	Axial T2-WI, coronal T2-WI, sagittal T2-WI, axial T1-WI	8.7% (N = 11)
		Axial T2-WI, coronal T2-WI, sagittal T2-WI, axial T1-WI supplemented with dynamic contrast-enhanced imaging	86.5% (N = 109)
		Axial T2-WI, coronal T2-WI, sagittal T2-WI, axial T1-WI supplemented with diffusion-weighted images (DWI)	4.8% (N = 6)
	Scanner magnetic field strength	1.5 Tesla	66.7% (N = 84)
		3.0 Tesla	33.3% (N = 42)
MRI findings		Tumor not visible	11.0% (N = 14)
		Largest diameter tumor	Mean 32.9 mm [SD 24.2]
		Volume tumor	Mean 24.5 mL [SD 74.3]
		Invasion junctional zone myometrium	67.5% (N = 85)
		Deep myometrial invasion ($\geq$50%)	62.7% (N = 79)
		No signs of cervical stromal invasion	91.3% (N = 115)
		Doubtful cervical stromal invasion	1.6% (N = 2)
		Obvious cervical stromal invasion	7.1% (N = 9)
		Myomas	48.4% (N = 61)
		No enlarged lymph nodes	92.8% (N = 117)
		Enlarged pelvic lymph nodes	4.0% (N = 5)
		Enlarged pelvic and para-aortic lymph nodes	3.2% (N = 4)
		Total	126

MRI-based T-staging was identical to pathological T-staging in 57.1% of cases (72/126), but the EC stage was understaged in 28.6% (36/126) and overstaged in 14.2% (18/126) of cases (Table 2).

Table 2. Pathological and MRI-based T-staging.

		pT Histopathology (n, %)						
		1a	1b	2	3a	3b	4	Total
iT MRI (n, %)	0 *	11 (8.7%)	1 (0.8%)	0	1 (0.8%)	1 (0.8%)	0	14 (11.1%)
	1a	44 (34.9%)	9 (7.1%)	3 (2.4%)	1 (0.8%)	2 (1.6%)	0	59 (46.8%)
	1b	9 (7.1%)	23 (18.3%)	1 (0.8%)	1 (0.8%)	2 (1.6%)	0	36 (28.6%)
	2	1 (0.8%)	3 (2.4%)	2 (1.6%)	0	2 (1.6%)	0	8 (6.3%)
	3a	1 (0.8%)	2 (1.6%)	0	2 (1.6%)	1 (0.8%)	0	6 (4.8%)
	3b	0	1 (0.8%)	1 (0.8%)	0	0	0	2 (1.6%)
	4	0	0	0	0	0	1 (0.8%)	1 (0.8%)
	Total	66 (52.4%)	39 (31.0%)	7 (5.6%)	5 (4.0%)	8 (6.3%)	1 (0.8%)	126

In green the identical iT MRI and pT Histopathology staging is highlighted, * No tumor visible on MRI.

For the detection of $\geq$pT1b disease, MRI had a sensitivity of 70.0%, a specificity of 83.3%, a PPV of 79.2%, an NPV of 75.3% and an accuracy of 77.0%.

An EC size (largest diameter measured) on MRI of >5 mm had a positive predictive value of $\geq$pT1b disease in 51.8%, irrespective of macroscopic visual EC extent in the outer half of the myometrium. Similarly, a maximum tumor diameter measured via MRI of >10, >20, >30, >40 and >50 mm had a positive predictive value of $\geq$pT1b disease in 52.3%, 58.0%, 60.3%, 78.3% and 88.0%, respectively (Table 3). Of the 14 invisible tumors on MRI, 11 (78.6%) were histologically pT1a. There were two tumors with a diameter between 0 and 5 mm on MRI, and they were both pT1a.

Table 3. Threshold EC tumor size (largest diameter measured on MRI) and presence of $\geq$pT1b disease.

		Sensitivity (%)	Specificity (%)	PPV (%)	NPV (%)	AUC (ROC-Analysis)
Threshold diameter	>5 mm	95.0	19.7	51.8	81.3	0.57
	>10 mm	93.3	22.7	52.3	78.9	0.57
	>20 mm	78.3	48.5	58.0	71.1	0.61
	>30 mm	63.3	62.1	60.3	65.1	0.63
	>40 mm	48.3	87.9	78.3	65.7	0.68
	>50 mm	36.7	95.5	88.0	62.8	0.66

In green the highest AUC is highlighted.

An EC volume of >3 mL had a positive predictive value of 61.0% for $\geq$pT1b disease, irrespective of macroscopically visible EC extent in the outer half of the myometrium. Similarly, an EC volume of >5, >10, >20 and >30 mL had a positive predictive value for $\geq$pT1b disease of 62.5%, 72.3%, 87.1% and 91.7%, respectively (Table 4).

The AUC of the ROC analysis for tumor size was highest at a threshold of 40 mm (0.77)) and 20 mL (0.70) (Figure 1).

When complete pathological staging (pT1a, pT1b, pT2, pT3a, pT3b, Tp4) was correlated with complete MRI-based staging (0, pT1a, pT1b, pT2, pT3a, pT3b, Tp4), a significant relationship was observed ($p < 0.05$). However, when the correlation was examined between binary pathological staging ($\geq$pT1b/$\leq$pT1a) and binary MRI staging ($\geq$pT1b/$\leq$pT1a), this correlation did not reach statistical significance ($p > 0.05$).

Table 4. Threshold EC tumor volume (calculated via MRI using the ellipsoid formula based on measurements in three directions) and presence of ≥pT1b disease.

		Sensitivity (%)	Specificity (%)	PPV (%)	NPV (%)	AUC (ROC-Analysis)
Threshold volume	>3 mL	78.3	54.5	61.0	73.5	0.66
	>5 mL	66.7	63.6	62.5	67.7	0.65
	>10 mL	56.7	80.3	72.3	67.1	0.69
	>20 mL	45.0	94.0	87.1	65.2	0.70
	>30 mL	36.7	97.0	91.7	62.7	0.67

In green the highest AUC is highlighted.

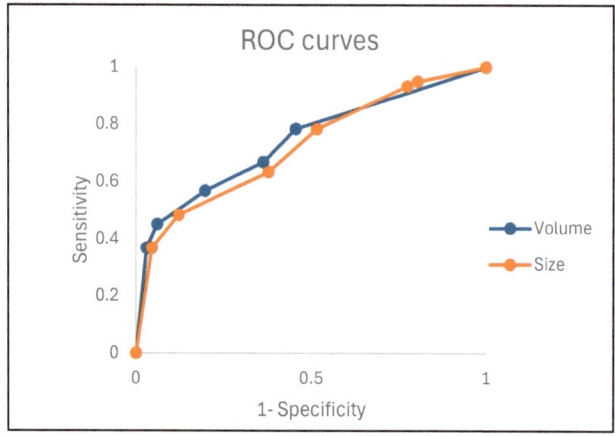

Figure 1. Receiver operator characteristic (ROC) curves for tumor size as determined by the greatest diameter (orange curve) and tumor volume (blue curve) in the assessment of ≥pT1b disease. The greatest area under the curve (AUC) was found with a threshold of 40 mm for tumor size (AUC 0.77) and a threshold of 20 mL for tumor volume (AUC 0.70).

The tumor diameters and volumes were significantly larger for patients with a disease stage of 1b or higher as compared to ≤pT1a (Table 5).

Table 5. Correlation of pathological T stage with Tumor Size and Volume.

Pathological T-Stage	N	Tumor Size (Largest Diameter)	Tumor Volume
≤pT1	66	23.2 mm (SD 17.1 mm)	7.4 mL (SD 17.3 mL)
≥pT1b	60	43.5 mm (SD 25.5 mm)	43.3 mL (SD 103.5 mL)
		p-value < 0.001	p-value < 0.001

4. Discussion

In this study, we evaluated the performance of MRI for the local staging of EC. We showed that MRI had good performance for the detection of ≥pT1b disease and that a larger tumor diameter and volume were predictive for ≥pT1b disease, irrespective of imaging signs of tumor invasion into the outer half of the myometrium, the cervical stroma or outside the uterus upon MRI. We grouped the T-staging in a binary manner with threshold ≥pT1b disease, which included all ECs with ≥50% myometrial invasion (i.e., the real pT1b tumors) but also all stage pT2 or higher tumors (i.e., cervical stromal invasion or spread outside the uterus) that are not necessarily associated with EC invasion in the outer half of the myometrium. This was reasonable because the ≥pT1b threshold is the most relevant clinical factor in T-staging. It has important prognostic value and direct implications for the decision to perform lymphadenectomy in addition to hysterectomy. After diagnosing EC through a biopsy (pipelle or curettage), the most determining factors for management are aggressive histological type, ≥pT1b disease and the presence of metastatic lymph nodes. They are associated with a poorer prognosis, and therefore lymphadenectomy is recommended in addition to hysterectomy in these cases [2,7,10,12–16,21,25]. Pelvic and para-aortic lymph node resection holds a risk of lymphocele and/or lower limb oedema [23]. The sentinel lymph node (SLN) has now become the new standard procedure as it may eliminate the need for extensive lymphadenectomy without risks of suboptimal treatment. When the SLN is not found, the decision to perform lymphadenectomy is based on the histological aggressiveness of the tumor or the presence of ≥pT1b disease [2,7,8,10,12–16,21,25]. We found in our study that an EC size of at least 5 mm measured via preoperative MRI was associated with ≥pT1b disease in more than 50% of cases, which supports the strategy of performing an SLN procedure in all patients with EC.

MRI has long been established as a valuable imaging method in the preoperative staging of EC. MRI can assess the depth of myometrial invasion, but histological type and grade can only be determined with endometrial tumor sampling (Figure 2). Preoperative staging with MRI may be advantageous to predict ≥pT1b disease preoperatively to avoid a second surgical procedure for lymphadenectomy [12], but there is ongoing discussion regarding the value of routine MRI in the preoperative assessment of EC [18,26].

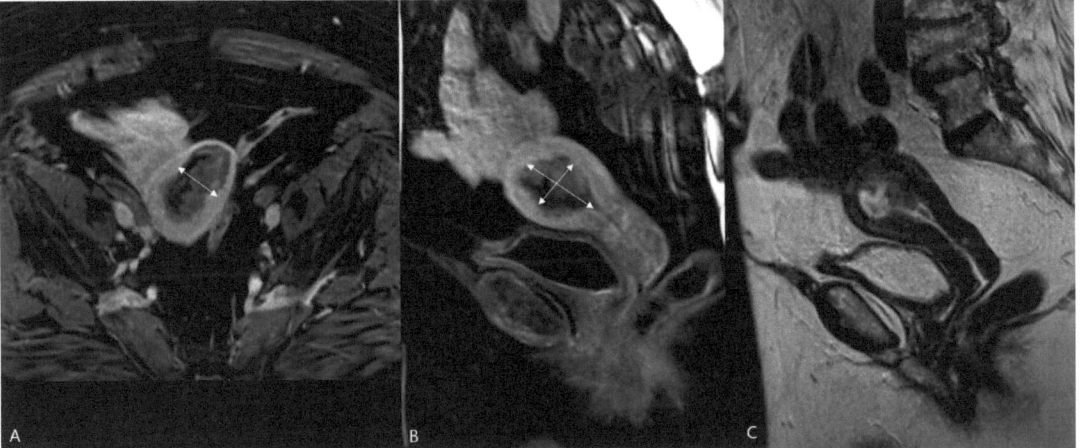

Figure 2. MRI of a pT1b endometrial cancer. T1-weighted images after Gadolinium administration in the axial (**A**) and sagittal plane (**B**). Sagittal T2-weighted image (**C**). The tumor is demonstrated as a heterogenous mass in the uterine cavity, with heterogenous contrast enhancement lower than the surrounding myometrium. The tumor is macroscopically invading the outer half of the myometrium, staged iT1b and confirmed histopathologically pT1b at hysterectomy. The size of the tumor was measured in three directions (white arrows) via MRI. The largest tumor diameter was assessed, and the tumor volume was calculated by the ellipsoid formula (AP × CC × LL × 0.52).

The British Gynaecological Cancer Society recommends pelvic MRI in patients with histologically high-risk EC but considers MRI as optional in patients with lower-risk tumors [9]. They state that MRI should be performed according to dedicated scan protocols and should ideally be interpreted by radiologists with expertise in gynecological oncological imaging. The ESGO-ESTRO-ESP (European Society of Gynaecological Oncology–European Society for Radiotherapy and Oncology–European Society of Pathology) guidelines mention MRI as alternative for TVU but report that both imaging techniques have similar performance for detecting myometrial invasion [27]. The European Society of Urogenital Radiology (ESUR) recommends performing MRI for the local staging of EC and published guidelines describing the indications and prerequisites for a high-quality MRI exam protocol and radiological report [12,19]. In the recent 2023 update of the FIGO staging guidelines, MRI is not mentioned [10]. In the clinical practice guidelines of the Society of Gynaecologic Oncology [28], MRI is not recommended for local invasiveness but is only mentioned as an alternative imaging technique to CT or PET-CT for the identification of metastatic lymph nodes or distant metastasis. In clinical practice, the use of MRI for staging EC appears to be limited, according to two recently published papers based on online surveys completed by expert radiologists and radiology residents [29,30]. In the meta-analyses of Bi et al. [16] and Alcazar et al. [26], both evaluating the diagnostic accuracy of MRI in local staging of EC, only 14 and 8 studies, respectively, could be included, again indicating a rather low use of MRI for the staging of EC worldwide.

Reasons for the ongoing discussion and limited use of MRI in clinical practice may be the costs and limited availability of MRI in many institutions. It is also argued that local staging is sufficient with TVU and that MRI may have no added value. TVU has the advantage that it is cheaper than MRI and is readily available for the gynecologist, but the quality is dependent on the skills of the examiner [27]. The reported sensitivities, specificities and accuracies for detection of deep myometrial invasion with TVU are 71–85%, 72–90% and 72–84%, respectively [18]. The reported sensitivities, specificities and accuracies of MRI for the detection of deep myometrial invasion vary largely in the literature between 33 and 100%, 44 and 100% and 58 and 100%, respectively [15,18]. In the meta-analysis of Bi et al., a pooled sensitivity of 83% and pooled specificity of 82% were reported [16]. In the meta-analysis of Alcazar et al., a sensitivity of 79% and a specificity of 81% were reported [26]. Hashimoto et al. [15] reported a sensitivity of MRI for deep myometrial invasion of 65.1%. These numbers are in line with the results of our study where we found a sensitivity of 70.0%, a specificity of 83.3% and an accuracy of 77.0% for the detection of $\geq$pT1b disease with MRI.

In the meta-analysis of Alcazar et al. [26], the sensitivity for detecting deep myometrial invasion was higher with MRI as compared to TVU (83% vs. 75%), but it was not statistically significant, and the specificity was similar (82%) for both techniques.

Hashimoto et al. [15] reported that preoperative MRI-based cancer stages and postoperative histopathological cancer stages were concordant in 70.0% of patients. The EC stage was underdiagnosed in MRI in 21.7% and overstaged in 8.2% of patients. This larger risk of understaging than overstaging with MRI was also observed in our study: the MRI-based T-stage was identical to the pathological T-stage in 57.1%, but the EC stage was underdiagnosed via MRI in 28.6% of patients and overstaged in 14.2% of patients. There are several causes reducing the accuracy of MRI in the local staging of EC. First, estimation of the depth of myometrial invasion is often difficult using MRI as the uterus grows atrophic in postmenopausal patients with an ill-defined junctional zone, hampering measurement of myometrial depth invasion. Moreover, in case of large or polypoid EC, or in the presence of concomitant leiomyomas or adenomyosis, myometrial compression by mass effect may further reduce the tumor-to-myometrium contrast, hampering image interpretation [8,11]. A polypoid EC bulging into the endocervical canal may be mistaken for a cervical stromal invasion, or an EC located intracavitary in the cornu may resemble tumor invasion in the outer half of the myometrium (Figures 3 and 4).

The secondary aim of our study was to investigate the correlation between the size and volume of EC measured via MRI and pathological staging. Our results showed that the PPV for $\geq$pT1b disease increased with increasing tumor diameter and volume, independent of imaging signs of deep myometrial invasion, cervical stromal invasion or spread outside the uterus. An EC diameter of 40 mm was predictive of $\geq$pT1b disease in 78.3% of cases, and an EC volume of >20 mL was predictive of $\geq$pT1b disease in 87% of cases. It was also observed that $\geq$pT1b disease was present in 51.8% of the cases in which EC size in MRI was only 5 mm. Our data support the results that have been reported in the literature indicating that tumor size is relevant and may be an independent prognostic factor of EC. Chattopadhyay et al. [21] showed that in stage I tumors, size is an independent and even a better predictor than myometrial invasion for distant failure and death of EC. A size cutoff of 3.75 cm was a prognostic indicator for distant failure with a sensitivity of 67%, specificity of 72% and high negative predictive value of 98%. Canlorbe et al. [22] reported that a threshold of 35 mm in diameter had the strongest correlation with nodal metastases and relapse-free survival in women with low-risk EC but not in women with intermediate/high-risk EC. Tumor size in these studies was, however, measured using the pathology specimen and not using MRI. Ytre-Hauge et al. [20] showed that tumor volume, based on the three-dimensional measurements from the preoperative MRI, equally had predictive value for myometrial and lymph node invasion and was a prognostic factor for EC. They reported that an anteroposterior tumor diameter >2 cm significantly predicted deep myometrial invasion and that a craniocaudal tumor diameter >4 cm significantly predicted lymph node metastases. Both size parameters were significantly associated with recurrence- and progression-free survival. Lopez-Gonzalez [24] analyzed tumor volume using MRI in 127 patients with type I EC and showed that tumor volume was significantly higher for deep myometrial invasion, cervical stromal involvement, infiltrated serosa, lymph node metastases, high-grade EC, lymphovascular invasion, advanced FIGO stage and recurrence ($p < 0.001$). A tumor volume of 10 cm^3 predicted deep myometrial invasion with a sensitivity of 82% and a specificity of 74%. ROC analysis showed that a tumor volume >25 cm^3 predicted lymph node metastases. A volume >17 cm^3 was associated with reduced disease-free survival and overall survival. Coronado et al. [23] reported that EC tumor volume measured via MRI was associated with aggressive histological types, deep myometrial invasion, metastatic lymph nodes and advanced FIGO stage. Five-year disease-free survival and overall survival were significantly lower at a tumor volume cut-off of $\geq$10 cm^3 (69.3% vs. 84.5% and 75.4% vs. 96.1%, respectively).

The prognostic impact of tumor size in EC is thus consistently reported with cut-off values of unfavorable tumor size and volume measured via preoperative MRI in the range of our own results, around 35–40 mm and 20–25 mL, respectively. Despite this evidence, it is remarkable that the FIGO guidelines and TNM staging systems do not take the size of EC into account for staging, management or prognosis. Tumor size is, however, a factor that determines the stage and is taken into account for management in many other types of cancer, such as breast, uterine cervix and lung, to name a few [31]. The most recent FIGO guidelines of 2023 [10] are increasingly focused on molecular biology and emphasize the pathological histological classification of tumors, but staging based on tumor size or tumor volume is neither recommended nor discussed. They retain the importance of the percentage of depth of myometrial invasion, although it can be questioned why EC would suddenly behave different once it invades more than half of the myometrium [10]. Tumor size is a relatively easy and reproducible parameter to measure, and it is easier than determining the 50% threshold of myometrial invasion via MRI as well as via histopathology. A single size diameter cannot always accurately describe the exact size of a tumor; therefore, like other researchers [23,24], we estimated tumor volume in our study by applying the ellipsoid formula based on three perpendicular maximum diameters. There are currently many technological advancements available to allow for more fast, easy and accurate automatic calculations of tumor volumes in 3D. In our opinion, it should be considered to implement the long-standing suggestions regarding the use of tumor dimensions in future updates of the FIGO EC guidelines. Based on our study results and in accordance with the above-mentioned evidence in the literature [20–24], it could be recommended to include a tumor diameter larger than 40 mm or tumor volume larger than 20 mL as additional criteria in the selection of patients for pelvic lymph node dissection. Tumor size may be measured via TVU or MRI, but MRI may have added value in the case of small tumors with doubtful findings on TVU or for more accurately measuring tumor size and detection of imaging signs of $\geq$pT1b disease. In the case of larger tumors with extensive invasion outside the uterus, MRI may have added value over TVU for surgical planning and lymph node detection. Currently, there is rapidly increasing interest in the use of artificial intelligence that may have the potential to improve the imaging of endometrial cancer, e.g., to automatically delineate and measure EC or to discriminate benign conditions from EC. Radiomic analysis has been reported to have value in MRI and is currently being investigated in transvaginal ultrasound [32,33].

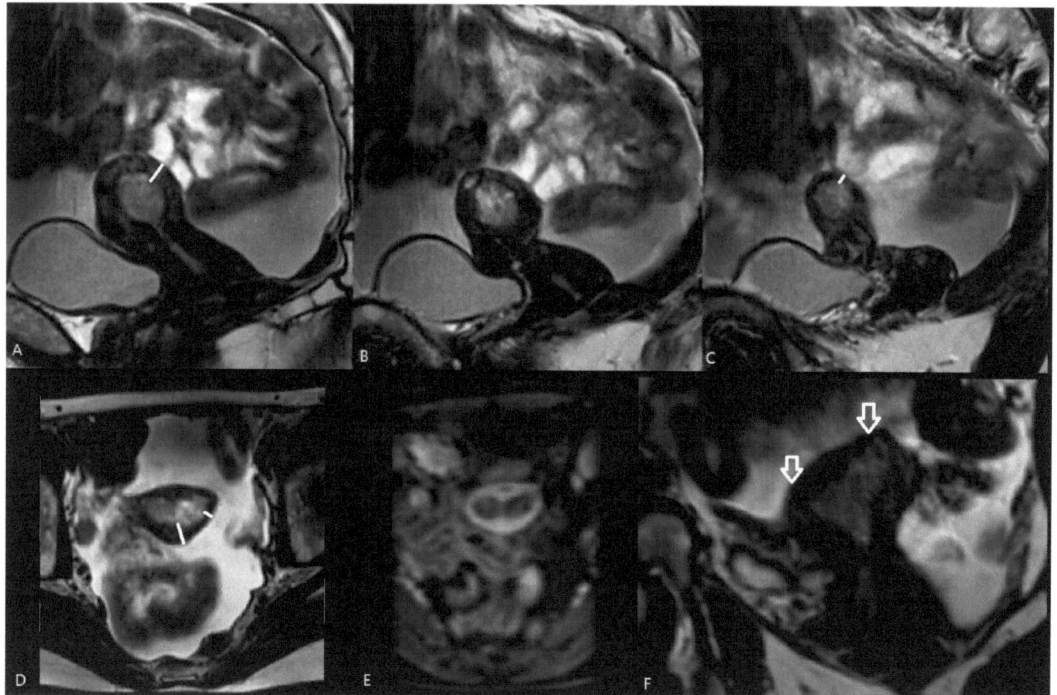

Figure 3. MRI of endometrial cancer. Sagittal T2-WI (**A–C**), axial T2-WI (**D**), axial T1-WI after Gadolinium administration (**E**) and coronal T2-WI (**F**). The tumor is extending intraluminal into the left and right cornu (white arrows on (**F**)). In the cornua, the myometrium is anatomically thinner (short white line in (**C,D**)) than in the uterine corpus (long white line in (**A,D**)), which may result in overstaging because intracavitary growth in the cornu (pT1a) may mimic tumor invasion in the outer half of the myometrium (iT1b).

Our study has some limitations. First, this is a retrospective study with different scanning protocols and magnetic field strengths as used over the years. The most frequently used protocol in our study was T2-WI in three planes combined with sagittal DCE. According to the ESUR guidelines [12], the recommended scanning protocol for staging local disease in EC includes T2, DCE and DWI, but equal accuracies have been reported with protocols omitting DCE or DWI [2,7,8,11–13,16,17,26,34]. It has been advocated that DCE may be safely omitted when including DWI in patients in whom Gadolinium is contraindicated [18], which was the case in 4.8% (6/126) of the patients in our study. Secondly, this was a single-center study, and patients were only included if MRI was performed at our institution, but this had the advantage that all the images were readily available and could be reassessed by a local expert reader. We made an effort to have all the MRI scans reviewed by this expert urogenital radiologist in order to harmonize the radiological interpretation and size measurement, instead of just relying on the findings as described in the initial radiological report. Nevertheless, another reader may have mild variation in image interpretation and measuring the tumor diameters; therefore, a suggestion for future research is to include more readers, preferably experts but equally less-experienced readers to quantify interobserver variability.

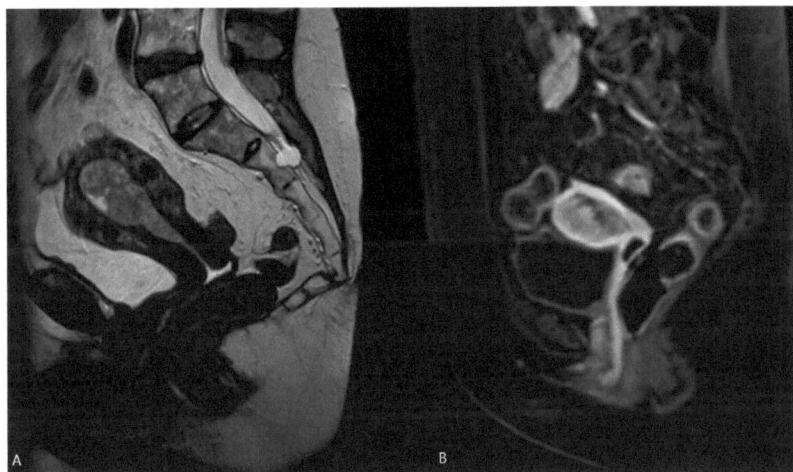

Figure 4. MRI of EC with bulging in the endocervical canal. Sagittal T2-WI (**A**) and sagittal T1-WI after Gadolinium administration (**B**). Histopathologically, this was pT1b disease, but in MRI there is risk of overstaging because tumor extension into the endocervical canal does not account for stage T2, which is preserved for cervical stromal invasion.

A final limitation of our study is that we had no prognostic features such as time to recurrence or survival rates available to directly correlate the MRI imaging interpretation and size measurements with prognostic factors. One of the reasons is that the patients were scanned between 2009 and 2022 and that long-term follow up is lacking. Future research should evaluate the direct prognostic value of tumor size and volume, preferably in a multivariate analysis.

5. Conclusions

MRI had good performance for the detection of ≥pT1b disease in the local staging of EC.

A tumor diameter of ≥40 mm and volume of ≥20 mL measured via MRI were predictive for ≥pT1b disease in 78.3% and 87.1% of patients, respectively. An EC size of at least 5 mm upon MRI was associated with ≥pT1b disease in more than 50% of cases. Our results support the use of MRI in the preoperative staging of patients with EC and suggest including size criteria in EC staging guidelines.

Author Contributions: Conceptualization, L.V.V. and P.J.L.D.V.; methodology, L.V.V., P.J.L.D.V., P.T. and G.M.V.; software, P.J.L.D.V.; validation, L.V.V. and P.J.L.D.V.; formal analysis, L.V.V. and P.J.L.D.V.; investigation, L.V.V.; resources, P.J.L.D.V.; data curation, L.V.V.; writing—original draft preparation, L.V.V., P.J.L.D.V. and P.T.; writing—review and editing, L.V.V., P.T., H.D., M.G., S.H., E.N., R.S., K.V.d.V., G.H.v.R., D.V.W., K.V., G.M.V. and P.J.L.D.V.; visualization, L.V.V. and P.J.L.D.V.; supervision, P.J.L.D.V., P.T. and G.M.V.; project administration, P.J.L.D.V.; funding acquisition, P.J.L.D.V. All authors have read and agreed to the published version of the manuscript.

Funding: This research received no external funding.

Institutional Review Board Statement: The study was conducted in accordance with the Declaration of Helsinki and approved by the Institutional Review Board (or Ethics Committee) of Ghent University Hospital (ONZ-2022-0167, approval date: 4 July 2022).

Informed Consent Statement: Informed consent was obtained from all subjects involved in the study.

Data Availability Statement: The data presented in this study are available on request from the corresponding author. The data are not publicly available due to privacy and ethical restrictions.

Conflicts of Interest: The authors declare no conflicts of interest.

References

1. Braun, M.M.; Overbeek-Wager, E.A.; Grumbo, R.J. Diagnosis and Management of Endometrial Cancer. *Am. Fam. Physician* **2016**, *93*, 468–474.
2. Bonatti, M.; Stuefer, J.; Oberhofer, N.; Negri, G.; Tagliaferri, T.; Schifferle, G.; Messini, S.; Manfredi, R.; Bonatti, G. MRI for local staging of endometrial carcinoma: Is endovenous contrast medium administration still needed? *Eur. J. Radiol.* **2015**, *84*, 208–214. [CrossRef]
3. Crosbie, E.J.; Kitson, S.J.; McAlpine, J.N.; Mukhopadhyay, A.; Powell, M.E.; Singh, N. Endometrial cancer. *Lancet (Lond. Engl.)* **2022**, *399*, 1412–1428. [CrossRef]
4. Amant, F.; Moerman, P.; Neven, P.; Timmerman, D.; Van Limbergen, E.; Vergote, I. Endometrial cancer. *Lancet (Lond. Engl.)* **2005**, *366*, 491–505. [CrossRef]
5. Passarello, K.; Kurian, S.; Villanueva, V. Endometrial Cancer: An Overview of Pathophysiology, Management, and Care. *Semin. Oncol. Nurs.* **2019**, *35*, 157–165. [CrossRef]
6. Koyama, T.; Tamai, K.; Togashi, K. Staging of carcinoma of the uterine cervix and endometrium. *Eur. Radiol.* **2007**, *17*, 2009–2019. [CrossRef]
7. Faria, S.C.; Devine, C.E.; Rao, B.; Sagebiel, T.; Bhosale, P. Imaging and Staging of Endometrial Cancer. *Semin. Ultrasound CT MR* **2019**, *40*, 287–294. [CrossRef]
8. Lin, M.Y.; Dobrotwir, A.; McNally, O.; Abu-Rustum, N.R.; Narayan, K. Role of imaging in the routine management of endometrial cancer. *Int. J. Gynaecol. Obs.* **2018**, *143* (Suppl S2), 109–117. [CrossRef] [PubMed]
9. Sundar, S.; Balega, J.; Crosbie, E.; Drake, A.; Edmondson, R.; Fotopoulou, C.; Gallos, I.; Ganesan, R.; Gupta, J.; Johnson, N.; et al. BGCS uterine cancer guidelines: Recommendations for practice. *Eur. J. Obstet. Gynecol. Reprod. Biol.* **2017**, *213*, 71–97. [CrossRef]
10. Berek, J.S.; Matias-Guiu, X.; Creutzberg, C.; Fotopoulou, C.; Gaffney, D.; Kehoe, S.; Lindemann, K.; Mutch, D.; Concin, N.; Endometrial Cancer Staging Subcommittee, F.W.s.C.C. FIGO staging of endometrial cancer: 2023. *Int. J. Gynaecol. Obstet. Off. Organ. Int. Fed. Gynaecol. Obstet.* **2023**, *162*, 383–394. [CrossRef]
11. Deng, L.; Wang, Q.P.; Chen, X.; Duan, X.Y.; Wang, W.; Guo, Y.M. The Combination of Diffusion- and T2-Weighted Imaging in Predicting Deep Myometrial Invasion of Endometrial Cancer: A Systematic Review and Meta-Analysis. *J. Comput. Assist. Tomogr.* **2015**, *39*, 661–673. [CrossRef]
12. Nougaret, S.; Horta, M.; Sala, E.; Lakhman, Y.; Thomassin-Naggara, I.; Kido, A.; Masselli, G.; Bharwani, N.; Sadowski, E.; Ertmer, A.; et al. Endometrial Cancer MRI staging: Updated Guidelines of the European Society of Urogenital Radiology. *Eur. Radiol.* **2019**, *29*, 792–805. [CrossRef]
13. Pintican, R.; Bura, V.; Zerunian, M.; Smith, J.; Addley, H.; Freeman, S.; Caruso, D.; Laghi, A.; Sala, E.; Jimenez-Linan, M. MRI of the endometrium—from normal appearances to rare pathology. *Br. J. Radiol.* **2021**, *94*, 20201347. [CrossRef]
14. Pecorelli, S. Revised FIGO staging for carcinoma of the vulva, cervix, and endometrium. *Int. J. Gynaecol. Obstet. Off. Organ. Int. Fed. Gynaecol. Obstet.* **2009**, *105*, 103–104. [CrossRef]
15. Hashimoto, C.; Shigeta, S.; Shimada, M.; Shibuya, Y.; Ishibashi, M.; Kageyama, S.; Sato, T.; Tokunaga, H.; Takase, K.; Yaegashi, N. Diagnostic Performance of Preoperative Imaging in Endometrial Cancer. *Curr. Oncol.* **2023**, *30*, 8233–8244. [CrossRef]
16. Bi, Q.; Chen, Y.; Wu, K.; Wang, J.; Zhao, Y.; Wang, B.; Du, J. The Diagnostic Value of MRI for Preoperative Staging in Patients with Endometrial Cancer: A Meta-Analysis. *Acad. Radiol.* **2020**, *27*, 960–968. [CrossRef]
17. Meissnitzer, M.; Forstner, R. MRI of endometrium cancer—how we do it. *Cancer Imaging Off. Publ. Int. Cancer Imaging Soc.* **2016**, *16*, 11. [CrossRef]
18. Haldorsen, I.S.; Salvesen, H.B. What Is the Best Preoperative Imaging for Endometrial Cancer? *Curr. Oncol. Rep.* **2016**, *18*, 25. [CrossRef]
19. Kinkel, K.; Forstner, R.; Danza, F.M.; Oleaga, L.; Cunha, T.M.; Bergman, A.; Barentsz, J.O.; Balleyguier, C.; Brkljacic, B.; Spencer, J.A.; et al. Staging of endometrial cancer with MRI: Guidelines of the European Society of Urogenital Imaging. *Eur. Radiol.* **2009**, *19*, 1565–1574. [CrossRef]
20. Ytre-Hauge, S.; Husby, J.A.; Magnussen, I.J.; Werner, H.M.; Salvesen, O.O.; Bjorge, L.; Trovik, J.; Stefansson, I.M.; Salvesen, H.B.; Haldorsen, I.S. Preoperative tumor size at MRI predicts deep myometrial invasion, lymph node metastases, and patient outcome in endometrial carcinomas. *Int. J. Gynecol. Cancer Off. J. Int. Gynecol. Cancer Soc.* **2015**, *25*, 459–466. [CrossRef]
21. Chattopadhyay, S.; Cross, P.; Nayar, A.; Galaal, K.; Naik, R. Tumor size: A better independent predictor of distant failure and death than depth of myometrial invasion in International Federation of Gynecology and Obstetrics stage I endometrioid endometrial cancer. *Int. J. Gynecol. Cancer Off. J. Int. Gynecol. Cancer Soc.* **2013**, *23*, 690–697. [CrossRef]
22. Canlorbe, G.; Bendifallah, S.; Laas, E.; Raimond, E.; Graesslin, O.; Hudry, D.; Coutant, C.; Touboul, C.; Bleu, G.; Collinet, P.; et al. Tumor Size, an Additional Prognostic Factor to Include in Low-Risk Endometrial Cancer: Results of a French Multicenter Study. *Ann. Surg. Oncol.* **2016**, *23*, 171–177. [CrossRef]
23. Coronado, P.J.; Santiago-Lopez, J.; Santiago-Garcia, J.; Mendez, R.; Fasero, M.; Herraiz, M.A. Tumoral volume measured preoperatively by magnetic resonance imaging is related to survival in endometrial cancer. *Radiol. Oncol.* **2021**, *55*, 35–41. [CrossRef]

24. Lopez-Gonzalez, E.; Rodriguez-Jimenez, A.; Gomez-Salgado, J.; Daza-Manzano, C.; Rojas-Luna, J.A.; Alvarez, R.M. Role of tumor volume in endometrial cancer: An imaging analysis and prognosis significance. *Int. J. Gynaecol. Obs.* **2023**, *163*, 840–846. [CrossRef]
25. Burg, L.C.; Kruitwagen, R.; de Jong, A.; Bulten, J.; Bonestroo, T.J.J.; Kraayenbrink, A.A.; Boll, D.; Lambrechts, S.; Smedts, H.P.M.; Bouman, A.; et al. Sentinel Lymph Node Mapping in Presumed Low- and Intermediate-Risk Endometrial Cancer Management (SLIM): A Multicenter, Prospective Cohort Study in The Netherlands. *Cancers* **2022**, *15*, 271. [CrossRef] [PubMed]
26. Alcazar, J.L.; Gaston, B.; Navarro, B.; Salas, R.; Aranda, J.; Guerriero, S. Transvaginal ultrasound versus magnetic resonance imaging for preoperative assessment of myometrial infiltration in patients with endometrial cancer: A systematic review and meta-analysis. *J. Gynecol. Oncol.* **2017**, *28*, e86. [CrossRef] [PubMed]
27. Concin, N.; Matias-Guiu, X.; Vergote, I.; Cibula, D.; Mirza, M.R.; Marnitz, S.; Ledermann, J.; Bosse, T.; Chargari, C.; Fagotti, A.; et al. ESGO/ESTRO/ESP guidelines for the management of patients with endometrial carcinoma. *Int. J. Gynecol. Cancer Off. J. Int. Gynecol. Cancer Soc.* **2021**, *31*, 12–39. [CrossRef]
28. Group, S.G.O.C.P.E.C.W.; Burke, W.M.; Orr, J.; Leitao, M.; Salom, E.; Gehrig, P.; Olawaiye, A.B.; Brewer, M.; Boruta, D.; Villella, J.; et al. Endometrial cancer: A review and current management strategies: Part I. *Gynecol. Oncol.* **2014**, *134*, 385–392. [CrossRef]
29. Nougaret, S.; Lakhman, Y.; Gourgou, S.; Kubik-Huch, R.; Derchi, L.; Sala, E.; Forstner, R.; European Society of Radiology (ESR); The European Society of Urogenital Radiology (ESUR). MRI in female pelvis: An ESUR/ESR survey. *Insights Into Imaging* **2022**, *13*, 60. [CrossRef] [PubMed]
30. Stanzione, A.; Hornia, E.A.; Moreira, A.S.L.; Russo, L.; Andrieu, P.C.; Carnelli, C.; Cuocolo, R.; Brembilla, G.; Zawaideh, J.P.; Committee, E.J.N. Dissemination of endometrial cancer MRI staging guidelines among young radiologists: An ESUR Junior Network survey. *Insights Into Imaging* **2023**, *14*, 143. [CrossRef] [PubMed]
31. Lee, S.I.; Atri, M. 2018 FIGO Staging System for Uterine Cervical Cancer: Enter Cross-sectional Imaging. *Radiology* **2019**, *292*, 15–24. [CrossRef]
32. Bogani, G.; Chiappa, V.; Lopez, S.; Salvatore, C.; Interlenghi, M.; D'Oria, O.; Giannini, A.; Leone Roberti Maggiore, U.; Chiarello, G.; Palladino, S.; et al. Radiomics and Molecular Classification in Endometrial Cancer (The ROME Study): A Step Forward to a Simplified Precision Medicine. *Healthcare* **2022**, *10*, 2464. [CrossRef] [PubMed]
33. Zhang, J.; Zhang, Q.; Wang, T.; Song, Y.; Yu, X.; Xie, L.; Chen, Y.; Ouyang, H. Multimodal MRI-Based Radiomics-Clinical Model for Preoperatively Differentiating Concurrent Endometrial Carcinoma From Atypical Endometrial Hyperplasia. *Front. Oncol.* **2022**, *12*, 887546. [CrossRef] [PubMed]
34. Moreira, A.S.L.; Ribeiro, V.; Aringhieri, G.; Fanni, S.C.; Tumminello, L.; Faggioni, L.; Cioni, D.; Neri, E. Endometrial Cancer Staging: Is There Value in ADC? *J. Pers. Med.* **2023**, *13*, 728. [CrossRef] [PubMed]

Disclaimer/Publisher's Note: The statements, opinions and data contained in all publications are solely those of the individual author(s) and contributor(s) and not of MDPI and/or the editor(s). MDPI and/or the editor(s) disclaim responsibility for any injury to people or property resulting from any ideas, methods, instructions or products referred to in the content.

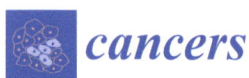

Systematic Review

Imaging of Peritoneal Metastases in Ovarian Cancer Using MDCT, MRI, and FDG PET/CT: A Systematic Review and Meta-Analysis

Athina C. Tsili [1,*], George Alexiou [2], Martha Tzoumpa [1], Timoleon Siempis [3] and Maria I. Argyropoulou [1]

1. Department of Clinical Radiology, Faculty of Medicine, School of Health Sciences, University of Ioannina, University Campus, 45110 Ioannina, Greece; martz_me@hotmail.com (M.T.); margyrop@uoi.gr (M.I.A.)
2. Department of Neurosurgery, Faculty of Medicine, School of Health Sciences, University of Ioannina, University Campus, 45110 Ioannina, Greece; galexiou@uoi.gr
3. ENT Department, Ulster Hospital, Upper Newtownards Rd., Dundonald, Belfast BT16 1RH, UK; timoleon.siempis@setrust.hscni.net
* Correspondence: atsili@uoi.gr

Simple Summary: Ovarian cancer is the leading cause of death due to gynecologic malignancies. Peritoneal metastases represent the most common pathway for the spread of OC, both at the time of initial diagnosis and at recurrence. Accurate mapping of peritoneal metastases helps in planning the appropriate therapeutic strategy, predicting the likelihood of optimal cytoreduction, and identifying potentially unresectable or difficult disease sites that may require surgical technique modifications. Preoperative diagnostic work-up with multidetector CT (MDCT), MRI, including diffusion-weighted imaging (DWI), or FDG PET/CT plays a vital role in the accurate assessment of the extent of peritoneal carcinomatosis. In this article, the aim was to update the role of MDCT, MRI, including DWI, and FDG PET/CT in the detection of peritoneal metastases in ovarian cancer by conducting a systematic review and meta-analysis of the existing literature.

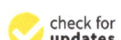

Citation: Tsili, A.C.; Alexiou, G.; Tzoumpa, M.; Siempis, T.; Argyropoulou, M.I. Imaging of Peritoneal Metastases in Ovarian Cancer Using MDCT, MRI, and FDG PET/CT: A Systematic Review and Meta-Analysis. *Cancers* **2024**, *16*, 1467. https://doi.org/10.3390/cancers16081467

Academic Editor: Edward J. Pavlik

Received: 7 February 2024
Revised: 5 April 2024
Accepted: 6 April 2024
Published: 11 April 2024

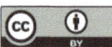

Copyright: © 2024 by the authors. Licensee MDPI, Basel, Switzerland. This article is an open access article distributed under the terms and conditions of the Creative Commons Attribution (CC BY) license (https://creativecommons.org/licenses/by/4.0/).

Abstract: This review aims to compare the diagnostic performance of multidetector CT (MDCT), MRI, including diffusion-weighted imaging, and FDG PET/CT in the detection of peritoneal metastases (PMs) in ovarian cancer (OC). A comprehensive search was performed for articles published from 2000 to February 2023. The inclusion criteria were the following: diagnosis/suspicion of PMs in patients with ovarian/fallopian/primary peritoneal cancer; initial staging or suspicion of recurrence; MDCT, MRI and/or FDG PET/CT performed for the detection of PMs; population of at least 10 patients; surgical results, histopathologic analysis, and/or radiologic follow-up, used as reference standard; and per-patient and per-region data and data for calculating sensitivity and specificity reported. In total, 33 studies were assessed, including 487 women with OC and PMs. On a per-patient basis, MRI ($p = 0.03$) and FDG PET/CT ($p < 0.01$) had higher sensitivity compared to MDCT. MRI and PET/CT had comparable sensitivities ($p = 0.84$). On a per-lesion analysis, no differences in sensitivity estimates were noted between MDCT and MRI ($p = 0.25$), MDCT and FDG PET/CT ($p = 0.68$), and MRI and FDG PET/CT ($p = 0.35$). Based on our results, FDG PET/CT and MRI are the preferred imaging modalities for the detection of PMs in OC. However, the value of FDG PET/CT and MRI compared to MDCT needs to be determined. Future research to address the limitations of the existing studies and the need for standardization and to explore the cost-effectiveness of the three imaging modalities is required.

Keywords: peritoneal carcinomatosis; ovarian cancer; computed tomography; multidetector; magnetic resonance imaging; diffusion weighted MRI; PET/CT scan

1. Introduction

Ovarian cancer (OC) represents the fifth most commonly diagnosed cancer among women, the fifth cause of cancer death, and the commonest cause of death due to gynecologic malignancies [1–8]. An estimated number of 19,680 new cases of OC are expected to be diagnosed in the US and 12,740 women are expected to die from the disease in 2024 [2]. Most cases (90%) are epithelial ovarian carcinomas and the majority are high-grade serous carcinomas. The most important revision in the last FIGO staging classification is that ovarian, fallopian, and primary peritoneal cancers are considered as one entity [9].

Ovarian cancer has a poor prognosis, with a 5-year relative survival rate of 48%, mainly because most women are diagnosed with advanced-stage disease [2]. Moreover, the percentage of recurrence in OC is very high. The standard of care in OC includes either primary debulking surgery (PDS) followed by adjuvant chemotherapy or neoadjuvant chemotherapy (NAC) prior to interval debulking surgery (IDS) and postoperative chemotherapy [10–12].

Peritoneal metastases (PMs) represent the commonest pathway for the spread of OC and are often seen either at the time of initial diagnosis or at recurrence [3,13–22]. The peritoneal cancer index (PCI) introduced by Jacquet and Sugarbaker combined the distribution of PMs in 13 abdominopelvic regions (ARs) with the tumor size providing a measurement of the volume of peritoneal carcinomatosis (PC) and also a valuable prognostic index (Table 1, Figure 1) [23].

Table 1. The Sugarbaker Peritoneal Carcinomatosis Index (ARs: abdominopelvic regions; PCI: peritoneal carcinomatosis index) [23].

ARs	Sugarbaker's PCI
AR0	midline abdominal incision, greater omentum, and transverse colon
AR1	superior surface of the right lobe of the liver, undersurface of the right hemidiaphragm, and right retrohepatic space
AR2	epigastric fat pad, left lobe of the liver, lesser omentum, and falciform ligament
AR3	undersurface of the left hemidiaphragm, spleen, pancreatic tail, and anterior and posterior surfaces of the stomach
AR4	descending colon and left paracolic gutter
AR5	pelvic side wall lateral to the sigmoid colon and sigmoid colon
AR6	female internal genitalia with ovaries, tubes and uterus, urinary bladder, cul-de-sac of Douglas, and rectosigmoid colon
AR7	right pelvic side wall and base of the cecum, including the appendix
AR8	right paracolic gutter and ascending colon
AR9–12	small bowel (AR9: upper jejunum; AR10: lower jejunum; AR11: upper ileum; and AR12: lower ileum)

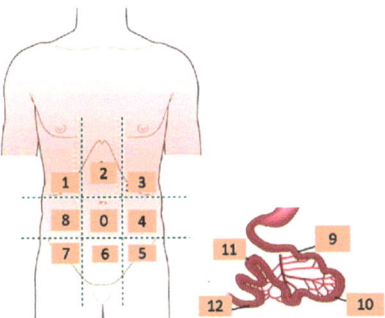

Figure 1. Coronal schematic drawing showing the Sugarbaker peritoneal carcinomatosis index.

Imaging has a fundamental role in the accurate diagnosis of PMs in OC, helping to plan the appropriate therapeutic strategy, predict the likelihood of optimal cytoreduction, and identify potentially unresectable or difficult disease sites, which may require either IDS following chemotherapy or surgical technique modifications during PDS [3,13–22].

Multidetector CT (MDCT) is considered the examination of choice for the initial staging of OC and for the evaluation of the extent of the disease in suspected recurrence [1]. However, CT has limitations, mainly low soft-tissue resolution, and difficulty in depicting small peritoneal implants or implants at certain anatomic areas, including the root of mesentery, lesser omentum, and serosal surfaces of the small bowel, especially in the absence of ascites [1,3,18,21,24–30].

MRI represents another reliable imaging tool for the assessment of PC. The efficacy of the technique in the detection of PMs has been improved by using fat-suppressed delayed contrast-enhanced imaging and diffusion-weighted imaging (DWI) [16,21,30–35]. Specifically, DWI improves the detection of small peritoneal hypercellular implants, even in the absence of ascites, due to their high signal against the hypointense background of normal tissues. However, MRI is recommended in specific circumstances, such as women with borderline ovarian tumors or OCs that have been previously staged with fertility preservation and also in cases with inconclusive CT findings [1].

The hypermetabolic activity of PMs increases their conspicuity using FDG PET/CT. CT and FDG PET/CT are considered equivalent alternatives for the detection of recurrent OC [1,17,30,36–44]. Based on the results of a recently published meta-analysis, FDG PET/CT had high diagnostic accuracy, with 88% sensitivity and 89% specificity in the detection of recurrent OC [45]. Up to now, FDG PET or FDG PET/CT may be used as an adjunct tool in the initial staging of OC, in cases of indeterminate CT findings [1].

Systematic reviews on the role of cross-sectional imaging in the detection of PC in women with OC are lacking. A few recently published meta-analyses assessed the diagnostic accuracy of imaging modalities in the detection of PMs from various primary malignancies, including OC [46–48].

The purpose of this systematic review and meta-analysis was to compare the diagnostic performance of MDCT, MRI, including DWI, and FDG PET/CT in the detection of peritoneal metastases in ovarian cancer.

2. Materials and Methods

This systematic review and meta-analysis was conducted in accordance with the preferred reporting items for systematic reviews and meta-analysis (PRISMA) guidelines [49]. The systematic review has not been registered.

2.1. Search Strategy

A systematic and comprehensive literature search was performed for all publications that reported the diagnostic performance of MDCT, MRI, and FDG PET/CT in the detection of PMs in OC. Data extraction was independently performed by two researchers (ACT and MT) from the PubMed/MEDLINE database and included articles published from 2000 to February 2023.

The following keywords were used: "ovarian cancer" OR "peritoneal metastases" OR "peritoneal carcinomatosis" OR "multidetector CT" OR "MDCT" OR "magnetic resonance imaging" OR "MRI" OR "diffusion-weighted imaging" OR "DWI" OR "fluorine-18-fluorodeoxyglucose (FDG) positron emission tomography (PET)/computed tomography (CT)" and "FDG PET/CT".

Articles found to be suitable on the basis of their title and abstract were subsequently selected to further determine appropriateness for inclusion in this meta-analysis. Only papers in the English language were assessed. Full-text studies were further evaluated, and exclusion criteria were applied to identify final papers for inclusion. References were manually screened to identify additional studies.

2.2. Eligibility Criteria

The inclusion criteria were as follows: diagnosis/suspicion of PMs in patients with ovarian/fallopian/primary peritoneal cancer; initial staging or suspicion of recurrence (primary outcome); MDCT, MRI, and/or FDG PET/CT performed for the detection of PMs; population of at least 10 patients; surgical results, histopathologic analysis, and/or radiologic follow-up, used as a reference standard; per-patient and per-region data included; and data for calculating sensitivity and specificity reported. Discrepancies regarding potential eligibility and inclusion were resolved by consensus.

Studies were excluded if results for different imaging modalities were presented in combination and if data on the performance of each individual technique were unavailable. Studies including patients with the diagnosis of PMs from tumors other than OC were considered eligible only if it was possible to extrapolate results obtained on PC from OC.

2.3. Data Extraction

From each study, the following design characteristics were recorded: first author and year of publication; study design (prospective or retrospective); primary outcome; characteristics of study population, including number of patients with ovarian/fallopian/primary peritoneal cancer, age, number of patients with PMs, number and size of PMs, location of PMs; imaging modality, including MDCT, MRI or FDG PET/CT; report of reference test; time interval between imaging modalities; and time interval between imaging and reference standard.

Imaging characteristics included detailed information on the following: imaging equipment (type of scanner for MDCT and FDG PET/CT, magnetic field strength); imaging technique (phases and reformations for MDCT, type of coil, sequences, section thickness, and b-values for MRI); bowel preparation (laxatives and spasmolytic drugs), and use of luminal and/or intravenous contrast medium.

The numbers of true-positive (TP), false-negative (FN), false-positive (FP), and true-negative (TN) results for the detection of PMs were extracted on a per-patient and per-region basis. When cumulative data on the detection of PMs were not reported, the results from the abdominopelvic region with the best diagnostic performance were included in the analysis.

Regarding the per-patient analysis, the diagnostic odds ratios (DORs) were also estimated. A bivariate random effect meta-analytic method was used to estimate pooled sensitivity, specificity, and summary receiver operating characteristic (SROC) curves. Via the percentage of heterogeneity between the studies, computing I^2 values were calculated. I^2 values equal to 25%, 50%, and 75% were assumed to represent low, moderate, and high heterogeneity, respectively. Study heterogeneity was also assessed visually via funnel plots.

When at least three datasets were available for the three imaging modalities, subgroup analyses were performed for the different ARs, including AR0 (central abdomen), AR1 (right hypochondrium), AR2 (epigastrium), AR3 (left hypochondrium), AR4 (left lumbar region), AR5–7 and AR6 (pelvis), AR8 (right lumbar region), small bowel (AR9–12), colon and mesentery (Table 1, Figure 1), on a per-patient and a per-region basis [23].

2.4. Quality Assessment

Analyses were performed using the RevMan software (ReviewManager, version 5.3; The Nordic Cochrane Centre, The Cochrane Collaboration, Copenhagen, Denmark). To assess the methodological quality of the included primary studies and to detect potential bias, we used the quality assessment of diagnostic accuracy studies-2 (QUADAS-2) tool [50].

3. Results

The initial search in the electronic database resulted in 848 articles. Following a review of the titles and abstracts, 187 studies were selected as potentially relevant, and their references were cross-checked. Thirty-three publications eventually fulfilled the inclusion criteria and were selected for quantitative synthesis (Table 2) [26,27,30,42,44,51–78]. The flow chart of the selection process is shown in Figure 2.

Table 2. Characteristics of the eligible studies (OC: ovarian cancer; PMs: peritoneal metastases, ARs: abdominopelvic regions; n/a: non-applicable).

Author	Year	Type of Study	Primary Outcome	No of pts with OC	Mean Age/Age Range (Years)	FIGO Stage (No. of pts)	No. of pts with PMs	No. of ARs with PMs	Mean Size-Size Range of PMs (cm) (No. of PMs)
Tempany et al. [51]	2000	prospective	suspected advanced OC	118	57 (19–79)	III and IV (73)	70	250	<2 (8) >2 (57) n/a (5)
Pannu et al. [52]	2003	retrospective	suspected primary or recurrent OC/ peritoneal cancer	17	58.1 (41–84)	IB (1) III (13) IV (3)	13	63	n/a
Ricke et al. [53]	2003	prospective	suspected primary or recurrent OC	57	58 (35–90)	I (11) II (2) III (36) IV (4) n/a (4)	n/a	204	n/a
Pannu et al. [54]	2004	retrospective	suspected recurrent OC	16	50.8 (17–77)	n/a	11	31	<1 (23) >1 (8)
Kim et al. [55]	2007	retrospective	suspected recurrent OC	36	51.3 (25–75)	I (2) II (5) III (27) IV (2)	n/a	14	2.2 (0.4–3.5)
Kitajima et al. [56]	2008	retrospective	suspected recurrent OC	132	56 (34–79)	I (20) II (10) III (81) IV (21)	n/a	45	n/a
Kitajima et al. [57]	2008	retrospective	primary OC	40	55.4 (38–77)	I (18) II (7) III (14) IV (1)	n/a	46	0.2–2.3
Choi et al. [58]	2011	prospective	primary OC	57	53.1 (30–72)	I (6) II (5) III (38) IV (8)	50	251	<1 >1
Metser et al. [59]	2011	retrospective	primary OC	76	58.2 (24–87)	I (11) II (3) III (55) IV (7)	n/a	414	<1 (142) ≥1 (272)
De Iaco et al. [60]	2011	retrospective	suspected OC	40	65 ± 7.9 (46–78)	III (22) IV (18)	40	308	≤0.5 (135) 0.5–5 (38) >5 (135)
Sanli et al. [61]	2012	retrospective	suspected recurrent OC	47	57.5 ± 8.4 (38–78)	n/a	n/a	n/a	<0.5 0.5–1 1–2 2–3 >3
Espada et al. [62]	2013	prospective	suspected advanced OC	34	53.08 ± 11.9	III (28) IV (6)	n/a	n/a	n/a
Hynninen et al. [63]	2013	prospective	suspected advanced ovarian/ fallopian/ peritoneal cancer	41	65 (45–79)	I (2) II (2) III (21) IV (16)	41	246	n/a
Kim et al. [64]	2013	retrospective	suspected primary or recurrent OC	46	54 (29–80)	I (12) II (4) III (28) IV (2)	26	n/a	n/a
Mazzei et al. [65]	2013	retrospective	advanced primary or recurrent OC	43	58.5 (30–72)	III (42) IV (1)	43	195	<0.5 0.5–5 >5
Michielsen et al. [66]	2014	prospective	suspected OC	32	61.9 (20–83)	n/a	32	208	<1 (75) >1 (60) confluent disease (73)
Schmidt et al. [67]	2015	prospective	suspected OC	15	65 (31–89)	III (4) IV (6)	10	74	≤0.5 (13) 0.5–5 (40) >5 cm (21)

Table 2. Cont.

Author	Year	Type of Study	Primary Outcome	No of pts with OC	Mean Age/Age Range (Years)	FIGO Stage (No. of pts)	No. of pts with PMs	No. of ARs with PMs	Mean Size-Size Range of PMs (cm) (No. of PMs)
Lopez-Lopez et al. [68]	2016	retrospective	suspected primary or recurrent OC	59	54 (27–78)	I (3) II (44) III (12)	55	278	<0.5 (110) ≥0.5–5 (53) >5 cm or confluent (115)
Nasser et al. [26]	2016	retrospective	suspected primary or recurrent OC	155	62.5 (31–85)	I (4) II (3) III (106) IV (42)	n/a	n/a	n/a
Rodolfino et al. [69]	2016	retrospective	suspected recurrent OC	40	48.5 (32–73)	III (33) IV (7)	29	182	<0.5 (38) ≥0.5–5 (81) >5 cm or confluent (63)
Tawakol et al. [70]	2016	prospective	suspected recurrent OC	111	54 (13–76)	n/a	n/a	75	n/a
Cerci et al. [71]	2016	retrospective	primary OC	114	59 (28–91)	I (21) II (4) III (47) IV (39)	n/a	n/a	n/a
Bagul et al. [72]	2017	prospective	suspected advanced ovarian/fallopian tube/primary peritoneal cancer	36	51 (39–74)	IIIc	n/a	n/a	n/a
Michielsen et al. [73]	2017	prospective	suspected OC	94	61 (14–88)	I (19) II (2) III (38) IV (35)	n/a	n/a	n/a
Rajan et al. [74]	2018	prospective	advanced OC	40	59.5 (43–87)	IIIc IV	40	115	<0.5 0.5–5 >5
Alcazar et al. [75]	2019	retrospective	suspected OC	93	57.6 ± 11.4 (18–84)	I (26) II (11) IIIA (1) IIIB (6) IIIC (40) IVA (6) IVB (3)	n/a	n/a	n/a
Abdalla Ahmed et al. [76]	2019	prospective	primary OC	85	55 (27–82)	II (5) III (80)	n/a	930	8.4 (1–13) <0.5 (280) 0.5–5 (605) >5 (45)
Tsoi et al. [77]	2020	retrospective	primary or recurrent ovarian/peritoneal cancer	49	49 ± 15	I (15) II (12) III (18) IV (1) n/a (3)	27	58	<1 (9) ≥1 (44)
An et al. [27]	2020	retrospective	recurrent advanced OC	58	57 (23–84)	III (31) IV (27)	n/a	315	3.7 (1–15)
Mikkelsen et al. [30]	2021	prospective	advanced OC	50	65 (32–78)	III (32) IV (18)	n/a	n/a	n/a
Feng et al. [42]	2021	prospective	advanced OC	43	57 (38–76)	III (32) IV (11)	n/a	286	n/a
Mallet et al. [44]	2021	retrospective	advanced OC	84	65 (44–89)	III (28) IV (56)	n/a	n/a	<0.5 0.5–5 >5
Fischerova et al. [78]	2022	prospective	suspected primary advanced ovarian/tubal/peritoneal cancer	67	61.4 ± 10.5	I (14) II (2) III (44) IV (7)	n/a	n/a	n/a

A total of 2025 women with OC were included in the meta-analysis, with a mean age of 57.4 years (range, 19–91 years). The primary outcome included 19 studies with initial diagnosis of ovarian/fallopian/peritoneal cancer, 7 reports with recurrent cancer, and 7 studies with primary or recurrent OC. Advanced OC (FIGO stages III and IV) was reported in 1453 patients (Table 2). The presence of PMs was reported in 487 women and included 4.588 ARs (Tables 2 and 3).

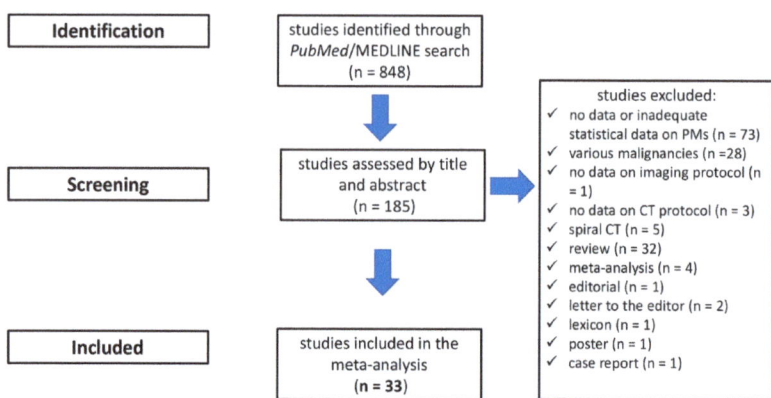

Figure 2. Flowchart depicting study selection.

Table 3. Location of PMs (ARs: abdominopelvic regions; n/a: non-applicable).

Study	Location of PMs (n = Number of Patients or ARs with PMs)
Tempany et al. [51] (n = number of ARs)	anterior part of the abdomen (37) RT, LT paracolic gutters AR4,8 (35) RT, LT subdiaphragmatic spaces AR1,3 (45) mesentery (small bowel/transverse/sigmoid colon) (38) hepatic surface AR1,2 (25) omentum (gastrocolic and infracolic) AR0 (70)
Pannu et al. [52] (n = number of patients)	diaphragm AR1,3 (11) liver AR1,2 (6) splenic surface AR3 (2) porta hepatis/gallbladder fossa AR1 (4) stomach AR3 (2) lesser sac AR2 (3) mesenteric root (3) infracolic omentum AR0 (7) paracolic gutters AR4,8 (8) bowel (5) pelvis AR5–7 (12)
Ricke et al. [53] (n = number of ARs)	pouch of Douglas AR6 (18) cervix/vaginal stump AR6 (9) uterus AR6 (11) bladder/ureter AR6 (10) pelvic wall AR5,7 (23) abdominal wall (18) small bowel/mesentery (22) large bowel (39) greater omentum AR0 (21) lesser sac AR2 (7) stomach AR3 (6) diaphragm AR1,3 (15) liver capsule AR1,2 (5)
Pannu et al. [54] (n = number of ARs)	pelvis AR5–7 (17) bowel/omentum (7) LT upper quadrant AR3 (2) paracolic gutters AR4,8 (4) RT upper quadrant AR1 (1)

Table 3. *Cont.*

Study	Location of PMs (*n* = Number of Patients or ARs with PMs)
Kim et al. [55] (*n* = number of ARs)	cul de sac AR6 (4) paracolic gutter AR4,8 (3) subphrenic/perihepatic/perisplenic (6) bowel (1)
Kitajima et al. [56] (n/a)	cul de sac AR6 paracolic gutter AR4,8 mesentery serosa of large and small bowel anterior part of the abdomen hepatic surface AR1,2 splenic hilum AR3 diaphragm AR1,3
Kitajima et al. [57] (*n* = number of ARs)	cul de sac AR6 (8) urinary bladder AR6 (2) rectosigmoid colon AR6 (4) peritoneum of anterior abdomen (6) paracolic gutter AR4,8 (3) diaphragm AR1,3 (1) omentum AR0 (9) mesentery (7) serous membrane of large and small bowel (4) liver surface AR1,2 (2)
Choi et al. [58] (*n* = number of ARs)	RT subdiaphragmatic area AR1 (35) LT subdiaphragmatic area AR3 (34) porta hepatis AR1 (10) lesser sac AR2 (18) small bowel mesentery (14) splenic hilar area AR3 (38) omentum AR0 (20) RT paracolic gutter AR8 (22) LT paracolic gutter AR4 (20) RT pelvic cavity AR7 (4) LT pelvic cavity AR5 (8) sigmoid mesentery (12) bladder dome area AR6 (16)
Metser et al. [59] (n/a)	RT diaphragm AR1 liver capsule AR1,2 liver parenchymal invasion gallbladder fossa AR1 RT paracolic gutter AR8 LT diaphragm AR3 omentum AR0 LT paracolic gutter AR4 bladder peritoneum AR6 porta hepatis AR1 root of small bowel mesentery mesentery ascending colon, serosa AR8 cecum, serosa AR7 appendix AR7 stomach, serosa AR3 small bowel, serosa transverse colon, serosa AR0 descending colon, serosa AR4 spleen, capsule AR3 spleen, hilum AR3 spleen, parenchymal invasion rectosigmoid mesentery RT pelvic sidewall AR7 LT pelvic sidewall AR5 cul-de-sac, posterior AR6 rectosigmoid, serosa AR6 rectosigmoid, invasion AR6

Table 3. Cont.

Study	Location of PMs (n = Number of Patients or ARs with PMs)
De Iaco et al. [60] (n = number of ARs)	central AR0 (37) RT upper AR1 (34) epigastrium AR2 (26) LT upper AR3 (28) LT flank AR4 (35) LT lower AR5 (36) pelvis AR6 (40) RT lower AR7 (38) RT flank AR8 (34)
Espada et al. [62] (n/a)	small and/or large bowel mesentery (8) hepatic parenchyma, hepatic hilum or surface implants > 2 cm AR1,2 (10) omental extension: spleen parenchyma, splenic hilum, stomach, lesser sac AR2,3 (11) diaphragm AR1,3 (5) peritoneal
Hynninen et al. [63] (n = number of patients)	diaphragm AR1,3 (34) omentum AR0 (34) small bowel mesentery (25) large bowel mesentery (30) small bowel serosae AR9–12 (14) large bowel serosae (64) RT 'high risk upper abdomen': dorsal subdiaphragmatic peritoneum, dorsal liver surface AR1 (31) LT 'high risk upper abdomen': ventricle, bursa omentalis, spleen, tail of pancreas AR3 (14)
Mazzei et al. [65] (n/a)	central AR0 RT upper AR1 epigastrium AR2 LT upper AR3 LT flank AR4 LT left AR5 pelvis AR6 RT lower AR7 RT flank AR8 upper jejunum AR9 lower jejunum AR10 upper ileum AR11 lower ileum AR12
Michielsen et al. [66] (n = number of ARs)	bladder peritoneal surface AR6 (17) Douglas pouch AR6 (19) RT peritoneal pelvic surface AR7 (20) RT lateroconal area AR8 (15) subhepatic space/Morrison's pouch AR1 (10) RT diaphragm AR1 (12) hepatic surface AR1,2 (4) LT diaphragm AR3 (9) splenic surface AR3 (1) LT lateroconal area AR4 (16) LT peritoneal pelvic surface AR5 (21) omentum AR0 (23) small bowel serosa AR9–12 (6) small bowel mesentery (12) colonic serosa (11) colonic mesentery (12)
Schmidt et al. [67] (n/a)	central AR0 RT upper AR1 epigastrium AR2 LT upper AR3 LT flank AR4 LT lower AR5 pelvis AR6 RT lower AR7 RT flank AR8
Lopez-Lopez et al. [68] (n/a)	upper region middle region lower region small intestine

Table 3. Cont.

Study	Location of PMs (n = Number of Patients or ARs with PMs)
Nasser et al. [26] (n = number of patients)	diaphragmatic involvement AR1,3 (55) splenic involvement AR3 (19) large bowel involvement (37) small bowel involvement (15) rectal involvement AR6 (38) porta hepatis involvement AR1 (6) mesenteric involvement (35)
Rodolfino et al. [69] (n/a)	central AR0 RT upper AR1 epigastrium AR2 LT upper AR3 LT flank AR4 LT lower AR5 pelvis AR6 RT lower AR7 RT flank AR8 upper jejunum AR9 lower jejunum AR10 upper ileum AR11 lower ileum AR12
Cerci et al. [71] (n = number of patients)	peritoneal carcinomatosis (61) omentum AR0 (53) ascites (61) perivesical-perirectal fat AR6 (54) diaphragm AR1,3 (20) liver AR1,2 (30) bladder AR6 (22) small and large bowel (47) mesentery (49)
Bagul et al. [72] (n = number of patients)	diffuse peritoneal thickening (17) RT subdiaphragm AR1 (35) LT subdiaphragm AR3 (27) porta hepatis AR1 (24) liver AR1,2 (25) spleen AR3 (11) lesser sac AR2 (15) omentum AR0 (35) omental cake extension (to splenic hilum, stomach, colon, or lesser sac) (24) RT paracolic region AR8 (33) LT paracolic region AR4 (27) small bowel serosa (20) large bowel serosa (29) small bowel mesentery (21) large bowel mesentery (32) uterus and ovary AR6 (34) pelvic peritoneum AR5–7 (34) urinary bladder peritoneum AR6 (32) parietal peritoneum (19)
Michielsen et al. [73] (n = number of patients)	duodenum, stomach, celiac trunk carcinomatosis AR2 (16) diffuse serosal carcinomatosis (34) superior mesenteric artery, mesenteric root (8)
Rajan et al. [74] (n = number of patients)	central AR0 (24) RT upper AR1 (4) epigastrium AR2 (6) LT upper AR3 (1) LT flank AR4 (7) LT lower AR5 (12) pelvis AR6 (36) RT lower AR7 (5) RT flank AR8 (8) upper jejunum AR9 (3) lower jejunum AR10 (2) upper ileum AR11 (2) lower ileum AR12 (5)

Table 3. Cont.

Study	Location of PMs (n = Number of Patients or ARs with PMs)
Alcazar et al. [75] (n = number of patients)	rectosigmoid AR6 (27) pelvic peritoneum AR5–7 (59) major omentum AR0 (46) upper abdominal peritoneum (43) small bowel (12) mesentery (4) mesogastrium AR2 (12) hepatic hilum AR1 (10) spleen AR3 (5)
Abdalla Ahmed et al. [76] (n/a)	central AR0 RT upper AR1 LT upper AR3 LT flank AR4 LT lower AR5 pelvis AR6 Douglas pouch, rectosigmoid colon AR6 RT lower AR7 RT flank AR8 upper jejunum AR9 lower jejunum AR10 upper ileum AR11 lower ileum AR12
Tsoi et al. [77] (n = number of patients)	RT subphrenic space AR1 (3) RT subhepatic space AR1 (2) gastric serosa AR2 (1) lesser sac AR2 (0) LT subphrenic space AR3 (1) LT perihepatic space AR2 (0) RT paracolic gutter AR8 (2) LT paracolic gutter AR4 (2) pouch of Douglas AR6 (6) bladder flap AR6 (6) mesentery (5) omentum AR0 (6) large bowel serosa (9) small bowel serosa (1) pelvis AR5–7 (14)
An et al. [27] (n = number of ARs)	subdiaphragmatic space AR1,3 (24) perihepatic space/Morrison pouch AR1 (24) porta hepatis AR1 (2) upper abdominal peritoneum/stomach serosa, lesser sac AR2 (33) splenic hilum AR3 (2) paracolic gutters AR4,8 (27) bowel serosa (45) bowel mesentery (35) omentum AR0 (48) pelvic peritoneum AR5–7 (75)
Mikkelsen et al. [30] (n = number of patients)	liver/duodenum/pancreas/gastric ventricle (7) porta hepatis/hepatoduodenal ligament AR1 (17) celiac trunk/superior mesenteric artery/bowel mesentery root (47)
Feng et al. [42] (n = number of ARs)	central AR0 (29) RT upper AR1 (31) epigastrium AR2 (11) LT upper AR3 (16) LT flank AR4 (19) LT lower AR5 (32) pelvis AR6 (43) RT lower AR7 (29) RT flank AR8 (21) upper jejunum AR9 (10) lower jejunum AR10 (10) upper ileum AR11 (18) lower ileum AR12 (17)

Table 3. Cont.

Study	Location of PMs (n = Number of Patients or ARs with PMs)
Mallet et al. [44] (n = number of patients)	central AR0 (73) RT upper AR1 (67) epigastrium AR2 (58) LT upper AR3 (56) LT flank AR4 (58) LT lower AR5 (77) pelvis AR6 (78) RT lower AR7 (71) RT flank AR8 (62) upper jejunum AR9 (19) lower jejunum AR10 (22) upper ileum AR11 (31) lower ileum AR12 (35)
Fischerova et al. [78] (n/a)	pelvic involvement: anterior and posterior compartment AR5–7 rectosigmoid AR6 upper abdominal involvement: LT diaphragm, spleen, RT diaphragm, liver, and lesser omentum greater omentum: supracolic and infracolic omentum AR0 colon infiltration by omentum RT and LT paracolic gutter AR4,8 anterior abdominal wall bowel serosal and mesenterial peritoneal involvement: small and large bowel serosa and small and large bowel mesentery

3.1. Study Characteristics

The studies selected for meta-analysis included 15 prospective and 18 retrospective articles (Table 2). In total, 23 datasets evaluated the presence of PMs in OC with MDCT [26,27,30,52,56–59,63–76,78] (Table 4); 2, 3, and 8 studies were performed on a 4-row [52,58], 16-row [56,57,74], and 64-row [27,30,59,63,67,70,72,75] MDCT scanner, respectively, 4 studies used both a 16-row and a 64-row CT [64,66,73,76], and 1 report used a 4-row, a 16-row, and a 64-row [65] CT machine (Table 5). Overall, 20 studies [27,30,52,56–59,63–74,76,78] reported the intravenous administration of iodinated contrast medium; 10 of them used the portal phase [27,56–59, 66–68,73,78], 4 used both the arterial and the portal phase [52,65,74,76], 1 used the arterial phase [72], and 1 study used both the portal and the delayed phase [69]. The use of luminal contrast was reported in 15 studies [30,52,64–74,76,78]; 8 studies reported the oral administration of H_2O and diluted contrast medium, including iodinated contrast material in 4 reports [30,66,74,78], gastrografin in 2 studies [69,72], mannitol in 1 study [70], Macrogol in 1 report [65], and 2 studies used H_2O, administered orally in 1 report [52] and as a rectal enema in 1 study [67]. Multiplanar reformations (MPRs) used for data interpretation were reported in 11 studies [27,52,56,57,59,65,67,69,70,73,78]; the application of coronal and sagittal reformations was reported in 4 studies [27,56,57,78]; coronal, sagittal, and oblique MPRs were used in 2 studies [52,65]; coronal plane in 2 reports [59,73]; and in 1 report [70] combined MPRs with three-dimensional maximum intensity projection reformations were performed (Table 5).

Table 4. Characteristics of imaging modalities (MDCT: multidetector CT; DWI: diffusion-weighted imaging; 18F FDG-PET/CT: fluorine-18-fluorodeoxyglucose positron emission tomography/CT, PDS: primary debulking surgery; SLL: second-look laparotomy; IDS: interval debulking surgery; EL: exploratory laparotomy; CECT: contrast-enhanced CT, WB-MRI: whole-body MRI; n/a: non-applicable).

Study	Standard of Reference	MDCT (n = 23)	MRI (n = 4)	DWI (n = 6)	18F FDG-PET/CT (n = 16)	Mean Time Interval between Imaging Modalities/Range (Days)	Mean Time Interval between Imaging and Surgery/Range (Days)
Tempany et al. [51]	surgical (PDS) and histopathologic findings		YES			-	28
Pannu et al. [52]	surgical findings (PDS or SLL)	YES				-	16 (2–108)

Table 4. Cont.

Study	Standard of Reference	MDCT (n = 23)	MRI (n = 4)	DWI (n = 6)	18F FDG-PET/CT (n = 16)	Mean Time Interval between Imaging Modalities/Range (Days)	Mean Time Interval between Imaging and Surgery/Range (Days)
Ricke et al. [53]	surgical (laparotomy) and histopathologic findings		YES			-	56
Pannu et al. [54]	surgical (laparotomy) and histopathologic findings				YES	-	31.7 (6–110)
Kim et al. [55]	surgical and/or histopathologic findings (SLL or biopsy), radiological and clinical follow-up		YES		YES	10 (1–20)	18 (2–35)
Kitajima et al. [56]	surgical and/or histopathologic findings (SLL or biopsy), radiological and clinical follow-up of at least 6 months	YES			YES (CECT)	concurrent	n/a
Kitajima et al. [57]	surgical (PDS) and histopathologic findings	YES			YES (CECT)	concurrent	14
Choi et al. [58]	surgical findings (PDS)	YES				-	17.6 (2–44)
Metser et al. [59]	surgical (PDS or IDS) and histopathologic findings, follow-up (mean time: 19 months)	YES				-	24 (1–67)
De Iaco et al. [60]	surgical (laparoscopy) and histopathologic findings				YES	-	n/a
Sanli et al. [61]	surgical and histopathologic findings (surgical exploration or biopsy), clinical follow-up of at least 6 months		YES		YES	≤30	n/a
Espada et al. [62]	surgical (EL) and histopathologic findings			YES		-	15
Hynninen et al. [63]	surgical (PDS, laparotomy or laparoscopy + IDS) and histopathologic findings	YES			YES (CECT)	concurrent	14
Kim et al. [64]	surgical (PDS or IDS) and histopathologic findings	YES			YES	17 (1–60)	PET/CT: 23 (1–54) MDCT: 26 (4–61)
Mazzei et al. [65]	surgical (PDS) and histopathologic findings	YES				-	45
Michielsen et al. [66]	surgical (PDS or IDS) and histopathologic findings, imaging follow-up	YES		YES (WB-MRI)	YES (CECT)	n/a	n/a
Schmidt et al. [67]	surgical and histopathologic findings	YES		YES	YES	1 ± 4 (0–14)	8.1 ± 2.4 (1–29)
Lopez-Lopez et al. [68]	surgical findings	YES			YES	n/a	<42
Nasser et al. [26]	surgical (debulking surgery) and histopathologic findings	YES				-	n/a
Rodolfino et al. [69]	imaging follow-up for a minimum of 12 months	YES				-	n/a
Tawakol et al. [70]	surgical and histopathologic findings (surgical exploration, biopsy), imaging and clinical follow-up for at least 6 months	YES			YES (CECT)	concurrent	n/a
Cerci et al. [71]	surgical and histopathologic findings	YES				-	28
Bagul et al. [72]	surgical (PDS) and histopathologic findings	YES				-	14
Michielsen et al. [73]	surgical (PDS or IDS) and histopathologic findings, imaging follow-up	YES		YES (WB-MRI)		n/a	n/a
Rajan et al. [74]	surgical (PDS or IDS) and histopathologic findings	YES				-	n/a

Table 4. Cont.

Study	Standard of Reference	MDCT (n = 23)	MRI (n = 4)	DWI (n = 6)	18F FDG-PET/CT (n = 16)	Mean Time Interval between Imaging Modalities/Range (Days)	Mean Time Interval between Imaging and Surgery/Range (Days)
Alcazar et al. [75]	surgical and histopathologic findings (surgical exploration, biopsy)	YES				-	15
Abdalla Ahmed et al. [76]	surgical (laparoscopy and laparotomy, PDS) and histopathologic findings	YES				-	10 (12 ± 5)
Tsoi et al. [77]	surgical (debulking surgery) and histopathologic findings				YES (CECT)	-	19 ± 16
An et al. [27]	surgical (IDS) and histopathologic findings or imaging follow-up in 6–12 months	YES				-	13 (2–43)
Mikkelsen et al. [30]	surgical (PDS) and histopathologic findings	YES (PET/CT)		YES	YES (CECT)	n/a	DWI: 15 (6–28) PET/CT: 14 (1–27)
Feng et al. [42]	surgical (PDS) and histopathologic findings				YES	-	14
Mallet et al. [44]	surgical (laparoscopy) and histopathologic findings				YES	-	28
Fischerova et al. [78]	surgical (laparoscopy or laparotomy, PDS) and histopathologic findings	YES		YES (WB-MRI)		few	28

Table 5. Description of MDCT features (n/a: non-applicable; cm: contrast medium; mgI/mL: iodine content; kV: kilovolt; MIP: maximum-intensity projection; CECT: contrast-enhanced CT).

	Summary of MDCT Features								
Study	Number of Rows	Type of Intravenous cm (mgI/mL)	Amount of cm	Type of Luminal cm	Phases	Slice Thickness (mm)	Slice Reconstruction (mm)	kV	MPRs
Pannu et al. [52]	4	non-ionic	120 mL	750–1000 mL H$_2$O	arterial, portal	3	2	n/a	coronal, sagittal, oblique
Kitajima et al. [PET/CECT] [56]	16	Iomeprole 300	2 mL/kg (150 mL max)	No	portal	2	n/a	140	coronal, sagittal
Kitajima et al. PET/CECT [57]	16	Iomeprole 300	2 mL/kg (150 mL max)	No	portal	2	n/a	140	coronal, sagittal
Choi et al. [58]	4	Ultravist 300	140 mL	n/a	portal	3.2	3	n/a	n/a
Metser et al. [59]	64	Omnipaque 300	2 mL/kg (180 mL max)	n/a	portal	5	2	120	coronal
Hynninen et al. [PET/CECT] [63]	64	Yes, n/a	n/a	n/a	n/a	n/a	n/a	120	n/a
Kim et al. [64]	16 or 64	Yes, n/a	130 mL	450 mL n/a	n/a	n/a	3	120	n/a

Table 5. Cont.

				Summary of MDCT Features					
Study	Number of Rows	Type of Intravenous cm (mgI/mL)	Amount of cm	Type of Luminal cm	Phases	Slice Thickness (mm)	Slice Reconstruction (mm)	kV	MPRs
Mazzei et al. [65]	4 or 16 or 64	Iopamiro 370	2 mL/kg	H$_2$O + Macrogol (7 patients)	late arterial, portal	3.75 (4-row) 3.75/2.5 (16-row) 3.75/1.25/2.5 (64-row)	1.5 (4-row) 0.8 (16-row) 0.8 (64-row)	120–140	coronal, sagittal, oblique
Michielsen et al. [66]	16 or 64	Visipaque 320	120 mL	30 mL Telebrix + 900 mL H$_2$O	portal	5	n/a	120	n/a
Schmidt et al. [67]	64	Iohexol 300	body weight + 30 mL	1 L H$_2$O (rectal enema)	portal	2	2	120	Yes, n/a
Lopez-Lopez et al. [68]	n/a	Yes, n/a	130 mL	450 mL n/a	portal	n/a	3	120	n/a
Nasser et al. [26]	n/a	n/a	n/a	n/a	n/a	n/a	n/a	n/a	n/a
Rodolfino et al. [69]	n/a	Iopromide 370	2 mL/kg	Gastrografin 15 mL + 300 mL H$_2$O	portal, delayed	1	n/a	n/a	Yes, n/a
Tawakol et al. [PET/CECT] [70]	64	non-ionic	1–2 mL/kg (150 mL max)	400–600 mL diluted mannitol	n/a	1.5	n/a	120	axial, coronal, sagittal, MIP
Cerci et al. [71]	n/a	Yes, n/a	n/a	Yes, n/a	n/a	n/a	n/a	n/a	n/a
Bagul et al. [72]	64	non-ionic	80 mL	Gastrografin 2%, 40 mL + 2 L H$_2$O	arterial	3–5	n/a	n/a	n/a
Michielsen et al. [73]	16 or 64	Yes, n/a	n/a	Yes, n/a	portal	n/a	3–5	n/a	transverse, coronal
Rajan et al. [74]	16	non-ionic	50 mL	1000 mL diluted contrast 2%	arterial, portal	5	2–3	n/a	n/a
Alcazar et al. [75]	64	n/a	n/a	n/a	n/a	n/a	n/a	n/a	n/a
Abdalla Ahmed et al. [76]	16 or 64	Ultravist 300	140 mL	500–750 mL n/a	arterial, portal	1.25	0.8	120	n/a
An et al. [27]	64	n/a	1.5 mL/kg	No	portal	2.5	2.5	120	coronal, sagittal
Mikkelsen et al. [30]	64	Iomeron	0.8 mL/kg	diluted Omnipaque	n/a	n/a	2.5 mm	n/a	n/a
Fischerova et al. [78]	n/a	non-ionic	n/a	1 L H$_2$O or diluted iodine contrast	portal	n/a	n/a	n/a	coronal, sagittal, axial

MRI was used in 10 studies [30,51,53,55,61,62,66,67,73,78], 5 performed on a 1.5 T [30,51,53,55,61] and 5 on a 3.0 T system [62,66,67,73,78] (Tables 4 and 6). DWI was applied in six studies [30,62,66,67,73,78], including three reports with whole-body DWI (WB-DWI) [66,73,78] (Table 6). Gadolinium chelate was administered intravenously in nine studies [51,53,55,61,62,66,67,73,78]; two studies reported the use of the portal phase [66,67] and one study used three post-contrast phases (arterial, portal, and delayed) [61]. The administration of luminal contrast prior to the MRI was reported in four studies [66,67,73,78]; two of them reported the use of pineapple juice [66,73], one study used both H_2O and pineapple juice [78], and, in one study, H_2O was given via the rectum [67]. Bowel preparation with intravenous or intramuscular administration of spasmolytic agents was reported in eight studies [30,51,53,55,66,67,73,78] (Table 6).

Table 6. Description of MRI features (T: Tesla; cm: contrast medium; WB-DWI: whole-body diffusion-weighted imaging; im: intramuscularly; iv: intravenously; n/a: non-applicable; DCE: dynamic contrast-enhanced).

	Summary of MRI Features								
Study	Magnetic Field Strength (T)	Type of Coil	Type of Intra-venous cm	Amount of cm (mg/mL)	Phases	Type of Luminal Contrast	Bowel Preparation	Section Thickness (mm)	b-Value (s/mm^2)
Tempany et al. [51]	1.5	multicoil array or body	Gadolinium	n/a	n/a	n/a	1 mg GlucaGen (im)	8–10	No
Ricke et al. [53]	1.5	body	Magnevist	0.2 mL/kg	n/a	n/a	2 × 20 mg Buscopan (iv)	8	No
Kim et al. [55]	1.5	phased array or body	Magnevist	0.1 mmol/kg	n/a	No	20 mg Buscopan (im)	5–8	No
Sanli et al. [61]	1.5	phased array	n/a	n/a	arterial, venous, delayed	n/a	n/a	4–8	No
Espada et al. [62]	3	phased array	Gadolinium	n/a	n/a	n/a	n/a	5	600
Michielsen et al. [66]	3	phased array	Gadolinium-DOTA	15 mL	portal	1 L pineapple juice	20 mg Buscopan (iv)	1.5–6	WB-DWI 0, 1000
Schmidt et al. [67]	3	phased array + spine clusters	Gadolinium-DOTA	0.2 mmol/kg	portal	1 L H_2O rectal enema	20 mg Buscopan/1 mg GlucaGen (iv)	3–6	0, 300, 600
Michielsen et al. [73]	3	phased array	Gadolinium	n/a	n/a	1 L pineapple juice	20 mg Buscopan (iv)	2.5–6	WB-DWI 0, 1000
Mikkelsen et al. [30]	1.5	multi-channel	No	n/a	n/a	No	1 mg glucagon im	5–8	0, 1000
Fischerova et al. [78]	3	phased array	Gadolinium	n/a	n/a	1 L pineapple juice or H_2O	Buscopan (iv)	5	WB-DWI 50, 1000

FDG PET/CT was used in 16 studies [30,42,44,54–57,60,61,63,64,66–68,70,77], including 7 reports with diagnostic contrast-enhanced CT (CECT) [30,56,57,63,66,70,77] (Tables 4 and 7). Six studies were performed on a 16-row [42,56,57,64,67,68] scanner, four on a 64-row [30,63,70,77] system, and three studies, each one used a 4-row [54], an 8-row [55], and a spiral [66] CT machine (Table 7).

Table 7. Description of FDG PET/CT features (n/a: non-applicable; cm; contrast medium; mgI/mL: iodine content; kV: kilovolt).

	Summary of FDG PET/CT Features								
	PET						CT		
Study	System (Covered Area)	Tracer Amount	Scanning Time (min)	Scanning Time (min) per Bed Position	Number of Rows	Slice Thickness (mm)	Type of Intravenous cm (mgI/mL)	Type of Luminal cm	kV
Pannu et al. [54]	caudal to cranial direction	0.22 mCi/kg	n/a	5	4	n/a	No	Readi-cat 1.3%	140
Kim et al. [55]	head-pelvic floor	260–485 MBq	n/a	5	8	5	No	No	140
Kitajima et al. [56]	ear-mid thigh	4 MBq/kg	18–21	3	16	2	Iomeprole 300, 2 mL/kg (150 mL max)	No	140
Kitajima et al. [57]	ear-mid thigh	4 MBq/kg	18–21	3	16	2	Iomeprole 300, 2 mL/kg (150 mL max)	No	140
De Iaco et al. [60]	n/a	5.3 MBq/kg	n/a	4	n/a	5	No	n/a	120
Sanli et al. [61]	skull-upper thigh	370–550 MBq	18–24	3	n/a	n/a	No	Yes, n/a	140
Hynninen et al. [63]	skull-mid thigh	4 MBq/kg	n/a	n/a	64	n/a	Yes, n/a	n/a	120
Kim et al. [64]	skull to upper thigh	350 MBq	n/a	3	16	3.75	No	No	120
Michielsen et al. [66]	whole-body	303 MBq (220–388)	n/a	n/a	spiral	5	Yes, n/a	Yes, n/a	120
Schmidt et al. [67]	skull base-mid thigh	5.5 MBq/kg	n/a	n/a	16	5	No	n/a	140
Lopez-Lopez et al. [68]	skull base-upper thigh	370 MBq	n/a	3	16	5	No	No	120
Tawakol et al. [70]	skull base-mid thigh	3.7–5.2 MBq/kg	18	2	64	5	non-ionic, 1–2 mL/kg, 150 mL max	400–600 mL mannitol	120
Tsoi et al. [77]	skull base-proximal thigh	298 + 53 MBq	15	2.5	64	2.5	±iodinated	No	120
Mikkelsen et al. [30]	n/a	4 MBq/kg	n/a	n/a	64	2.5	Iomeron 0.8 mL/kg	dilute Omnipaque	n/a
Feng et al. [42]	inguinal region-head	7.4 MBq/kg	n/a	2–3	16	n/a	n/a	n/a	120
Mallet et al. [44]	head to midthighs	2–4 MBq/kg	n/a	n/a	n/a	n/a	n/a	n/a	n/a

The following reference tests were used: surgical and histopathologic results ($n = 21$) [26,30,42,44,51,53,54,57,60,62–65,67,71,72,74–78], surgical findings ($n = 3$) [52,58,68], surgical and histopathologic results or follow-up ($n = 8$) [27,55,56,59,61,66,70,73], and follow-up ($n = 1$) [69] (Table 4).

3.2. Quality Assessment

Study quality grading using QUADAS II scores showed that in terms of risk bias and regarding patient selection, index test, reference standard, flow, and timing, the majority of studies included in the analysis were of high to good quality (Figure 3). In terms of applicability, the quality of reporting on patient selection, index test, and the gold standard was good (Figure 3).

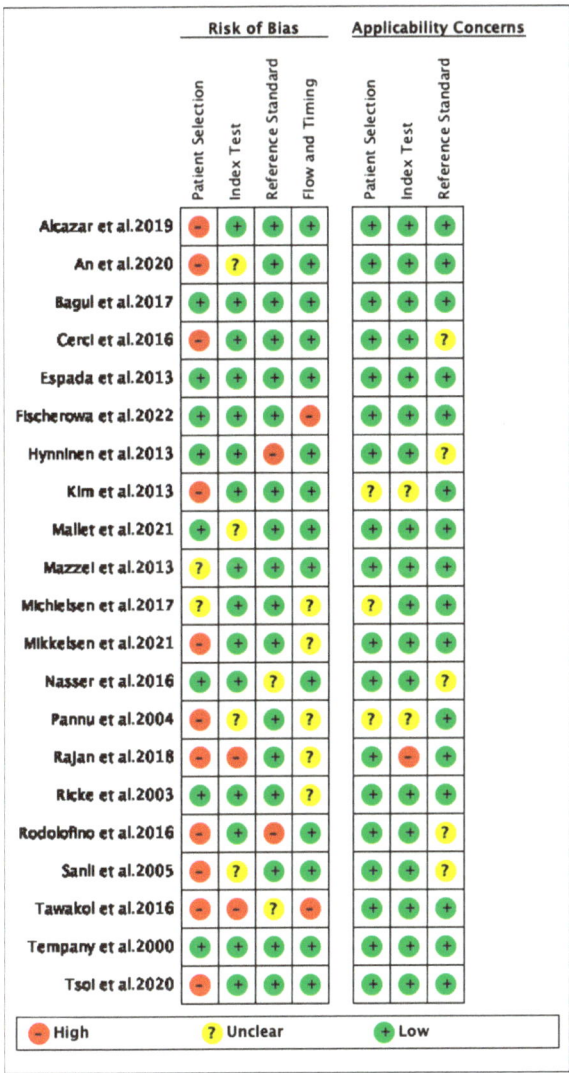

Figure 3. The quality assessment of the included studies [26,27,44,50–53,61–66,69–75,77,78].

3.3. Diagnostic Performance

3.3.1. Per-Patient Analysis

In total, 15, 7, and 8 datasets for MDCT [26,27,30,52,63–65,69–75,78], MRI, including DWI [30,51,53,61,62,73,78], and FDG PET/CT [30,44,54,61,63,64,70,77], respectively, were included in the per-patient analysis. The sensitivity estimates for MDCT, MRI, and FDG

PET/CT on a per-patient basis were 79.7% (95% confidence interval [CI], 75.6–83.4%, I^2 = 82.6%), 82.7% (95% CI, 76.0–88.2%, I^2 = 87.9%), and 93.7% (95% CI, 90.0–96.3%, I^2 = 20.4%), respectively. The specificity estimates for MDCT, MRI, and FDG PET/CT on a per-patient basis were 92.1% (95% CI, 89.6–94.2%, I^2 = 85.1%), 90.3% (95% CI, 86.7–93.1%, I^2 = 86.4%), and 91.5% (95% CI, 86.8–95.0%, I^2 = 84.6%), respectively (Figures 4 and 5). Figure 6 shows study heterogeneity via funnel plots.

Summary Sensitivity

Study	Sensitivity	[95% CI]	TP/(TP+FN)	TN/(TN+FP)
Pannu et al.	1.000	0.590 - 1.000	7/7	10/10
Hynninen et al.	0.571	0.289 - 0.823	8/14	8/8
Kim et al.	0.885	0.698 - 0.976	23/26	13/20
Mazzei et al.	1.000	0.907 - 1.000	38/38	2/5
Nasser et al.	0.571	0.184 - 0.901	4/7	147/148
Rodolfino et al.	0.931	0.772 - 0.992	27/29	8/11
Tawakol et al.	0.693	0.576 - 0.795	52/75	52/61
Cerci et al.	0.574	0.441 - 0.700	35/61	47/51
Bagul et al.	1.000	0.805 - 1.000	17/17	19/19
Michielsen et al.	0.688	0.413 - 0.890	11/16	77/78
Rajan et al.	1.000	0.025 - 1.000	1/1	38/39
Alcazar et al.	0.761	0.612 - 0.874	35/46	44/47
An et al.	0.922	0.811 - 0.978	47/51	4/7
Mikkelsen et al.	0.429	0.099 - 0.816	3/7	43/43
Fischerova et al.	0.953	0.842 - 0.994	41/43	14/24
Pooled Sensitivity	**0.797**	**0.756 - 0.834**		

Heterogeneity chi-squared = 80.42 (d.f.= 14) p = 0.000
Inconsistency (I-square) = 82.6 %
No. studies = 15
Filter OFF
Add 1/2 to all cells of the studies with zero

Summary Specificity

Study	Specificity	[95% CI]	TP/(TP+FN)	TN/(TN+FP)
Pannu et al.	1.000	0.692 - 1.000	7/7	10/10
Hynninen et al.	1.000	0.631 - 1.000	8/14	8/8
Kim et al.	0.650	0.408 - 0.846	23/26	13/20
Mazzei et al.	0.400	0.053 - 0.853	38/38	2/5
Nasser et al.	0.993	0.963 - 1.000	4/7	147/148
Rodolfino et al.	0.727	0.390 - 0.940	27/29	8/11
Tawakol et al.	0.852	0.738 - 0.930	52/75	52/61
Cerci et al.	0.922	0.811 - 0.978	35/61	47/51
Bagul et al.	1.000	0.824 - 1.000	17/17	19/19
Michielsen et al.	0.987	0.931 - 1.000	11/16	77/78
Rajan et al.	0.974	0.865 - 0.999	1/1	38/39
Alcazar et al.	0.936	0.825 - 0.987	35/46	44/47
An et al.	0.571	0.184 - 0.901	47/51	4/7
Mikkelsen et al.	1.000	0.918 - 1.000	3/7	43/43
Fischerova et al.	0.583	0.366 - 0.779	41/43	14/24
Pooled Specificity	**0.921**	**0.896 - 0.942**		

Heterogeneity chi-squared = 93.95 (d.f.= 14) p = 0.000
Inconsistency (I-square) = 85.1 %
No. studies = 15
Filter OFF
Add 1/2 to all cells of the studies with zero

(a)

Summary Sensitivity

Study	Sensitivity	[95% CI]	TP/(TP+FN)	TN/(TN+FP)
Tempany et al.	0.951	0.835 - 0.994	39/41	107/134
Ricke et al.	0.381	0.181 - 0.616	8/21	34/36
Sanli et al.	0.938	0.698 - 0.998	15/16	31/31
Espada et al.	1.000	0.715 - 1.000	11/11	23/23
Michielsen et al.	0.938	0.698 - 0.998	15/16	77/78
Mikkelsen et al.	0.429	0.177 - 0.711	6/14	33/33
Fischerova et al.	0.930	0.809 - 0.985	40/43	19/24
Pooled Sensitivity	**0.827**	**0.760 - 0.882**		

Heterogeneity chi-squared = 49.42 (d.f.= 6) p = 0.000
Inconsistency (I-square) = 87.9 %
No. studies = 7
Filter OFF
Add 1/2 to all cells of the studies with zero

Summary Specificity

Study	Specificity	[95% CI]	TP/(TP+FN)	TN/(TN+FP)
Tempany et al.	0.799	0.721 - 0.863	39/41	107/134
Ricke et al.	0.944	0.813 - 0.993	8/21	34/36
Sanli et al.	1.000	0.888 - 1.000	15/16	31/31
Espada et al.	1.000	0.852 - 1.000	11/11	23/23
Michielsen et al.	0.987	0.931 - 1.000	15/16	77/78
Mikkelsen et al.	1.000	0.894 - 1.000	6/14	33/33
Fischerova et al.	0.792	0.578 - 0.929	40/43	19/24
Pooled Specificity	**0.903**	**0.867 - 0.931**		

Heterogeneity chi-squared = 44.06 (d.f.= 6) p = 0.000
Inconsistency (I-square) = 86.4 %
No. studies = 7
Filter OFF
Add 1/2 to all cells of the studies with zero

(b)

Summary Sensitivity

Study	Sensitivity	[95% CI]	TP/(TP+FN)	TN/(TN+FP)
Pannu et al.	0.727	0.390 - 0.940	8/11	2/5
Sanli et al.	1.000	0.782 - 1.000	15/15	32/32
Hynninen et al.	0.912	0.763 - 0.981	31/34	6/7
Kim et al.	0.962	0.804 - 0.999	25/26	18/20
Tawakol et al.	0.960	0.888 - 0.992	72/75	61/61
Tsoi et al.	0.926	0.757 - 0.991	25/27	18/22
Mikkelsen et al.	0.857	0.421 - 0.996	6/7	42/43
Mallet et al.	0.945	0.866 - 0.985	69/73	5/11
Pooled Sensitivity	**0.937**	**0.900 - 0.963**		

Heterogeneity chi-squared = 8.80 (d.f.= 7) p = 0.267
Inconsistency (I-square) = 20.4 %
No. studies = 8
Filter OFF
Add 1/2 to all cells of the studies with zero

Summary Specificity

Study	Specificity	[95% CI]	TP/(TP+FN)	TN/(TN+FP)
Pannu et al.	0.400	0.053 - 0.853	8/11	2/5
Sanli et al.	1.000	0.891 - 1.000	15/15	32/32
Hynninen et al.	0.857	0.421 - 0.996	31/34	6/7
Kim et al.	0.900	0.683 - 0.988	25/26	18/20
Tawakol et al.	1.000	0.941 - 1.000	72/75	61/61
Tsoi et al.	0.818	0.597 - 0.948	25/27	18/22
Mikkelsen et al.	0.977	0.877 - 0.999	6/7	42/43
Mallet et al.	0.455	0.167 - 0.766	69/73	5/11
Pooled Specificity	**0.915**	**0.868 - 0.950**		

Heterogeneity chi-squared = 45.51 (d.f.= 7) p = 0.000
Inconsistency (I-square) = 84.6 %
No. studies = 8
Filter OFF
Add 1/2 to all cells of the studies with zero

(c)

Figure 4. Forest plots for the pooled sensitivity and specificity calculation for (**a**) MDCT [26,27,30,52,63–65,69–75,78], (**b**) MRI [30,51,53,61,62,73,78], and (**c**) FDG PET/CT [30,44,54,61,63,64,70,77] in the detection of peritoneal metastases in ovarian cancer, on a per-patient basis (CI: confidence interval; TP: true positive; FN: false negative; TN: true negative).

The per-patient diagnostic performance, including TP, FN, FP, and TN findings; sensitivity; specificity; positive predictive value (PPV); and negative predictive value (NPV) for each imaging modality are presented in Tables S1–S3. The DOR estimates for MDCT, MRI, and FDG PET/CT on a per-patient basis were 29.55% (95% CI, 17.54–49.78%), 93.95% (95%CI, 27.41–321.97%), and 84.15% (95%CI, 17.62–401.8%), respectively. The summary area-under-the-curve (SAUC) for MDCT, MRI, and FDG PET/CT was determined to be 0.91, 0.96, and 0.97, respectively (Figure 7). The sensitivity estimates for MRI ($p = 0.03$) and FDG PET/CT ($p < 0.01$) were higher than that for MDCT, on a per-patient basis. FDG PET/CT had higher sensitivity compared to MRI, although non-significant ($p = 0.84$).

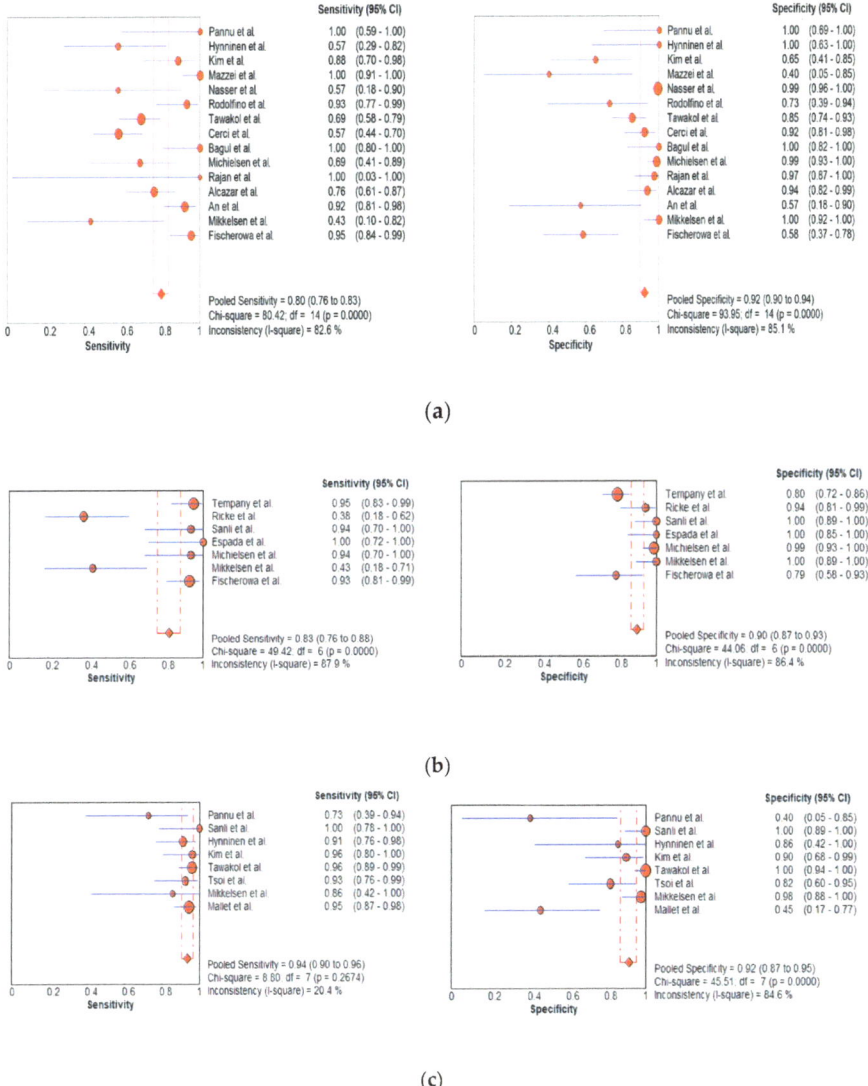

Figure 5. Foster plots for sensitivity and specificity for (**a**) MDCT [26,27,30,52,63–65,69–75,78], (**b**) MRI [30,44,54,61,63,64,70,77], and (**c**) FDG PET/CT [30,51,53,61,62,73,78] in the detection of peritoneal metastases in ovarian cancer, on a per-patient basis (CI: confidence interval).

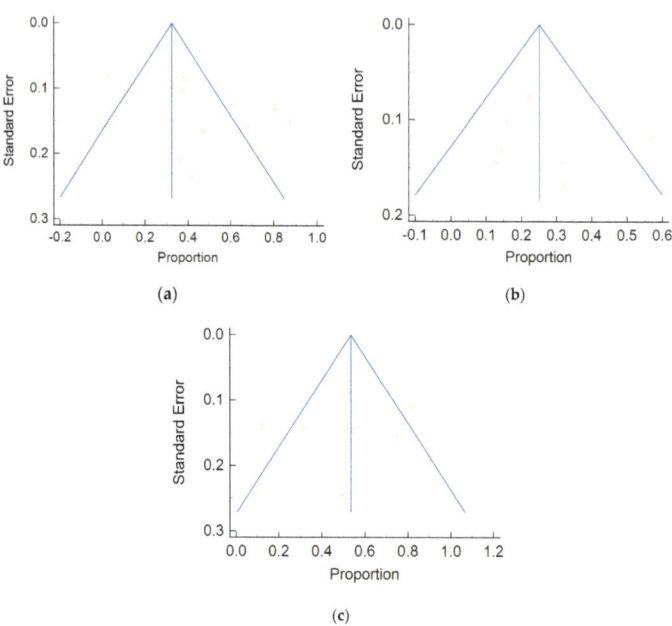

Figure 6. Funnel plots of the (**a**) MDCT, (**b**) MRI, and (**c**) FDG PET/CT data on a per-patient basis.

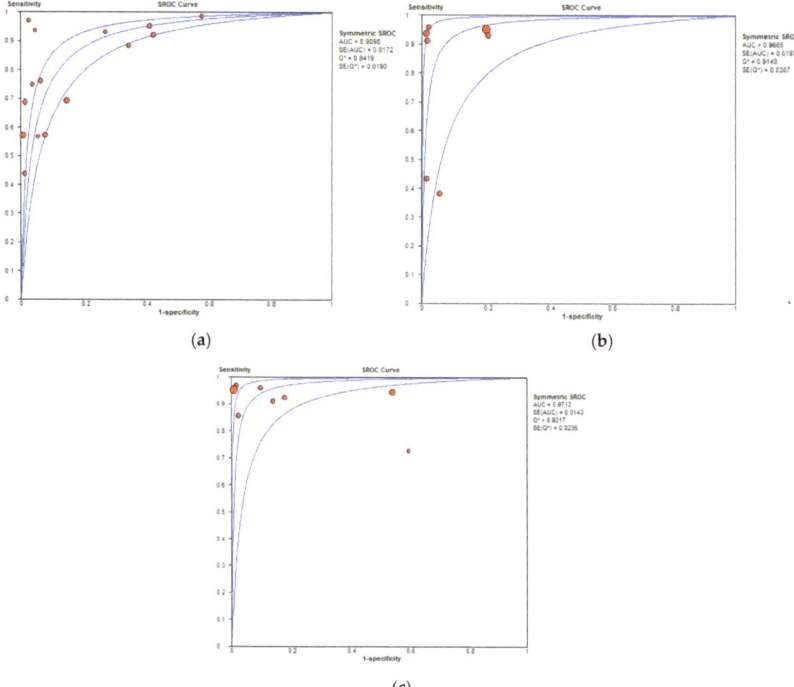

Figure 7. Summary receiver operating characteristic curves depicting the diagnostic performance of (**a**) MDCT, (**b**) MRI, and (**c**) FDG PET/CT in the detection of peritoneal metastases in ovarian cancer, on a per-patient basis.

3.3.2. Per-Region Analysis

Per-region data were analyzed for 338 women with advanced OC and 3.881 ARs (Tables S4–S6). Overall, 12, 3 and 11 datasets for MDCT [27,56–59,63,65–69,76], MRI, including DWI [55,66,67], and FDG PET/CT [42,54–57,60,63,66–68,77], respectively, were included in the per-region analysis. On a per-region basis, comparison between MDCT, MRI, and FDG PET/CT for detecting PMs revealed a sensitivity of 70.1% (95% CI, 68.5–71.6% I^2 = 98.9%), 92.6% (95% CI, 89.0–95.3%, I^2 = 73.2%), and 58.3% (95% CI, 56–60.6%, I^2 = 96.8%), respectively. The specificity estimates for MDCT, MRI, and FDG PET/CT were 90.2% (95% CI, 89.3–91.1%, I^2 = 97.4%), 90.3% (95% CI, 86.7–93.2%, I^2 = 72.6%), and 92.6% (95% CI, 91.4–93.7%, I^2 = 92.6%), respectively (Figures 8 and 9). The per-region diagnostic performances are presented in Tables S4–S6. MDCT, MRI, and FDG PET/CT had an AUC of 0.92, 0.96, and 0.89, respectively, on a per-region analysis (Figure 10). No differences in sensitivity estimates were found between MDCT and MRI (p = 0.25), MDCT and FDG PET/CT (p = 0.68), and MRI and FDG PET/CT (p = 0.35), on a per-region basis.

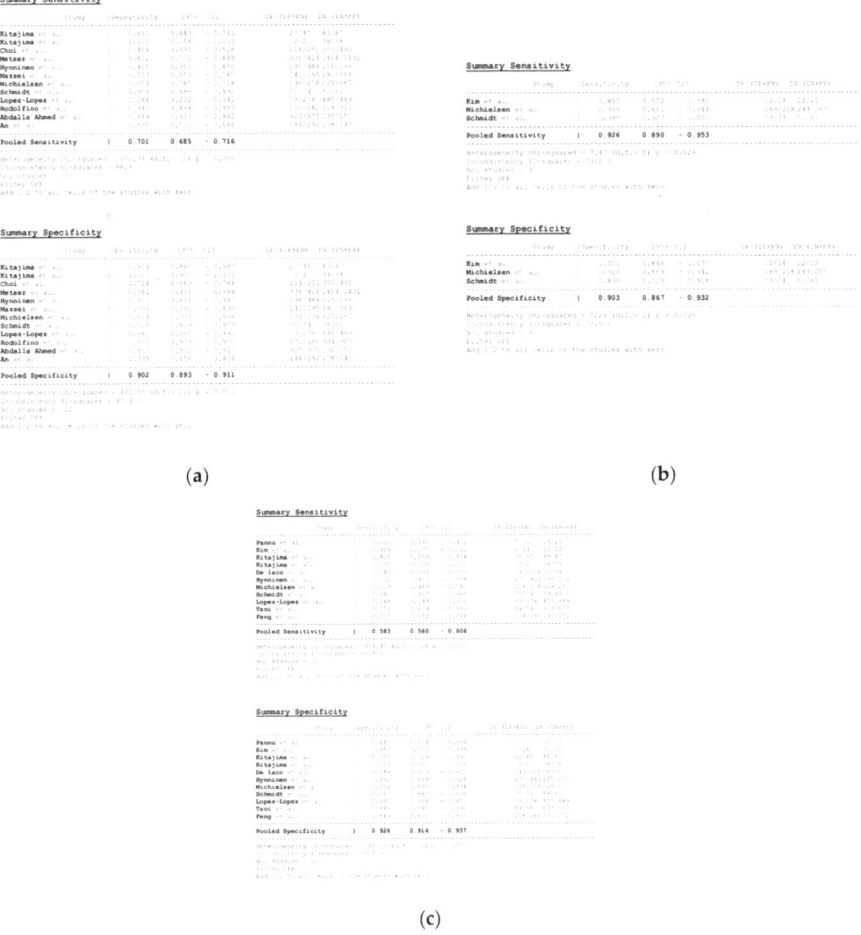

Figure 8. Forest plots for the pooled sensitivity and specificity calculation for (**a**) MDCT [27,56–59,63,65–69,76], (**b**) MRI [55,66,67], and (**c**) FDG PET/CT [42,54–57,60,63,66–68,77] in the detection of peritoneal metastases in ovarian cancer, on a per-region basis (CI: confidence interval; TP: true positive; FN: false negative; TN: true negative).

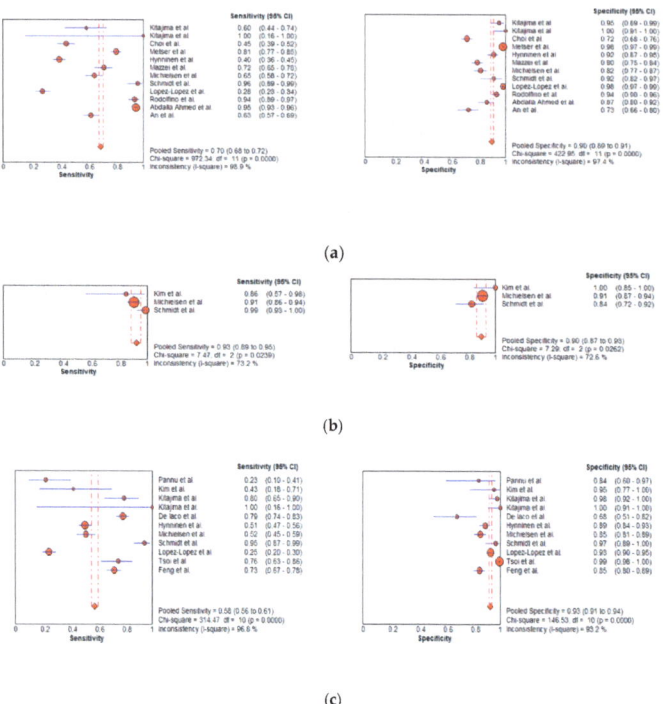

Figure 9. Foster plots for sensitivity and specificity for (**a**) MDCT [27,56–59,63,65–69,76], (**b**) MRI [55,66,67], and (**c**) FDG PET/CT [42,54–57,60,63,66–68,77] in the detection of peritoneal metastases in ovarian cancer, on a per-region basis (CI: confidence interval).

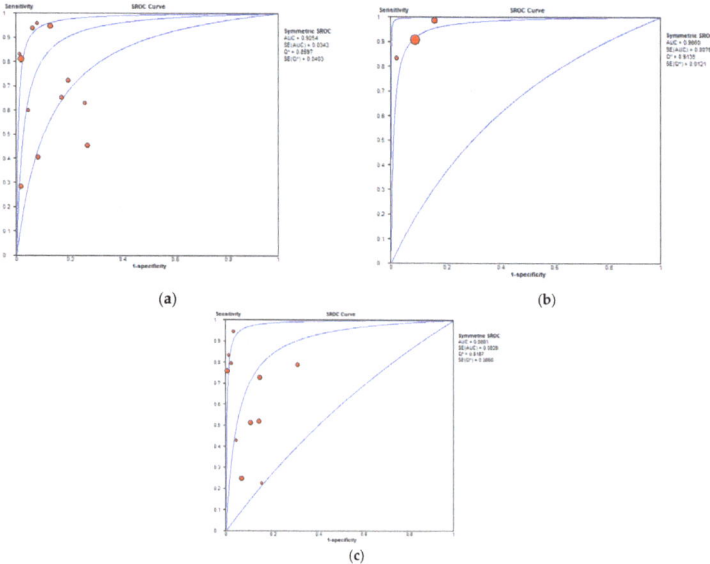

Figure 10. Summary receiver operating characteristic curves depicting the diagnostic performance of (**a**) MDCT, (**b**) MRI, and (**c**) FDG PET/CT in the detection of peritoneal metastases in ovarian cancer, on a per-region basis.

3.3.3. Subgroup Analysis: Abdominopelvic Regions
Per-Patient Analysis

Tables 8–10 show sensitivity and specificity estimates for the three imaging modalities in different ARs, on a per-patient basis.

Datasets for assessing per-patient diagnostic accuracy of MDCT were available for all ARs, including AR0 [52,63,71,72,74,75,78], AR1 [26,30,52,63,72,74,75,78], AR2 [52,72,74,78], AR3 [26,52,63,72,74,75,78], AR4 [72,74,78], AR5–7 [26,52,63,71,72,74,75,78], AR6 [26,52,71,72,74,75,78], AR8 [72,74,78], diaphragm [26,52,63,71,72,78], small bowel [26,63,65,72,74,75,78], colon [26,63,72,78], and mesentery [26,30,52,63,71–73,75,78] (Table S7). The accuracy of MDCT in the detection of PMs on a per-patient basis was higher in six ARs: the left hypochondrium (AR3), including the undersurface of the left hemidiaphragm, spleen, pancreatic tail of the pancreas, and anterior and posterior surfaces of the stomach, with sensitivity estimates of 61.8% (95% CI, 50.9–71.9%), specificity estimates 97.9% (95% CI, 95.8–99.2%), and an AUC of 0.93; the diaphragm, with a sensitivity of 49.7% (95% CI, 42.6–56.9%), a specificity of 97.7% (95% CI, 94.8–99.3%), and an AUC of 0.91; the pelvis–hypogastrium (AR6), including the female internal genitalia, the urinary bladder, the cul-de-sac of Douglas, and the rectosigmoid colon, with a sensitivity of 66.2% (95% CI, 59.7–72.3%), a specificity of 93.3% (95% CI, 89.7–95.9%), and an AUC of 0.92; and the central abdomen (AR0), including the midline abdominal incision, the greater omentum, and the transverse colon, with sensitivity estimates of 80.1% (95% CI, 74.5–84.9%), specificity estimates 89% (95% CI, 83.1–93.3%), and an AUC of 0.91; left lumbar region (AR4), including the descending colon and the left paracolic gutter, with sensitivity estimates of 73% (95% CI, 60.3–83.4%), specificity estimates 86.3% (95% CI, 76.7–92.9%), and an AUC of 0.92; and pelvis (A5–7), with a sensitivity of 64.1% (95% CI, 58.4–69.4%), a specificity of 95.1% (95% CI, 91.6–97.4%), and an AUC of 0.90 (Table 8). MDCT had the lowest diagnostic performance on a per-patient basis in two regions: the colon, with a sensitivity of 30.5% (95% CI, 23.2–38.5%), a specificity of 95.8% (95% CI, 92.2–98.1%), and an AUC of 0.36, and the mesentery, with a sensitivity of 33.8% (95% CI, 27.2–41%), a specificity of 96.9% (95% CI, 94.9–98.3%), and an AUC of 0.66 (Table 8).

Datasets for assessing the per-patient diagnostic accuracy of MRI were available for only three ARs, including, AR0 [51,53,78], the diaphragm [51,53,62,78], and the mesentery [30,51,62,73,78] (Table S8). The sensitivity (59.2%) and specificity (75.7%) of MRI were higher in the mesentery, with an AUC of 0.90 (Table 9).

Table 8. Diagnostic accuracy of MDCT in different abdominopelvic regions on a per-patient basis (AR: abdominopelvic region; CI: confidence interval; AUC: area under the curve).

ARs	Pooled Sensitivity (%CI)	Pooled Specificity (%CI)	AUC
AR0	80.1 (74.5–84.9)	89 (83.1–93.3)	0.91
AR1	62.5 (54.1–70.4)	97.1 (94.8–98.6)	0.86
AR2	53.1 (34.7–70.9)	92.8 (86.8–96.7)	0.72
AR3	61.8 (50.9–71.9)	97.9 (95.8–99.2)	0.93
AR4	73 (60.3–83.4)	86.3 (76.7–92.9)	0.92
AR5–7	64.1 (58.4–69.4)	95.1 (91.6–97.4)	0.90
AR6	66.2 (59.7–72.3)	93.3 (89.7–95.9)	0.92
AR8	71 (58.8–81.3)	86.3 (76.2–93.2)	0.74
diaphragm	49.7 (42.6–56.9)	97.7 (94.8–99.3)	0.91
small bowel (AR9–12)	45.5 (35.4–55.8)	94.9 (92.2–96.9)	0.80
colon	30.5 (23.2–38.5)	95.8 (92.2–98.1)	0.36
mesentery	33.8 (27.2–41)	96.9 (94.9–98.3)	0.66

Table 9. Diagnostic accuracy of MRI in different abdominopelvic regions on a per-patient basis (AR: abdominopelvic region; CI: confidence interval; AUC: area under the curve).

ARs	Pooled Sensitivity (%CI)	Pooled Specificity (%CI)	AUC (SE)
AR0	64.7 (55.9–72.7)	67.2 (61.2–72.7)	0.82
diaphragm	67.3 (57.3–76.3)	66.5 (61.2–71.5)	0.66
mesentery	59.2 (48.8–69)	75.7 (71.3–79.7)	0.90

Table 10. Diagnostic accuracy of FDG PET-CT in different abdominopelvic regions on a per-patient basis (AR: abdominopelvic region; CI: confidence interval; AUC: area under the curve).

ARs	Pooled Sensitivity (%CI)	Pooled Specificity (%CI)	AUC (SE)
AR0	92.9 (86.5–96.9)	85.2 (73.8–93)	0.95
AR1	73.5 (64.5–81.2)	92.1 (85–96.5)	0.83
AR3	70.4 (58.4–80.7)	86.9 (77.8–93.3)	0.78
AR5–7	91.5 (85–95.9)	87.5 (74.8–95.3)	0.94
mesentery	45.5 (30.4–61.2)	98.9 (94–100)	0.9

Available data for assessing the diagnostic performance of FDG PET/CT on a per-patient basis included five ARs: AR0 [44,63,77], AR1 [30,44,63,77], AR3 [44,63,77], A5–7 [44,63,77], and mesentery [30,63,77] (Table S9). Detection rates for FDG PET/CT were higher in two regions: the central abdomen (AR0), with sensitivity estimates of 92.9% (95% CI, 86.5–96.9%), specificity estimates of 85.2% (95% CI, 73.8–93%), and an AUC of 0.95, and the pelvis (AR5–7), with sensitivity estimates of 91.5% (95% CI, 85–95.9%), specificity estimates of 87.5% (95% CI, 74.8–95.3%), and an AUC of 0.94 (Table 10).

Per-Region Analysis

On a per-region analysis, data assessing the diagnostic accuracy were available for MDCT in four regions, including AR0, AR5–7, and AR6, the diaphragm and mesentery [27,57,58,66], and for FDG PET/CT in six regions, including AR0 [42,57,60,66], AR1 [42,54,60,66], AR3 [42,54,60,66], AR4 [42,60,66], AR8 [42,60,66], and the pelvis (AR5–7) [42,54,57,60,66] (Tables S10 and S11). The assessment of MRI data in different ARs on a per-region basis was not possible due to the small number of studies.

The highest detection rates for MDCT on a per-region analysis were noted at the pelvis–hypogastrium [sensitivity, 24.4% (95% CI, 12.4–40.3%); specificity, 96.4% (95% CI, 89.9–99.3%); and, AUC, 0.99] and the lowest detection rates were found at the mesentery [sensitivity: 43.4% (95% CI, 29.8–57.7%); specificity, 90.7% (95% CI, 83.6–95.5%); and, AUC: 0.68] (Table 11). The sensitivity for detecting PMs in different ARs for FDG PET/CT on a per-region basis revealed better results in the right hypochondrium [sensitivity: 66.7% (95% CI, 54.8–77.1%); specificity, 81.8% (95% CI, 69.1–90.9%); and, AUC: 0.99] (Table 12).

Table 11. Diagnostic accuracy of MDCT in different abdominopelvic regions on a per-region basis (AR: abdominopelvic region; CI: confidence interval; AUC: area under the curve).

ARs	Pooled Sensitivity (%CI)	Pooled Specificity (%CI)	AUC
AR0	60.7 (49.7–70.9)	77 (66.8–85.4)	0.72
AR5–7	46.6 (35.9–57.5)	88.7 (81.4–93.8)	0.78
AR6	24.4 (12.4–40.3)	96.4 (89.9–99.3)	0.99
diaphragm	40.7 (28.1–54.3)	86 (73.3–94.2)	0.89
mesentery	43.4 (29.8–57.7)	90.7 (83.6–95.5)	0.68

Table 12. Diagnostic accuracy of FDG PET-CT in different abdominopelvic regions on a per-region basis (AR: abdominopelvic region; CI: confidence interval; AUC: area under the curve).

ARs	Pooled Sensitivity (%CI)	Pooled Specificity (%CI)	AUC
AR0	83.7 (74.8–90.4)	89.3 (78.1–96)	0.90
AR1	66.7 (54.8–77.1)	81.8 (69.1–90.9)	0.99
AR3	74.5 (59.7–86.1)	82.5 (70.1–91.3)	0.88
AR4	75.7 (64–85.2)	80.5 (65.1–91.2)	0.81
AR5–7	57.1 (47.4–66.5)	91.8 (81.9–97.3)	0.74
AR8	77.1 (65.6–86.3)	82.5 (67.2–92.7)	0.86

4. Discussion

According to our knowledge, this is an up-to-date systematic review and meta-analysis that exclusively compares the diagnostic performance of MDCT, MRI, including DWI, and FDG PET/CT in the detection of peritoneal metastases in women with ovarian cancer. In total, 33 studies, 23 using MDCT, 10 MRI (including three reports with DWI and three studies with WB-DWI), and 16 using FDG PET/CT (including seven studies with CECT), were evaluated. On a per-patient basis, FDG PET/CT had the highest sensitivity (93.7%) when compared to MRI (82.7%) and MDCT (79.7%). Specificity estimates were high for all imaging modalities (92.1%, 90.3%, and 91.5% for MDCT, MRI, and FDG PET/CT, respectively). Both FDG PET/CT and MRI have comparably higher per-patient diagnostic accuracy for the detection of PMs when compared to MDCT.

No differences in the diagnostic performance between MDCT, MRI, and FDG PET/CT were found on a per-lesion basis. MRI had the highest sensitivity (92.6%), when compared to MDCT (70.1%) and FDG PET/CT (58.3%), although our results are limited, due to the small number of MRI datasets ($n = 3$). Specificity estimates were comparably high for all imaging modalities (90.2%, 90.3%, and 92.6% for MDCT, MRI, and FDG PET/CT, respectively). Based on the results of this meta-analysis, FDG PET/CT and MRI had higher sensitivity compared to MDCT in the detection of PMs in OC.

Similar to our results, a recently published meta-analysis reported comparable diagnostic performance for DWI MRI and FDG PET/CT, higher than that of CT for the detection of PMs in ovarian and gastrointestinal cancer patients [47]. This review was based on 28 articles, including 20, 7, and 10 CT, DWI MRI, and FDG PET/CT datasets, respectively. The pooled sensitivity and specificity were 68% and 88% for CT, 92% and 85% for DWI MRI, and 80% and 90% for FDG PET/CT [47].

MDCT is routinely used for the preoperative imaging of primary OC, with a reported staging accuracy of up to 94% [1,3,5,6,18–21,69,79]. Portal venous phase and water density oral contrast usually provide detailed mapping of PMs [1,69]. MDCT is also used for the evaluation of any persistence of disease after CRS and during follow-up, with a sensitivity and specificity of 58–84% and 59–100%, respectively, in the detection of OC recurrence [1,69,70,80].

The main advantages of MDCT include the following: wide availability, rapid scanning, increased volume coverage, excellent spatial resolution, robustness, and reproducibility of image acquisition. CT is devoid of misregistration artifacts and allows the acquisition of thin sections and the creation of high-resolution MPRs, improving the detection of small PMs, especially when a large amount of ascites is present, and the detailed exploration of curved peritoneal surfaces [18–21,67,69,70,81–85]. Coronal reformations improve the assessment of hemidiaphragms, hepatic and splenic surfaces, and paracolic gutters and the evaluation of the extent of omental disease. Sagittal MPRs improve the assessment of the hemidiaphragms, the Douglas pouch, the vaginal cuff, the peritoneal surface of the bladder, and the rectosigmoid colon [83–85]. The use of multiplanar reformations was reported in 11 articles in this meta-analysis, although comparative studies on the diagnostic performance of axial images versus MPRs in the detection of PMs were not performed due to limited data [27,52,56,57,59,65,67,69,70,73,78].

However, CT has limitations, including poor soft tissue contrast and reduced sensitivity for the detection of small PMs (<5 mm) and those in certain anatomical locations (e.g., mesentery and bowel serosa), especially in the absence of ascites [3,13,18–21,25,26,66,67,69,70,73,81,82]. Subgroup analysis including PMs of different sizes was not performed in the present review, due to inadequate relevant data.

MDCT comprised the largest dataset in our meta-analysis, allowing a comprehensive assessment of the diagnostic accuracy of the technique in the detection of PMs in different abdominopelvic regions. The highest MDCT detection rates were noted at the left hypochondrium (AR3), the central abdomen (AR0), the diaphragm, the pelvis (AR5–7 and AR6), and the left lumbar region (AR4). Our observations are primarily related to the advantages of MDCT technology, namely, the acquisition of thin slices and the creation of high-resolution reformations, resulting in an improvement in the evaluation of curved structures, such as the undersurface of the diaphragms, the paracolic gutter, and the pelvis [3,19]. Similar to published data, this review confirmed the low diagnostic performance of CT in the colon and the mesentery [3,13,20,25,26,73,81]. The detection of early mesenteric involvement or small-sized serosal bowel PMs may be problematic, as CT signs may be subtle, especially in the absence of adequate bowel distention [3].

Based on the analysis of 10 datasets, MRI proved more accurate compared to MDCT for the detection of PMs, on a per-patient basis. The use of fat suppression, delayed contrast-enhanced sequences, and DWI contribute to the improvement in the accuracy of MRI in the detection of PMs [3,5,16,20,21,30–35,66,69,86–91]. MRI allows better detection of subcentimeter PMs and PC involving certain anatomic areas, such as the bowel serosal surface, the pelvis, the right hypochondrium, and the mesentery. The interobserver agreement of MRI has also been reported to be higher compared to CT in most ARs [31,81]. Although the diagnostic performance of MRI was only assessed in three ARs, including the central abdomen (AR0), the diaphragm, and the mesentery, our systematic review found that MRI was more accurate in the bowel mesentery.

Normal peritoneal enhancement is equal to or less than that of the liver. Contrast enhancement greater than the liver is abnormal and may represent the only finding suggestive of PC. This sign is not always detected by MDCT; however, it is readily appreciated by MRI on delayed fat-suppressed contrast-enhanced imaging [3,5,20,81,88]. The sensitivity of MRI for PMs has been reported to increase by using DWI in combination with conventional MRI sequences, even in the absence of ascites. The increased contrast between the hyperintense hypercellular implants against the surrounding hypointense normal tissues enhances the detectability of PC by DWI [5,20,21,31,81,86–89].

No direct comparison between the accuracy of conventional MRI sequences and DWI was performed in this analysis, due to limited data.

Limitations of MRI are related to the high cost and long examination time, motion artifacts, lack of routine use of intraluminal contrast agents, and need for experience in image acquisition and interpretation [1,20,81,92]. MRI is also limited by its ability to detect small, calcified PMs, which are easily detected by MDCT. Disadvantages related to DWI are due to the low spatial resolution; presence of false-positives, attributed to densely cellular tissue, such as fibrosis, bowel mucosa, endometrium, and abscess; and false-negatives, attributed to mucinous carcinomas and well-differentiated malignancies [1,20].

Similar to MRI, this meta-analysis showed that FDG PET/CT was more sensitive than MDCT in the assessment of PC in OC on a per-patient basis. The main advantage of the technique is the whole-body coverage. FDG PET/CT can detect small PMs; evaluate all peritoneal compartments, even those inaccessible during surgery, such as the subdiaphragmatic peritoneal surfaces and the bowel mesentery; better assess ascites; and discriminate nodular peritoneal implants from the intestinal loops [1,5,17,30,36–44,63,67–69,93–101]. The present review showed that FDG PET/CT had the highest detection rates in the central abdomen (AR0), the right hypochondrium (AR1), and the pelvis (AR5–7).

FDG PET/CT disadvantages are related to limited spatial resolution in the detection of small PMs (<5 mm), difficulty in the evaluation of diffuse peritoneal disease, presence of tissues with low FDG avidity, such as mucinous tumors, and possible discrepancy in lesion location between CT and PET/CT caused by respiratory movements and intestinal peristalsis. False positives may be due to inflammation, infection, and benign conditions or the normal physiological activity in the bowel, gallbladder, vessels, ureters, and urinary bladder. Shortcomings of PET/CT also include the limited availability and the high cost [5,67,68,101].

Complete resection of all macroscopic peritoneal implants has been proven to be the single most important independent prognostic factor in OC. Diagnostic laparoscopy can provide a definitive histologic diagnosis and detailed information on the extent of PC. However, up to 40% of women may be understaged surgically as small PMs in areas such as the subdiaphragmatic surfaces, the porta hepatis, or the hepatorenal fossa are not easily accessible. In addition, diagnostic laparoscopy has been associated with a high incidence of port-site metastases, although these do not worsen the patient's prognosis [1,79]. Preoperative diagnostic work-up with CT, MRI, or FDG PET/CT is vital in the assessment of the extent of PC in OC [1,79].

Tumor heterogeneity in OC at a cellular and genetic level is a well-known phenomenon that cannot be thoroughly evaluated using conventional imaging data. Quantitative semi-automated and automated methods based on artificial intelligence techniques have been developed, which can be applied to routine medical images to assess tumor heterogeneity. The use of radiomics and radiogenomics may be helpful in the future in predicting OC genotype and biology and in assessing treatment response, clinical outcome, and patient survival [102–106]. Based on preliminary data, MRI and CT-based radiomics have been reported to predict the presence of PMs in OC [107–110].

This meta-analysis has inherent limitations, mainly related to publication bias and study heterogeneity. Our systematic review was limited to the PubMed database, including published studies reporting a "positive effect" that might overestimate the actual magnitude of an effect. However, study quality grading showed that most of the studies included in the analysis were of high to good quality.

Heterogeneity among included patient groups is another shortcoming, due to differences in primary outcome (primary staging and recurrent disease). Subgroup analysis assessing the differences in the diagnostic performance of MDCT, MRI, and FDG PET/CT in the detection of PMs between primary and recurrent OC was not performed, due to the lack of relevant data. Heterogeneity in study design, imaging methodologies (including scanners, protocols, sequences, and intravenous/oral contrast), reader experience, and reference standards (ranging from histopathologic confirmation to surgical findings and imaging follow-up) is another limitation. The standardization of imaging techniques and consensus on the interpretation criteria for PMs across different centers would facilitate more accurate and reliable assessments. Finally, no data on the cost-effectiveness of MDCT, MRI, and FDG PET/CT were analyzed. Future research should focus on evaluating the cost-effectiveness of these imaging modalities in detecting peritoneal metastases and their impact on treatment decision making.

5. Conclusions

Peritoneal metastases represent a common finding in women with primary or recurrent OC. Preoperative diagnostic work-up with MDCT, MRI, or FDG PET/CT is mandatory to define the extent of the disease, predict the likelihood of optimal cytoreduction, identify potentially unresectable or difficult disease locations, requiring surgical technique modifications, and select patients who may benefit from adjuvant chemotherapy.

Based on the results of this meta-analysis, FDG PET/CT and MRI had a higher diagnostic performance in the detection of PMs compared to MDCT on a per-patient analysis. No differences between the three imaging modalities were found on a per-lesion basis.

In summary, while FDG PET/CT and MRI can be considered equivalent alternatives for the detection of peritoneal metastases in ovarian cancer, the limitations of the included studies and the need for standardization should be considered. Future research addressing these limitations and exploring cost-effectiveness would contribute to the improvement in clinical practice in the management of ovarian cancer.

Supplementary Materials: The following supporting information can be downloaded at https://www.mdpi.com/article/10.3390/cancers16081467/s1, Table S1: Results of the per-patient analysis for MDCT (TP: true positive, FN: false negative; FP: false positive; TN: true negative; PPV: positive-predictive value; NPV: negative-predictive value; MPR: multiplanar reformation); Table S2: Results of the per-patient analysis for MRI (TP: true positive, FN: false negative; FP: false positive; TN: true negative; PPV: positive-predictive value; NPV: negative-predictive value; PMs: peritoneal metastases); Table S3: Results of the per-patient analysis for FDG PET/CT (TP: true positive, FN: false negative; FP: false positive; TN: true negative; PPV: positive-predictive value; NPV: negative-predictive value); Table S4: Results of the per-region analysis for MDCT (TP: true positive, FN: false negative; FP: false positive; TN: true negative; PPV: positive-predictive value; NPV: negative-predictive value); Table S5: Results of the per-region analysis for MRI (TP: true positive, FN: false negative; FP: false positive; TN: true negative; PPV: positive-predictive value; NPV: negative-predictive value); Table S6: Results of the per-region analysis for FDG PET/CT (TP: true positive, FN: false negative; FP: false positive; TN: true negative; PPV: positive-predictive value; NPV: negative-predictive value); Table S7: Results of the per-patient analysis for MDCT in different abdominopelvic regions (TP: true positive, FN: false negative; FP: false positive; TN: true negative; PPV: positive-predictive value; NPV: negative-predictive value; ARs: abdominopelvic regions; MPR: multiplanar reformation); Table S8: Results of the per-patient analysis for MRI in different abdominopelvic regions (TP: true positive, FN: false negative; FP: false positive; TN: true negative; PPV: positive-predictive value; NPV: negative-predictive value); Table S9: Results of the per-patient analysis for FDG PET/CT in different abdominopelvic regions (TP: true positive, FN: false negative; FP: false positive; TN: true negative; PPV: positive-predictive value; NPV: negative-predictive value); Table S10: Results of the per-region analysis for MDCT in different abdominopelvic regions (TP: true positive, FN: false negative; FP: false positive; TN: true negative; PPV: positive-predictive value; NPV: negative-predictive value; ARs: abdominopelvic regions); Table S11: Results of the per-region analysis for FDG PET-CT in different abdominopelvic regions (TP: true positive, FN: false negative; FP: false positive; TN: true negative; PPV: positive-predictive value; NPV: negative-predictive value; ARs: abdominopelvic regions). References [26,27,30,42,44,51–78] are cited in the Supplementary Materials.

Author Contributions: A.C.T., M.T. and T.S. wrote the review. M.T. and T.S. prepared the figures. A.C.T., G.A. and M.I.A. reviewed and edited the draft. All authors have read and agreed to the published version of the manuscript.

Funding: This research received no external funding.

Data Availability Statement: The data presented in this study are available in this article.

Conflicts of Interest: The authors declare no conflicts of interest in the context of the present review.

Abbreviations

OC	ovarian cancer
PDS	primary debulking surgery
IDS	interval debulking surgery
NAC	neoadjuvant chemotherapy
PMs	peritoneal metastases
PCI	peritoneal carcinomatosis index
ARs	abdominopelvic regions
PC	peritoneal carcinomatosis
MDCT	multidetector CT
DWI	diffusion-weighted imaging
PRISMA	preferred reporting items for systematic reviews and meta-analysis

FDG	fluorodeoxyglucose
PET	positron emission tomography
TP	true-positive
FN	false-negative
FP	false-positive
TN	true-negative
QUADAS	quality assessment of diagnostic accuracy studies
MPR	multiplanar reformation
WB-DWI	whole-body DWI
CECT	contrast-enhanced CT
CI	confidence interval
PPV	positive predictive value
NPV	negative predictive value
AUC	area under the curve
DOR	diagnostic odds ratio
SROC	summary receiver operating characteristic curve

References

1. Expert Panel on Women's Imaging; Kang, S.K.; Reinhold, C.; Atri, M.; Benson, C.B.; Bhosale, P.R.; Jhingran, A.; Lakhman, Y.; Maturen, K.E.; Nicola, R.; et al. ACR Appropriateness Criteria® Staging and Follow-Up of Ovarian Cancer. *J. Am. Coll. Radiol.* **2018**, *15*, S198–S207. [CrossRef] [PubMed]
2. American Cancer Society. Cancer Facts & Figures 2024. Available online: https://www.cancer.org/content/dam/cancer-org/research/cancer-facts-and-statistics/annual-cancer-facts-and-figures/2024/2024-cancer-facts-and-figures-acs.pdf (accessed on 4 April 2024).
3. Nougaret, S.; Addley, H.C.; Colombo, P.E.; Fujii, S.; Al Sharif, S.S.; Tirumani, S.H.; Jardon, K.; Sala, E.; Reinhold, C. Ovarian carcinomatosis: How the radiologist can help plan the surgical approach. *Radiographics* **2012**, *32*, 1775–1800. [CrossRef] [PubMed]
4. Nam, E.J.; Yun, M.J.; Oh, Y.T.; Kim, J.W.; Kim, J.H.; Kim, S.; Jung, Y.W.; Kim, S.W.; Kim, Y.T. Diagnosis and staging of primary ovarian cancer: Correlation between PET/CT, Doppler US, and CT or MRI. *Gynecol. Oncol.* **2010**, *116*, 389–394. [CrossRef] [PubMed]
5. An, H.; Lee, E.Y.P.; Chiu, K.; Chang, C. The emerging roles of functional imaging in ovarian cancer with peritoneal carcinomatosis. *Clin. Radiol.* **2018**, *73*, 597–609. [CrossRef] [PubMed]
6. Forstner, R.; Meissnitzer, M.; Cunha, T.M. Update on Imaging of Ovarian Cancer. *Curr. Radiol. Rep.* **2016**, *4*, 31. [CrossRef] [PubMed]
7. Forstner, R.; Sala, E.; Kinkel, K.; Spencer, J.A. European Society of Urogenital Radiology, ESUR guidelines: Ovarian cancer staging and follow-up. *Eur. Radiol.* **2010**, *20*, 2773–2780. [CrossRef] [PubMed]
8. Shinagare, A.B.; Sadowski, E.A.; Park, H.; Brook, O.R.; Forstner, R.; Wallace, S.K.; Horowitz, J.M.; Horowitz, N.; Javitt, M.; Jha, P.; et al. Ovarian cancer reporting lexicon for computed tomography (CT) and magnetic resonance (MR) imaging developed by the SAR Uterine and Ovarian Cancer Disease-Focused Panel and the ESUR Female Pelvic Imaging Working Group. *Eur. Radiol.* **2022**, *32*, 3220–3235. [CrossRef] [PubMed]
9. Javadi, S.; Ganeshan, D.M.; Qayyum, A.; Iyer, R.B.; Bhosale, P. Ovarian Cancer, the Revised FIGO Staging System, and the Role of Imaging. *AJR Am. J. Roentgenol.* **2016**, *206*, 1351–1360. [CrossRef] [PubMed]
10. Ghirardi, V.; Fagotti, A.; Ansaloni, L.; Valle, M.; Roviello, F.; Sorrentino, L.; Accarpio, F.; Baiocchi, G.; Piccini, L.; De Simone, M.; et al. Diagnostic and Therapeutic Pathway of Advanced Ovarian Cancer with Peritoneal Metastases. *Cancers* **2023**, *15*, 407. [CrossRef] [PubMed]
11. Armbrust, R.; Ledwon, P.; Von Rüsten, A.; Schneider, C.; Sehouli, J. Primary Treatment Results in Patients with Ovarian, Fallopian or Peritoneal Cancer-Results of a Clinical Cancer Registry Database Analysis in Germany. *Cancers* **2022**, *24*, 4638. [CrossRef] [PubMed]
12. Pasqual, E.M.; Londero, A.P.; Robella, M.; Tonello, M.; Sommariva, A.; De Simone, M.; Bacchetti, S.; Baiocchi, G.; Asero, S.; Coccolini, F.; et al. Repeated Cytoreduction Combined with Hyperthermic Intraperitoneal Chemotherapy (HIPEC) in Selected Patients Affected by Peritoneal Metastases: Italian PSM Oncoteam Evidence. *Cancers* **2023**, *15*, 607. [CrossRef] [PubMed]
13. Kyriazi, S.; Kaye, S.B.; DeSouza, N.M. Imaging ovarian cancer and peritoneal metastases-current and emerging techniques. *Nat. Rev. Clin. Oncol.* **2010**, *7*, 381–393. [CrossRef] [PubMed]
14. Rizzo, S.; Del Grande, M.; Manganaro, L.; Papadia, A.; Del Grande, F. Imaging before cytoreductive surgery in advanced ovarian cancer patients. *Int. J. Gynecol. Cancer* **2020**, *30*, 133–138. [CrossRef] [PubMed]
15. Nougaret, S.; Sadowski, E.; Lakhman, Y.; Rousset, P.; Lahaye, M.; Worley, M.; Sgarbura, O.; Shinagare, A.B. The BUMPy road of peritoneal metastases in ovarian cancer. *Diagn. Interv. Imaging* **2022**, *103*, 448–459. [CrossRef]
16. Gagliardi, T.; Adejolu, M.; DeSouza, N.M. Diffusion-Weighted Magnetic Resonance Imaging in Ovarian Cancer: Exploiting Strengths and Understanding Limitations. *J. Clin. Med.* **2022**, *11*, 1524. [CrossRef] [PubMed]

17. Lee, E.Y.P.; An, H.; Tse, K.Y.; Khong, P.L. Molecular Imaging of Peritoneal Carcinomatosis in Ovarian Carcinoma. *AJR Am. J. Roentgenol.* **2020**, *215*, 305–312. [CrossRef]
18. Coakley, F.V.; Choi, P.H.; Gougoutas, C.A.; Pothuri, B.; Venkatraman, E.; Chi, D.; Bergman, A.; Hricak, H. Peritoneal metastases: Detection with spiral CT in patients with ovarian cancer. *Radiology* **2002**, *223*, 495–499. [CrossRef] [PubMed]
19. Tsili, A.C.; Naka, C.; Argyropoulou, M.I. Multidetector computed tomography in diagnosing peritoneal metastases in ovarian carcinoma. *Acta Radiol.* **2021**, *62*, 1696–1706. [CrossRef] [PubMed]
20. Patel, C.M.; Sahdev, A.; Reznek, R.H. CT, MRI and PET imaging in peritoneal malignancy. *Cancer Imaging* **2011**, *11*, 123–139. [CrossRef] [PubMed]
21. Iafrate, F.; Ciolina, M.; Sammartino, P.; Baldassari, P.; Rengo, M.; Lucchesi, P.; Sibio, S.; Accarpio, F.; Di Giorgio, A.; Laghi, A. Peritoneal carcinomatosis: Imaging with 64-MDCT and 3T MRI with diffusion-weighted imaging. *Abdom. Imaging* **2012**, *37*, 616–627. [CrossRef] [PubMed]
22. Qayyum, A.; Coakley, F.V.; Westphalen, A.C. Role of CT and MR imaging in predicting optimal cytoreduction of newly diagnosed primary epithelial ovarian cancer. *Gynecol. Oncol.* **2005**, *96*, 301–306. [CrossRef] [PubMed]
23. Jacquet, P.; Sugarbaker, P.H. Clinical research methodologies in diagnosis and staging of patients with peritoneal carcinomatosis. In *Peritoneal Carcinomatosis: Principles of Management*; Sugarbaker, P.H., Ed.; Kluwer Academic Publishers: Boston, MA, USA, 1996; Volume 82, pp. 359–374.
24. Abdalla Ahmed, S.; Abou-Taleb, H.; Ali, N.; Badary, D.M. Accuracy of radiologic- laparoscopic peritoneal carcinomatosis categorization in the prediction of surgical outcome. *Br. J. Radiol.* **2019**, *92*, 20190163. [CrossRef]
25. Rutten, I.J.; Van de Laar, R.; Kruitwagen, R.F.; Bakers, F.C.; Ploegmakers, M.J.; Pappot, T.W.; Beets-Tan, R.G.H.; Massuger, L.F.A.G.; Zusterzeel, P.L.M.; Gorp, T.V. Prediction of incomplete primary debulking surgery in patients with advanced ovarian cancer: An external validation study of three models using computed tomography. *Gynecol. Oncol.* **2016**, *140*, 22–28. [CrossRef]
26. Nasser, S.; Lazaridis, A.; Evangelou, M.; Jones, B.; Nixon, K.; Kyrgiou, M.; Gabra, H.; Rockall, A.; Fotopoulou, C. Correlation of pre-operative CT findings with surgical & histological tumor dissemination patterns at cytoreduction for primary advanced and relapsed epithelial ovarian cancer: A retrospective evaluation. *Gynecol. Oncol.* **2016**, *143*, 264–269. [PubMed]
27. An, H.; Chiu, K.W.H.; Tse, K.Y.; Ngan, H.Y.S.; Khong, P.L.; Lee, E.Y.P. The Value of Contrast-Enhanced CT in the Detection of Residual Disease After Neo-Adjuvant Chemotherapy in Ovarian Cancer. *Acad. Radiol.* **2020**, *27*, 951–957. [CrossRef]
28. Tozzi, R.; Traill, Z.; Valenti, G.; Ferrari, F.; Gubbala, K.; Campanile, R.G. A prospective study on the diagnostic pathway of patients with stage IIIC-IV ovarian cancer: Exploratory laparoscopy (EXL) + CT scan VS. CT scan. *Gynecol. Oncol.* **2021**, *161*, 188–193. [CrossRef] [PubMed]
29. Onda, T.; Tanaka, Y.O.; Kitai, S.; Manabe, T.; Ishikawa, M.; Hasumi, Y.; Miyamoto, K.; Ogawa, G.; Satoh, T.; Saito, T.; et al. Stage III disease of ovarian, tubal and peritoneal cancers can be accurately diagnosed with pre-operative CT. Japan Clinical Oncology Group Study JCOG0602. *Jpn. J. Clin. Oncol.* **2021**, *51*, 205–212. [CrossRef] [PubMed]
30. Mikkelsen, M.S.; Petersen, L.K.; Blaakaer, J.; Marinovskij, E.; Rosenkilde, M.; Andersen, G.; Bouchelouche, K.; Iversen, L.H. Assessment of peritoneal metastases with DW-MRI, CT, and FDG PET/CT before cytoreductive surgery for advanced stage epithelial ovarian cancer. *Eur. J. Surg. Oncol.* **2021**, *47*, 2134–2141. [CrossRef] [PubMed]
31. Fehniger, J.; Thomas, S.; Lengyel, E.; Liao, C.; Tenney, M.; Oto, A.; Yamada, S.D. A prospective study evaluating diffusion weighted magnetic resonance imaging (DW-MRI) in the detection of peritoneal carcinomatosis in suspected gynecologic malignancies. *Gynecol. Oncol.* **2016**, *142*, 169–175. [CrossRef] [PubMed]
32. Kyriazi, S.; Collins, D.J.; Morgan, V.A.; Giles, S.L.; DeSouza, N.M. Diffusion-weighted imaging of peritoneal disease for noninvasive staging of advanced ovarian cancer. *Radiographics* **2010**, *30*, 1269–1285. [CrossRef]
33. Sala, E.; Kataoka, M.Y.; Priest, A.N.; Gill, A.B.; McLean, M.A.; Joubert, I.; Graves, M.J.; Crawford, R.A.F.; Jimenez-Linan, M.; Earl, H.M.; et al. Advanced ovarian cancer: Multiparametric MR imaging demonstrates response- and metastasis-specific effects. *Radiology* **2012**, *263*, 149–159. [CrossRef] [PubMed]
34. Low, R.N.; Barone, R.M. Combined diffusion-weighted and gadolinium-enhanced MRI can accurately predict the peritoneal cancer index preoperatively in patients being considered for cytoreductive surgical procedures. *Ann. Surg. Oncol.* **2012**, *19*, 1394–1401. [CrossRef] [PubMed]
35. Engbersen, M.P.; Van' T Sant, I.; Lok, C.; Lambregts, D.M.J.; Sonke, G.S.; Beets-Tan, R.G.H.; Van Driel, W.J.; Lahaye, M.J. MRI with diffusion-weighted imaging to predict feasibility of complete cytoreduction with the peritoneal cancer index (PCI) in advanced stage ovarian cancer patients. *Eur. J. Radiol.* **2019**, *114*, 146–151. [CrossRef]
36. Pannu, H.K.; Bristow, R.E.; Cohade, C.; Fishman, E.K.; Wahl, R.L. PET-CT in recurrent ovarian cancer: Initial observations. *Radiographics* **2004**, *24*, 209–223. [CrossRef] [PubMed]
37. Risum, S.; Høgdall, C.; Loft, A.; Berthelsen, A.K.; Høgdall, E.; Nedergaard, L.; Lundvall, L.; Engelholm, S.A. The diagnostic value of PET/CT for primary ovarian cancer-A prospective study. *Gynecol. Oncol.* **2007**, *105*, 145–149. [CrossRef] [PubMed]
38. Thrall, M.M.; DeLoia, J.A.; Gallion, H.; Avril, N. Clinical use of combined positron emission tomography and computed tomography (FDG-PET/CT) in recurrent ovarian cancer. *Gynecol. Oncol.* **2007**, *105*, 17–22. [CrossRef] [PubMed]
39. Soussan, M.; Wartski, M.; Cherel, P.; Fourme, E.; Goupil, A.; Le Stanc, E.; Callet, N.; Alexandre, J.; Pecking, A.; Alberini, J. Impact of FDG PET-CT imaging on the decision making in the biologic suspicion of ovarian carcinoma recurrence. *Gynecol. Oncol.* **2008**, *108*, 160–165. [CrossRef] [PubMed]

40. Fulham, M.J.; Carter, J.; Baldey, A.; Hicks, R.J.; Ramshaw, J.E.; Gibson, M. The impact of PET-CT in suspected recurrent ovarian cancer: A prospective multi-centre study as part of the Australian PET Data Collection Project. *Gynecol. Oncol.* **2009**, *112*, 462–468. [CrossRef] [PubMed]
41. Boria, F.; Chiva, L.; Carbonell, M.; Gutierrez, M.; Sancho, L.; Alcazar, A.; Coronado, M.; Hernández Gutiérrez, A.; Zapardiel, I. ^{18}F-fluorodeoxyglucose positron emission tomography/computed tomography (^{18}F-FDG PET/CT) predictive score for complete resection in primary cytoreductive surgery. *Int. J. Gynecol. Cancer* **2022**, *32*, 1427–1432. [CrossRef] [PubMed]
42. Feng, Z.; Liu, S.; Ju, X.; Chen, X.; Li, R.; Bi, R.; Wu, X. Diagnostic accuracy of ^{18}F-FDG PET/CT scan for peritoneal metastases in advanced ovarian cancer. *Quant. Imaging Med. Surg.* **2021**, *11*, 3392–3398. [CrossRef]
43. Delvallée, J.; Rossard, L.; Bendifallah, S.; Touboul, C.; Collinet, P.; Bricou, A.; Huchon, C.; Lavoue, V.; Body, G.; Ouldamer, L. Accuracy of peritoneal carcinomatosis extent diagnosis by initial FDG PET CT in epithelial ovarian cancer: A multicentre study of the FRANCOGYN research group. *J. Gynecol. Obstet. Hum. Reprod.* **2020**, *49*, 101867. [CrossRef] [PubMed]
44. Mallet, E.; Angeles, M.A.; Cabarrou, B.; Chardin, D.; Viau, P.; Frigenza, M.; Navarro, A.S.; Ducassou, A.; Betrian, S.; Martínez-Gómez, C.; et al. Performance of Multiparametric Functional Imaging to Assess Peritoneal Tumor Burden in Ovarian Cancer. *Nucl. Med.* **2021**, *46*, 797–806. [CrossRef] [PubMed]
45. Wang, X.; Yang, L.; Wang, Y. Meta-analysis of the diagnostic value of ^{18}F-FDG PET/CT in the recurrence of epithelial ovarian cancer. *Front. Oncol.* **2022**, *12*, 1003465. [CrossRef] [PubMed]
46. Laghi, A.; Bellini, D.; Rengo, M.; Accarpio, F.; Caruso, D.; Biacchi, D.; Di Giorgio, A.; Sammartino, P. Diagnostic performance of computed tomography and magnetic resonance imaging for detecting peritoneal metastases: Systematic review and meta-analysis. *Radiol. Med.* **2017**, *122*, 1–15. [CrossRef] [PubMed]
47. Van 't Sant, I.; Engbersen, M.P.; Bhairosing, P.A.; Lambregts, D.M.J.; Beets-Tan, R.G.H.; Van Driel, W.J.; Aalbers, A.G.J.; Kok, N.F.M.; Lahaye, M.J. Diagnostic performance of imaging for the detection of peritoneal metastases: A meta-analysis. *Eur. Radiol.* **2020**, *30*, 3101–3112. [CrossRef] [PubMed]
48. Gu, P.; Pan, L.L.; Wu, S.Q.; Sun, L.; Huang, G. CA 125, PET alone, PET-CT, CT and MRI in diagnosing recurrent ovarian carcinoma: A systematic review and meta-analysis. *Eur. J. Radiol.* **2009**, *71*, 164–174. [CrossRef]
49. Page, M.J.; McKenzie, J.E.; Bossuyt, P.M.; Boutron, I.; Hoffmann, T.C.; Mulrow, C.D.; Shamseer, L.; Tetzlaff, J.M.; Akl, E.A.; Brennan, S.E.; et al. The PRISMA 2020 statement: An updated guideline for reporting systematic reviews. *BMJ* **2021**, *372*, n71. [CrossRef] [PubMed]
50. Whiting, P.F.; Rutjes, A.W.; Westwood, M.E.; Mallett, S.; Deeks, J.J.; Reitsma, J.B.; Leeflang, M.M.; Sterne, J.A.; Bossuyt, P.M. QUADAS-2 Group, QUADAS-2: A Revised Tool for the Quality Assessment of Diagnostic Accuracy Studies. *Ann. Intern. Med.* **2011**, *155*, 529–536. [CrossRef] [PubMed]
51. Tempany, C.M.; Zou, K.H.; Silverman, S.G.; Brown, D.L.; Kurtz, A.B.; McNeil, B.J. Staging of advanced ovarian cancer: Comparison of imaging modalities-report from the Radiological Diagnostic Oncology Group. *Radiology* **2000**, *215*, 761–767. [CrossRef] [PubMed]
52. Pannu, H.K.; Horton, K.M.; Fishman, E.K. Thin section dual-phase multidetector-row computed tomography detection of peritoneal metastases in gynecologic cancers. *J. Comput. Assist. Tomogr.* **2003**, *27*, 333–340. [CrossRef] [PubMed]
53. Ricke, J.; Sehouli, J.; Hach, C.; Hänninen, E.L.; Lichtenegger, W.; Felix, R. Prospective evaluation of contrast-enhanced MRI in the depiction of peritoneal spread in primary or recurrent ovarian cancer. *Eur. Radiol.* **2003**, *13*, 943–949. [CrossRef] [PubMed]
54. Pannu, H.K.; Cohade, C.; Bristow, R.E.; Fishman, E.K.; Wahl, R.L. PET-CT detection of abdominal recurrence of ovarian cancer: Radiologic-surgical correlation. *Abdom. Imaging* **2004**, *29*, 398–403. [CrossRef] [PubMed]
55. Kim, C.K.; Park, B.K.; Choi, J.Y.; Kim, B.G.; Han, H.J. Detection of recurrent ovarian cancer at MRI: Comparison with integrated PET/CT. *Comput. Assist. Tomogr.* **2007**, *31*, 868–875. [CrossRef]
56. Kitajima, K.; Murakami, K.; Yamasaki, E.; Kaji, Y.; Fukasawa, I.; Inaba, N.; Sugimura, K. Diagnostic accuracy of integrated FDG-PET/contrast-enhanced CT in staging ovarian cancer: Comparison with enhanced CT. *Eur. J. Nucl. Med. Mol. Imaging* **2008**, *35*, 1912–1920. [CrossRef] [PubMed]
57. Kitajima, K.; Murakami, K.; Yamasaki, E.; Domeki, Y.; Kaji, Y.; Fukasawa, I.; Inaba, N.; Suganuma, N.; Sugimura, K. Performance of integrated FDG-PET/contrast-enhanced CT in the diagnosis of recurrent ovarian cancer: Comparison with integrated FDG-PET/non-contrast-enhanced CT and enhanced CT. *Eur. J. Nucl. Med. Mol. Imaging* **2008**, *35*, 1439–1448. [CrossRef] [PubMed]
58. Choi, H.J.; Lim, M.C.; Bae, J.; Cho, K.S.; Jung, D.C.; Kang, S.; Yoo, C.W.; Seo, S.S.; Park, S.Y. Region-based diagnostic performance of multidetector CT for detecting peritoneal seeding in ovarian cancer patients. *Arch. Gynecol. Obstet.* **2011**, *283*, 353–360. [CrossRef] [PubMed]
59. Metser, U.; Jones, C.; Jacks, L.M.; Bernardini, M.Q.; Ferguson, S. Identification and quantification of peritoneal metastases in patients with ovarian cancer with multidetector computed tomography: Correlation with surgery and surgical outcome. *Int. J. Gynecol. Cancer* **2011**, *21*, 1391–1398. [CrossRef] [PubMed]
60. De Iaco, P.; Musto, A.; Orazi, L.; Zamagni, C.; Rosati, M.; Allegri, V.; Cacciari, N.; Al-Nahhas, A.; Rubello, D.; Venturoli, S.; et al. FDG-PET/CT in Advanced Ovarian Cancer Staging: Value and Pitfalls in Detecting Lesions in Different Abdominal and Pelvic Quadrants Compared with Laparoscopy. *Eur. J. Radiol.* **2011**, *80*, e98–e103. [CrossRef] [PubMed]
61. Sanli, Y.; Turkmen, C.; Bakir, B.; Iyibozkurt, C.; Ozel, S.; Has, D.; Yilmaz, E.; Topuz, S.; Yavuz, E.; Unal, S.N.; et al. Diagnostic value of PET/CT is similar to that of conventional MRI and even better for detecting small peritoneal implants in patients with recurrent ovarian cancer. *Nucl. Med. Commun.* **2012**, *33*, 509–515. [CrossRef]

62. Espada, M.; Garcia-Flores, J.R.; Jimenez, M.; Alvarez-Moreno, E.; De Haro, M.; Gonzalez-Cortijo, L.; Hernandez-Cortes, G.; Martinez-Vega, V.; De La Cuesta, R.S. Diffusion-weighted magnetic resonance imaging evaluation of intra-abdominal sites of implants to predict likelihood of suboptimal cytoreductive surgery in patients with ovarian carcinoma. *Eur. Radiol.* **2013**, *23*, 2636–2642. [CrossRef]
63. Hynninen, J.; Kemppainen, J.; Lavonius, M.; Virtanen, J.; Matomäki, J.; Oksa, S.; Carpén, O.; Grénman, S.; Seppänen, M.; Auranen, A. A prospective comparison of integrated FDG-PET/contrast-enhanced CT and contrast-enhanced CT for pretreatment imaging of advanced epithelial ovarian cancer. *Gynecol. Oncol.* **2013**, *131*, 389–394. [CrossRef]
64. Kim, W.H.; Won, K.S.; Zeon, S.K.; Ahn, B.C.; Gayed, I.W. Peritoneal carcinomatosis in patients with ovarian cancer. Enhanced CT versus 18F-FDG PET/CT. *Clin. Nucl. Med.* **2013**, *38*, 93–97.
65. Mazzei, M.A.; Khader, L.; Cirigliano, A.; Cioffi Squitieri, N.; Guerrini, S.; Forzoni, B.; Marrelli, D.; Roviello, F.; Mazzei, F.G.; Volterrani, L. Accuracy of MDCT in the preoperative definition of Peritoneal Cancer Index (PCI) in patients with advanced ovarian cancer who underwent peritonectomy and hyperthermic intraperitoneal chemotherapy (HIPEC). *Abdom. Imaging* **2013**, *38*, 1422–1430. [CrossRef] [PubMed]
66. Michielsen, K.; Vergote, I.; Op de Beeck, K.; Amant, F.; Leunen, K.; Moerman, P.; Deroose, C.; Souverijns, G.; Dymarkowski, S.; De Keyzer, F.; et al. Whole-body MRI with diffusion-weighted sequence for staging of patients with suspected ovarian cancer: A clinical feasibility study in comparison to CT and FDG-PET/CT. *Eur. Radiol.* **2014**, *24*, 889–901. [CrossRef] [PubMed]
67. Schmidt, S.; Meuli, R.A.; Achtari, C.; Prior, J.O. Peritoneal carcinomatosis in primary ovarian cancer staging: Comparison between MDCT, MRI, and 18F-FDG PET/CT. *Clin. Nucl. Med.* **2015**, *40*, 371–377. [CrossRef] [PubMed]
68. Lopez-Lopez, V.; Cascales-Campos, P.A.; Gil, J.; Frutos, L.; Andrade, R.J.; Fuster-Quiñonero, M.; Feliciangeli, E.; Gil, E.; Parrilla, P. Use of (18)F-FDG PET/CT in the preoperative evaluation of patients diagnosed with peritoneal carcinomatosis of ovarian origin, candidates to cytoreduction and hipec. A pending issue. *Eur. J. Radiol.* **2016**, *85*, 1824–1828. [CrossRef] [PubMed]
69. Rodolfino, E.; Devicienti, E.; Miccò, M.; Del Ciello, A.; Di Giovanni, S.E.; Giuliani, M.; Conte, C.; Gui, B.; Valentini, A.L.; Bonomo, L. Diagnostic accuracy of MDCT in the evaluation of patients with peritoneal carcinomatosis from ovarian cancer: Is delayed enhanced phase really effective? *Eur. Rev. Med. Pharmacol. Sci.* **2016**, *20*, 4426–4434.
70. Tawakol, A.; Abdelhafez, Y.G.; Osama, A.; Hamada, E.; El Refaei, S. Diagnostic performance of 18F-FDG PET/contrast-enhanced CT versus contrast-enhanced CT alone for post-treatment detection of ovarian malignancy. *Nucl. Med. Commun.* **2016**, *37*, 453–460. [CrossRef] [PubMed]
71. Cerci, Z.C.; Sakarya, D.K.; Yetimalar, M.H.; Bezircioglu, I.; Kasap, B.; Baser, E.; Yucel, K. Computed tomography as a predictor of the extent of the disease and surgical outcomes in ovarian cancer. *Ginekol. Pol.* **2016**, *87*, 326–332. [CrossRef] [PubMed]
72. Bagul, K.; Vijaykumar, D.K.; Rajanbabu, A.; Antony, M.A.; Ranganathan, V. Advanced Primary Epithelial Ovarian and Peritoneal Carcinoma-Does Diagnostic Accuracy of Preoperative CT Scan for Detection of Peritoneal Metastatic Sites Reflect into Prediction of Suboptimal Debulking? A Prospective Study. *Indian J. Surg. Oncol.* **2017**, *8*, 98–104. [CrossRef]
73. Michielsen, K.; Dresen, R.; Vanslembrouck, R.; De Keyzer, F.; Amant, F.; Mussen, E.; Leunen, K.; Berteloot, P.; Moerman, P.; Vergote, I.; et al. Diagnostic value of whole-body diffusion-weighted MRI compared to computed tomography for pre-operative assessment of patients suspected for ovarian cancer. *Eur. J. Cancer* **2017**, *83*, 88–98. [CrossRef] [PubMed]
74. Rajan, J.; Kuriakose, S.; Rajendran, V.R.; Sumangaladevi, D. Radiological and surgical correlation of disease burden in advanced ovarian cancer using peritoneal carcinomatosis index. *Indian. J. Gynecol. Oncol.* **2018**, *16*, 7. [CrossRef]
75. Alcázar, J.L.; Caparros, M.; Arraiza, M.; Mínguez, J.A.; Guerriero, S.; Chiva, L.; Jurado, M. Pre-operative Assessment of Intra-Abdominal Disease Spread in Epithelial Ovarian Cancer: A Comparative Study between Ultrasound and Computed Tomography. *Int. J. Gynecol. Cancer* **2019**, *29*, 227–233. [CrossRef] [PubMed]
76. Ahmed, S.A.; Abou-Taleb, H.; Yehia, A.; El Malek, N.A.A.; Siefeldein, G.S.; Badary, D.M.; Jabir, M.A. The accuracy of multi-detector computed tomography and laparoscopy in the prediction of peritoneal carcinomatosis index score in primary ovarian cancer. *Acad. Radiol.* **2019**, *26*, 1650–1658. [CrossRef] [PubMed]
77. Tsoi, T.T.; Chiu, K.W.H.; Chu, M.Y.; Ngan, H.Y.S.; Lee, E.Y.P. Metabolic active peritoneal sites affect tumor debulking in ovarian and peritoneal cancers. *J. Ovarian Res.* **2020**, *13*, 61. [CrossRef] [PubMed]
78. Fischerova, D.; Pinto, P.; Burgetova, A.; Masek, M.; Slama, J.; Kocian, R.; Frühauf, F.; Zikan, M.; Dusek, L.; Dundr, P.; et al. Preoperative staging of ovarian cancer: Comparison between ultrasound, CT and whole-body diffusion-weighted MRI (ISAAC study). *Ultrasound Obstet. Gynecol.* **2022**, *59*, 248–262. [CrossRef] [PubMed]
79. Colombo, N.; Sessa, C.; du Bois, A.; Ledermann, J.; McCluggage, W.G.; McNeish, I.; Morice, P.; Pignata, S.; Ray-Coquard, I.; Vergote, I.; et al. ESMO-ESGO consensus conference recommendations on ovarian cancer: Pathology and molecular biology, early and advanced stages, borderline tumours and recurrent disease. *Ann. Oncol.* **2019**, *30*, 672–705. [CrossRef] [PubMed]
80. Bae, H.; Jung, D.C.; Lee, J.Y.; Nam, E.J.; Kang, W.J.; Oh, Y.T. Patterns of initially overlooked recurrence of peritoneal lesions in patients with advanced ovarian cancer on postoperative multi-detector row CT. *Acta Radiol.* **2019**, *60*, 1713–1720. [CrossRef] [PubMed]
81. Gadelhak, B.; Tawfik, A.M.; Saleh, G.A.; Batouty, N.M.; Sobh, D.M.; Hamdy, O.; Refky, B. Extended abdominopelvic MRI versus CT at the time of adnexal mass characterization for assessing radiologic peritoneal cancer index (PCI) prior to cytoreductive surgery. *Abdom. Radiol.* **2019**, *44*, 2254–2261. [CrossRef] [PubMed]
82. Forstner, R. Radiological staging of ovarian cancer: Imaging findings and contribution of CT and MRI. *Eur. Radiol.* **2007**, *17*, 3223–3335. [CrossRef] [PubMed]

83. Pannu, H.K.; Bristow, R.E.; Montz, F.J.; Fishman, E.K. Multidetector CT of peritoneal carcinomatosis from ovarian cancer. *Radiographics* **2003**, *23*, 687–701. [CrossRef] [PubMed]
84. Franiel, T.; Diederichs, G.; Engelken, F.; Elgeti, T.; Rost, J.; Rogalla, P. Multi-detector CT in peritoneal carcinomatosis: Diagnostic role of thin slices and multiplanar reconstructions. *Abdom. Imaging* **2009**, *34*, 49–54. [CrossRef]
85. Marin, D.; Catalano, C.; Baski, M.; De Martino, M.; Geiger, D.; Di Giorgio, A.; Sibio, S.; Passariello, R. 64-Section multi-detector row CT in the preoperative diagnosis of peritoneal carcinomatosis: Correlation with histopathological findings. *Abdom. Imaging* **2010**, *35*, 694–700. [CrossRef]
86. Low, R.N.; Sebrechts, C.P.; Barone, R.M.; Muller, W. Diffusion-weighted MRI of peritoneal tumors: Comparison with conventional MRI and surgical and histopathologic findings: A feasibility study. *AJR Am. J. Roentgenol.* **2009**, *193*, 461–470. [CrossRef] [PubMed]
87. Namimoto, T.; Awai, K.; Nakaura, T.; Yanaga, Y.; Hirai, T.; Yamashita, Y. Role of diffusion-weighted imaging in the diagnosis of gynecological diseases. *Eur. Radiol.* **2009**, *19*, 745–760. [CrossRef] [PubMed]
88. Priest, A.N.; Gill, A.B.; Kataoka, M.; McLean, M.A.; Joubert, I.; Graves, M.J.; Griffiths, J.R.; Crawford, R.A.F.; Earl, H.; Brenton, J.D.; et al. Dynamic contrast-enhanced MRI in ovarian cancer: Initial experience at 3 tesla in primary and metastatic disease. *Magn. Reson. Med.* **2010**, *63*, 1044–1049. [CrossRef] [PubMed]
89. Low, R.N.; Barone, R.M. Imaging for Peritoneal Metastases. *Surg. Oncol. Clin. N. Am.* **2018**, *27*, 425–442. [CrossRef]
90. Guo, H.L.; He, L.; Zhu, Y.C.; Wu, K.; Yuan, F. Comparison between multi-slice spiral CT and magnetic resonance imaging in the diagnosis of peritoneal metastasis in primary ovarian carcinoma. *Oncol. Targets Ther.* **2018**, *11*, 1087–1094. [CrossRef] [PubMed]
91. Satoh, Y.; Ichikawa, T.; Motosugi, U.; Kimura, K.; Sou, H.; Sano, K.; Araki, T. Diagnosis of peritoneal dissemination: Comparison of 18F-FDG PET/CT, diffusion-weighted MRI, and contrast-enhanced MDCT. *AJR Am. J. Roentgenol.* **2001**, *196*, 447–453. [CrossRef] [PubMed]
92. Torkzad, M.R.; Casta, N.; Bergman, A.; Ahlström, H.; Påhlman, L.; Mahteme, H. Comparison between MRI and CT in prediction of peritoneal carcinomatosis index (PCI) in patients undergoing cytoreductive surgery in relation to the experience of the radiologist. *J. Surg. Oncol.* **2015**, *111*, 746–751. [CrossRef] [PubMed]
93. Sironi, S.; Messa, C.; Mangili, G.; Zangheri, B.; Aletti, G.; Garavaglia, E.; Vigano, R.; Picchio, M.; Taccagni, G.; Del Maschio, A.; et al. Integrated FDG PET/CT in patients with persistent ovarian cancer: Correlation with histologic findings. *Radiology* **2004**, *233*, 433–440. [CrossRef] [PubMed]
94. Hauth, E.A.; Antoch, G.; Stattaus, J.; Kuehl, H.; Veit, P.; Bockisch, A.; Kimmig, R.; Forsting, M. Evaluation of integrated whole-body PET/CT in the detection of recurrent ovarian cancer. *Eur. J. Radiol.* **2005**, *56*, 263–268. [CrossRef]
95. Nanni, C.; Rubello, D.; Farsad, M.; De Iaco, P.; Sansovini, M.; Erba, P.; Rampin, L.; Mariani, G.; Fanti, S. (18)F-FDG PET/CT in the evaluation of recurrent ovarian cancer: A prospective study on forty-one patients. *Eur. J. Surg. Oncol.* **2005**, *31*, 792–797. [CrossRef] [PubMed]
96. Mangili, G.; Picchio, M.; Sironi, S.; Vigano, R.; Rabaiotti, E.; Bornaghi, D.; Bettinardi, V.; Crivellaro, C.; Messa, C.; Fazio, F. Integrated PET/CT as a first-line re-staging modality in patients with suspected recurrence of ovarian cancer. *Eur. J. Nucl. Med. Mol. Imaging* **2007**, *34*, 658–666. [CrossRef] [PubMed]
97. Castellucci, P.; Perrone, A.M.; Picchio, M.; Ghi, T.; Farsad, M.; Nanni, C.; Messa, C.; Meriggiola, M.C.; Pelusi, G.; Al-Nahhas, A.; et al. Diagnostic accuracy of 18F-FDG PET/CT in characterizing ovarian lesions and staging ovarian cancer: Correlation with transvaginal ultrasonography, computed tomography, and histology. *Nucl. Med. Commun.* **2007**, *28*, 589–595. [CrossRef]
98. Sebastian, S.; Lee, S.I.; Horowitz, N.S.; Scott, J.A.; Fischman, A.J.; Simeone, J.F.; Fuller, A.F.; Hahn, P.F. PET-CT vs. CT alone in ovarian cancer recurrence. *Abdom. Imaging* **2008**, *33*, 112–118. [CrossRef] [PubMed]
99. Pfannenberg, C.; Konigsrainer, I.; Aschoff, P.; Oksüz, M.O.; Zieker, D.; Beckert, S.; Symons, S.; Nieselt, K.; Glatzle, J.; Weyhern, C.V.; et al. (18)F-FDG-PET/CT to select patients with peritoneal carcinomatosis for cytoreductive surgery and hyperthermic intraperitoneal chemotherapy. *Ann. Surg. Oncol.* **2009**, *16*, 1295–1303. [CrossRef] [PubMed]
100. Kumar Dhingra, V.; Kand, P.; Basu, S. Impact of FDG-PET and PET/CT imaging in the clinical decision-making of ovarian carcinoma: An evidence-based approach. *Womens Health* **2012**, *8*, 191–203. [CrossRef] [PubMed]
101. Rubini, G.; Altini, C.; Notaristefano, A.; Merenda, N.; Rubini, D.; Ianora, A.A.; Asabella, A.N. Role of 18F-FDG PET/CT in diagnosing peritoneal carcinomatosis in the restaging of patient with ovarian cancer as compared to contrast enhanced CT and tumor marker Ca-125. *Rev. Esp. Med. Nucl. Imagen Mol.* **2014**, *33*, 22–27. [PubMed]
102. Miceli, V.; Gennarini, M.; Tomao, F.; Cupertino, A.; Lombardo, D.; Palaia, I.; Curti, F.; Riccardi, S.; Ninkova, R.; Maccioni, F.; et al. Imaging of peritoneal carcinomatosis in advanced ovarian cancer: CT, MRI, radiomics features and resectability criteria. *Cancers* **2023**, *15*, 5827. [CrossRef] [PubMed]
103. Nougaret, S.; Tardieu, M.; Vargas, H.A.; Reinhold, C.; Vande Perre, S.; Bonanno, N.; Sala, E.; Thomassin-Naggara, I. Ovarian cancer: An update on imaging in the era of radiomics. *Diagn. Interv. Imaging* **2019**, *100*, 647–655. [CrossRef] [PubMed]
104. Nougaret, S.; McCague, C.; Tibermacine, H.; Vargas, H.A.; Rizzo, S.; Sala, E. Radiomics and radiogenomics in ovarian cancer: A literature review. *Abdom. Radiol.* **2021**, *46*, 2308–2322. [CrossRef] [PubMed]
105. Panico, C.; Avesani, G.; Zormpas-Petridis, K.; Rundo, L.; Nero, C.; Sala, E. Radiomics and Radiogenomics of Ovarian Cancer: Implications for Treatment Monitoring and Clinical Management. *Radiol. Clin. N. Am.* **2023**, *61*, 749–760. [CrossRef]

106. Beer, L.; Sahin, H.; Bateman, N.W.; Blazic, I.; Vargas, H.A.; Veeraraghavan, H.; Kirby, J.; Fevrier-Sullivan, B.; Freymann, J.B.; Jaffeet, C.C.; et al. Integration of proteomics with CT-based qualitative and radiomic features in high-grade serous ovarian cancer patients: An exploratory analysis. *Eur. Radiol.* **2020**, *30*, 4306–4316. [CrossRef] [PubMed]
107. Song, X.L.; Ren, J.L.; Yao, T.Y.; Zhao, D.; Niu, J. Radiomics based on multisequence magnetic resonance imaging for the preoperative prediction of peritoneal metastasis in ovarian cancer. *Eur. Radiol.* **2021**, *31*, 8438–8446. [CrossRef] [PubMed]
108. Wei, M.; Zhang, Y.; Ding, C.; Jia, J.; Xu, H.; Dai, Y.; Feng, G.; Qin, C.; Bai, G.; Chen, S.; et al. Associating peritoneal metastasis with T2-weighted MRI images in epithelial ovarian cancer using deep learning and radiomics: A multicenter study. *Magn. Reson. Imaging* **2024**, *59*, 122–131. [CrossRef] [PubMed]
109. Guo, Q.; Lin, Z.; Lu, J.; Li, R.; Wu, L.; Deng, L.; Qiang, J.; Wu, X.; Gu, Y.; Li, H. Preoperative prediction of miliary changes in the small bowel mesentery in advanced high-grade serous ovarian cancer using MRI radiomics nomogram. *Abdom. Radiol.* **2023**, *48*, 1119–1130. [CrossRef]
110. Li, J.; Zhang, J.; Wang, F.; Ma, J.; Cui, S.; Ye, Z. CT-based radiomics for the preoperative prediction of occult peritoneal metastasis in epithelial ovarian cancers. *Acad. Radiol.* **2023**. [CrossRef] [PubMed]

Disclaimer/Publisher's Note: The statements, opinions and data contained in all publications are solely those of the individual author(s) and contributor(s) and not of MDPI and/or the editor(s). MDPI and/or the editor(s) disclaim responsibility for any injury to people or property resulting from any ideas, methods, instructions or products referred to in the content.

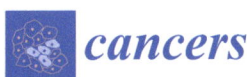

Review

Update on Renal Cell Carcinoma Diagnosis with Novel Imaging Approaches

Marie-France Bellin [1,2,3,*], Catarina Valente [1], Omar Bekdache [1], Florian Maxwell [1], Cristina Balasa [1], Alexia Savignac [1] and Olivier Meyrignac [1,2,3]

[1] Service de Radiologie Diagnostique et Interventionnelle, Hôpital de Bicêtre AP-HP, 78 Rue du Général Leclerc, 94275 Le Kremlin-Bicêtre, France; catarina.valente@aphp.fr (C.V.); omar.bekdache@aphp.fr (O.B.); florian.maxwell@aphp.fr (F.M.); alexia.savignac@aphp.fr (A.S.); olivier.meyrignac@aphp.fr (O.M.)
[2] Faculté de Médecine, University of Paris-Saclay, 63 Rue Gabriel Péri, 94276 Le Kremlin-Bicêtre, France
[3] BioMaps, UMR1281 INSERM, CEA, CNRS, University of Paris-Saclay, 94805 Villejuif, France
* Correspondence: marie-france.bellin@aphp.fr

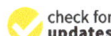

Citation: Bellin, M.-F.; Valente, C.; Bekdache, O.; Maxwell, F.; Balasa, C.; Savignac, A.; Meyrignac, O. Update on Renal Cell Carcinoma Diagnosis with Novel Imaging Approaches. *Cancers* **2024**, *16*, 1926. https://doi.org/10.3390/cancers16101926

Academic Editor: Athina C Tsili

Received: 21 March 2024
Revised: 6 May 2024
Accepted: 14 May 2024
Published: 18 May 2024

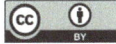

Copyright: © 2024 by the authors. Licensee MDPI, Basel, Switzerland. This article is an open access article distributed under the terms and conditions of the Creative Commons Attribution (CC BY) license (https://creativecommons.org/licenses/by/4.0/).

Simple Summary: The incidence of renal cell carcinoma (RCC) is increasing due to the expansion of cross-sectional imaging and advanced imaging techniques. They allow for the detection of tumors at an earlier stage, but there are often overlapping similarities in the appearance of benign and malignant renal tumors. This review presents and discusses the ever-evolving landscape of imaging techniques that can be used to detect and diagnose renal cell carcinoma, including its major histologic subtypes. It also provides insight into recently proposed or updated imaging algorithms and guidelines for the diagnosis of RCC. The review considers the major advances in spectral CT, photo- counting CT, multiparametric MRI, contrast-enhanced ultrasound, sestamibi SPECT/CT, PSMA PET/CT, radiomics, artificial intelligence, Bosniak classification version 2019, clear cell likelihood score, and AUA guidelines. The goal for radiologists is to be better equipped to guide the diagnosis and management of these patients.

Abstract: This review highlights recent advances in renal cell carcinoma (RCC) imaging. It begins with dual-energy computed tomography (DECT), which has demonstrated a high diagnostic accuracy in the evaluation of renal masses. Several studies have suggested the potential benefits of iodine quantification, particularly for distinguishing low-attenuation, true enhancing solid masses from hyperdense cysts. By determining whether or not a renal mass is present, DECT could avoid the need for additional imaging studies, thereby reducing healthcare costs. DECT can also provide virtual unenhanced images, helping to reduce radiation exposure. The review then provides an update focusing on the advantages of multiparametric magnetic resonance (MR) imaging performance in the histological subtyping of RCC and in the differentiation of benign from malignant renal masses. A proposed standardized stepwise reading of images helps to identify clear cell RCC and papillary RCC with a high accuracy. Contrast-enhanced ultrasound may represent a promising diagnostic tool for the characterization of solid and cystic renal masses. Several combined pharmaceutical imaging strategies using both sestamibi and PSMA offer new opportunities in the diagnosis and staging of RCC, but their role in risk stratification needs to be evaluated. Although radiomics and tumor texture analysis are hampered by poor reproducibility and need standardization, they show promise in identifying new biomarkers for predicting tumor histology, clinical outcomes, overall survival, and the response to therapy. They have a wide range of potential applications but are still in the research phase. Artificial intelligence (AI) has shown encouraging results in tumor classification, grade, and prognosis. It is expected to play an important role in assessing the treatment response and advancing personalized medicine. The review then focuses on recently updated algorithms and guidelines. The Bosniak classification version 2019 incorporates MRI, precisely defines previously vague imaging terms, and allows a greater proportion of masses to be placed in lower-risk classes. Recent studies have reported an improved specificity of the higher-risk categories and better inter-reader agreement. The clear cell likelihood score, which adds standardization to the characterization of solid renal masses on MRI, has been validated in recent studies with high interobserver agreement. Finally, the review discusses the key imaging implications of the 2017 AUA guidelines for renal masses and localized renal cancer.

Keywords: renal cell carcinoma; dual-energy CT; spectral CT; photon-counting detector CT; quantitative computed tomography; multiparametric MRI; contrast-enhanced ultrasound; sestamibi SPECT/CT; PSMA PET/CT; radiomics; artificial intelligence; Bosniak classification version 2019; clear cell likelihood score; AUA guidelines

1. Introduction

Kidney cancer is the 14th most common cancer worldwide, with more than 434,840 new cases diagnosed and 155,953 deaths in 2022 [1]. Renal cell carcinoma (RCC) accounts for 3.5% of all malignancies in Europe [2] and is the most common solid tumor of the kidney. Its incidence has been increasing until recently [3], primarily due to the increased incidental diagnosis of small renal lesions found during abdominal examinations for a variety of indications. Sixty-seven percent of cases are now diagnosed incidentally [4], resulting in a decreasing trend in tumor size and stage [5]. However, most incidentally discovered renal lesions are small and benign, the majority being renal cysts [6,7], while benign solid renal lesions are rarer and mainly represented by angiomyolipomas and oncytomas. The main goal of imaging is to differentiate RCC from benign disease, although in many cases this may not be possible. In fact, approximately 20% of surgically resected renal masses are reported to be benign [8], resulting in increased healthcare costs and exposing patients to surgical risks.

Radiologists play a key role in the diagnosis, characterization, and staging of RCC. In addition, the pretreatment identification of major histologic subtypes of RCC is important because they have different characteristics and clinical behaviors. Clear cell RCC, the most common subtype, accounts for 65–70% of cases and 94% of metastatic RCC and has a 5-year survival rate of 44–59%, whereas papillary RCC (10–15% of RCC) accounts for 4% of metastatic RCC with a survival rate of 82–92% and chromophobe RCC (5% of RCC) accounts for 2% of metastatic RCC with a survival rate of 78–87% [9,10]. Other malignant RCCs (collecting duct carcinoma, MiT family translocation renal cell carcinoma, tubulocystic carcinoma, etc.) are rare and account for 5 to 6% of cases.

CT is the first choice for the characterization of a renal mass and for staging because of its cost and availability [11]. MRI may also be indicated because it offers the added benefits of no radiation exposure and improved characterization of cystic lesions, lesions smaller than 2 cm, and histologic subtypes of RCC [12,13]. However, compared with CT, MRI is more expensive and time-consuming [14]. Based on the American Urological Association (AUA) guidelines, renal biopsy may be considered in patients with suspected renal hematologic or metastatic involvement and in patients with suspected benign renal masses [15] or before active surveillance of RCC.

In recent years, there have been remarkable advances in imaging technology [16]. Current novel imaging modalities include dual-energy CT (DECT) [17,18], photon-counting detector CT [19], radiomics, and high-resolution multiparametric MRI [20]. Compared to single-energy CT, DECT offers new capabilities and provides access to the iodine concentration within renal lesions. It provides images with improved diagnostic performance and a potential reduction in contrast and radiation doses. In addition, the recent introduction of photon-counting detector CT into clinical practice may dramatically change the imaging management of renal masses in the coming years. The introduction of the multi-step interpretation of multiparametric MRI for preoperative assessment of histologic subtypes of RCC and differentiation from benign lesions is also a major advance [20]. Recently, radiomics has been proposed to allow the in-depth assessment of tumor heterogeneity to facilitate precision medicine and better decision making [21]. In addition, due to recent developments, artificial intelligence (AI) has been adopted in the field of radiology and appears to be a useful tool for physicians to make more accurate diagnoses in less time.

Therefore, the purpose of this review is to provide an overview of the most promising novel imaging approaches in RCC diagnosis.

2. Novel Imaging Techniques

2.1. Dual-Energy CT

CT is currently the most widely used modality for the initial diagnosis and staging of renal cell carcinoma [11,14]. Over the past decade, there has been an increasing trend toward the use of DECT for the evaluation of renal lesions [17,22–24]. Several technical approaches are currently available, including dual-source DECT, single-source rapid kilovoltage switching (fast kVp-switch), single-source sequential ("rotate-rotate"), single-source dual-beam, single-source sequential, and dual-layer spectral multidetector CT. They offer different spectral contrast and dose efficiencies and different post-processing algorithms [22].

DECT systems allow essentially simultaneous acquisition of dual-energy images, typically acquired at 80 and 140 kVp, without a significant increase in radiation dose [16]. By acquiring images of the same object at different energies (typically 80 kVp and 140 kVp), DECT is able not only to reconstruct the anatomical structure of the imaged object (conventional CT), but also to approximate the composition of an element contained in the object (spectral CT). Each material has its own spectral response (variation in absorption coefficient) as a function of energy. Thus, two materials with close linear absorption coefficients in one energy band of the radiological spectrum can be completely distinguished from each other by performing measurements in two energy bands.

Post-processing algorithms play a crucial role in DECT. They generate several sets of images:

- Monoenergetic images. These images are produced at specific energy levels (e.g., 80 keV, 100 keV, and 140 keV). They provide different levels of contrast and are useful for specific diagnostic tasks, offering improved contrast and tissue visualization compared to conventional polychromatic images.
- Optimum contrast images. These result from the non-linear mixing of low-energy images, which enhance contrast, and high-energy images, which provide low noise.

DECT also facilitates the reduction in metal artifacts by post-processing the acquired data.

Differentiation algorithms facilitate the isolation or distinction of specific materials within the data set, often through color coding. Image post-processing algorithms can generate synthetic virtual unenhanced (VUE) images by removing the iodine signal from contrast-enhanced scans, reducing the need for additional scans and minimizing the radiation dose. In a series of 221 patients with 273 renal masses, the differences in renal mass attenuation between VUE and true unenhanced images were within 3 HU for enhancing masses (95% limits of agreement −3.1 HU to 2.7 HU) and non-enhancing cysts (95% limits of agreement −2.9 HU to 2.5 HU) [25]. In addition, the elimination of true enhanced acquisition would result in an estimated mean radiation dose savings of 24% (range 10–36%) for CT renal mass examinations [25]. A large, recently published retrospective study [26] confirmed that there is a strong agreement between VUE and true unenhanced images in the assessment of renal masses. This is important because unenhanced images provide essential information for the classification of renal cystic lesions and the detection of macroscopic fat, hemorrhage, and calcifications and serve as a baseline for comparison with contrast-enhanced images. Numerous studies have shown that CT numbers of virtual unenhanced images are reproducible and comparable to true non-contrast images, allowing the reliable assessment of precontrast renal lesion attenuation [26–28]. Nevertheless, Graser et al. [28] observed a difference in attenuation of ≥ 5 Hounsfield units (HU) between virtual and true unenhanced images in approximately 20% of patients in one study. In addition, significant interscanner variation in attenuation measurements and qualitative assessment of VUE images has been reported [29], particularly in patients scanned on different dual-energy CT scanner types during follow-up imaging. Chandarana et al. [30] also found variability in renal lesion attenuation between virtual and true unenhanced images. Given these findings, it cannot be definitively concluded that VUE images can replace true non-contrast scans. In fact, the effects of reconstruction algorithms, noise reduction techniques, and convolution kernels on the attenuation values of virtual unenhanced and weighted average data remain incompletely understood.

Along with unenhanced images, enhancement on multiphasic CT provides a simple, noninvasive means of suggesting the histologic type of a renal mass. It is defined by an increase of 20 HU or more between precontrast and contrast-enhanced images [11]. In daily practice, an enhancement of <10 HU is considered to be characteristic of a cyst, 10–19 HU of an indeterminate mass, and >20 HU suggestive of a renal tumor. Young et al. [9] showed that the mean enhancement of clear cell RCC (Figure 1) was significantly greater than that of oncocytoma (Figure 2) and chromophobe RCC (Figure 3) in the cortico-medullary and excretory phases, and significantly greater than that of papillary RCC (Figure 4) in the cortico-medullary, nephrographic, and excretory phases. In their series, the mean attenuation values during the corticomedullary phase were 125.0 HU for RCCs, 106.0 HU for oncocytomas, 53.6 HU for papillary RCCs, and 73.8 HU for chromophobe RCCs. However, this quantitative information does not necessarily translate into clinically meaningful measures in daily practice due to the variability and overlap in HU measurements. In a recently published study of 87 patients with 93 pathologically proven papillary RCCs [31], most papillary RCCs presented as a hypovascular, circumscribed, solid renal mass; a few (17%) papillary RCCs presented as the newly defined Bosniak class IIF subtype.

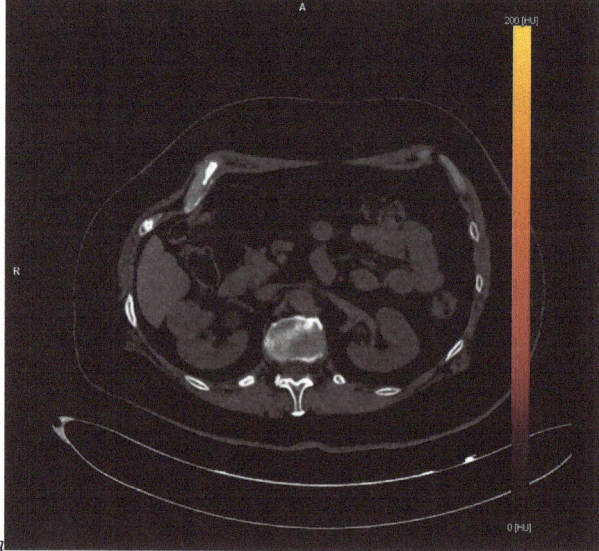

Figure 1. *Cont.*

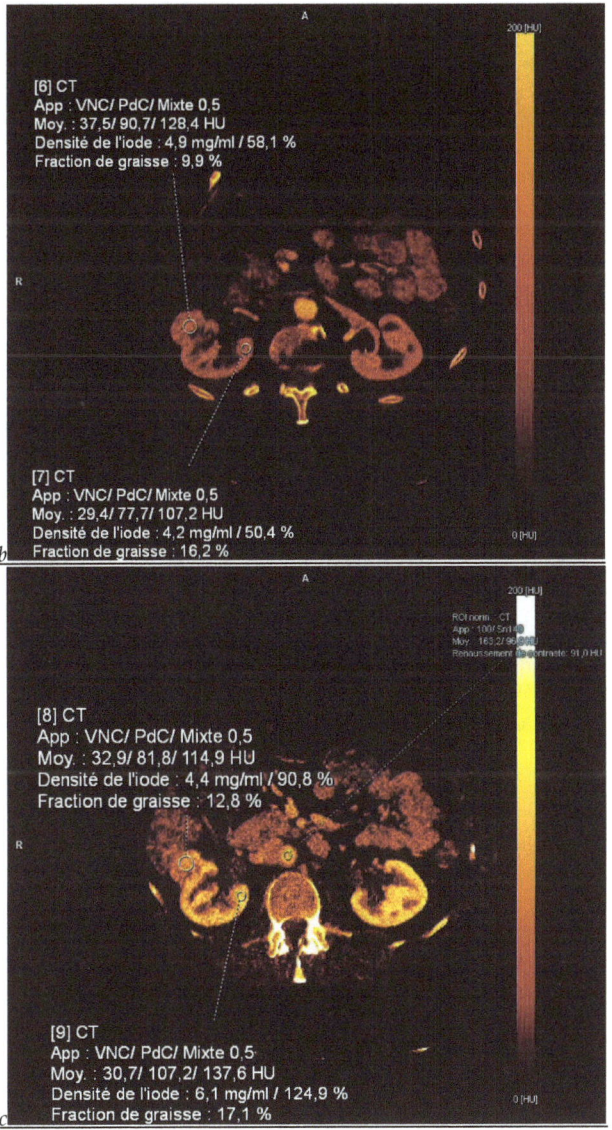

Figure 1. Cont.

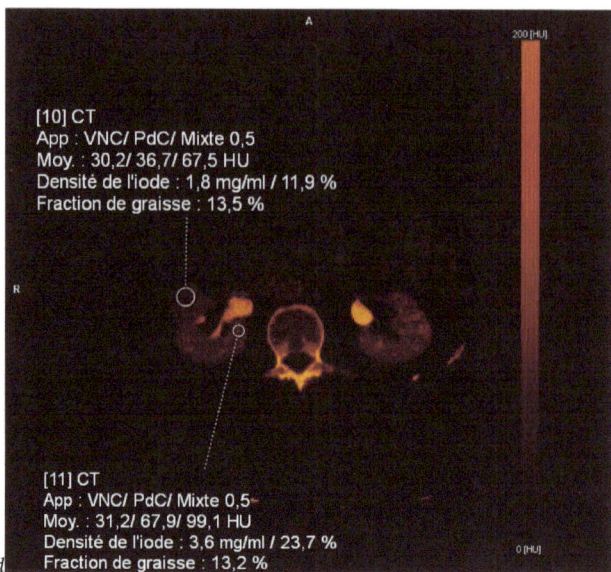

Figure 1. Dual-energy CT aspect of a hypervascularized clear cell renal cell carcinoma of the upper pole of the right kidney. (**a**) Virtual unenhanced image. Note the presence of a solid exophytic renal mass in the upper pole of the right kidney. (**b**) The lesion enhances during the corticomedullary phase; measurement of the iodine concentration of the lesion (4.9 mg/mL) compared to that of the renal cortex (4.2 mg/mL) during the corticomedullary phase. (**c**) Monoenergetic image obtained at 40 keV during the nephrographic phase. Note the decrease in iodine concentration of the lesion (4.42 mg/mL) compared to that of the renal cortex (6.1 mg/mL). (**d**) Monoenergetic image obtained at 70 keV during the excretory phase. Compared to the monoenergetic image at 40 keV, the contrast between the lesion and the adjacent renal cortex is reduced. Note the washout of the lesion (iodine content: 1.8 mg/mL).

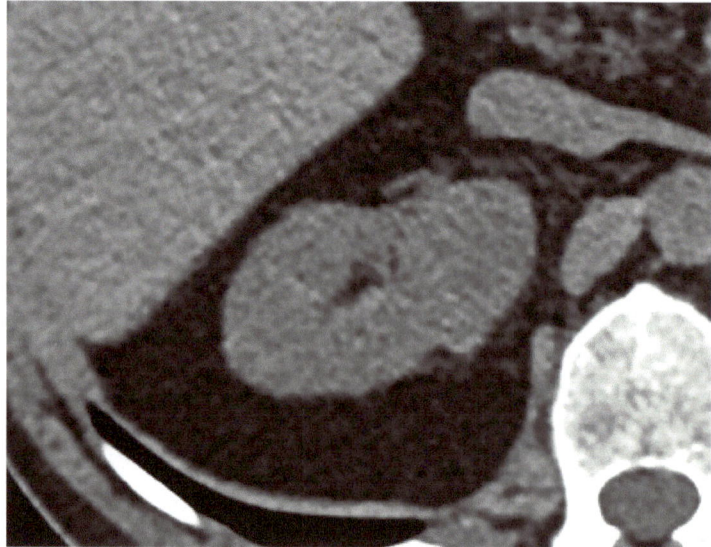

Figure 2. *Cont.*

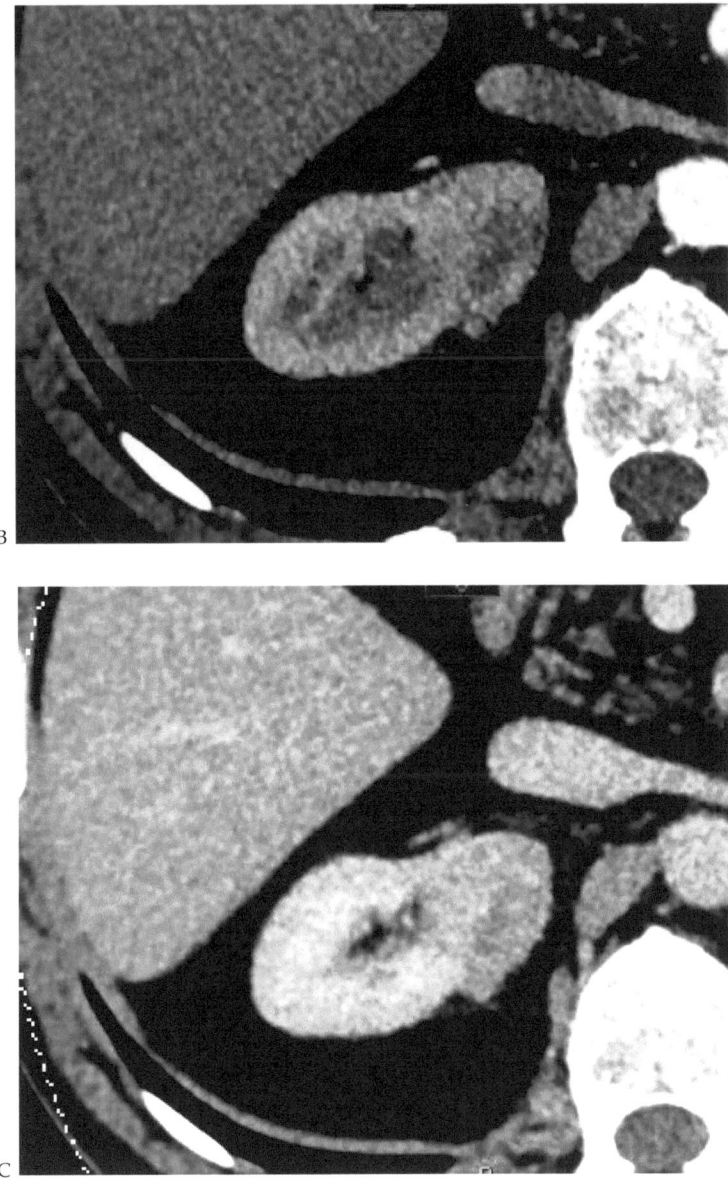

Figure 2. Cont.

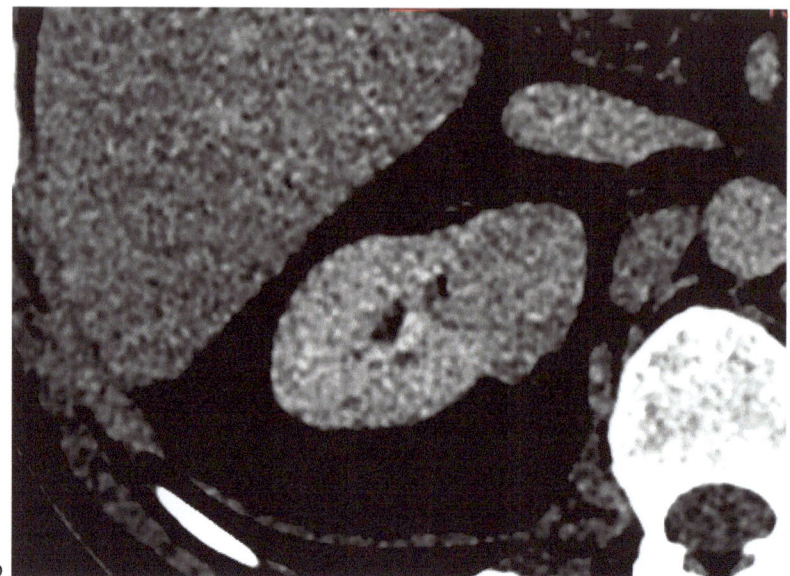

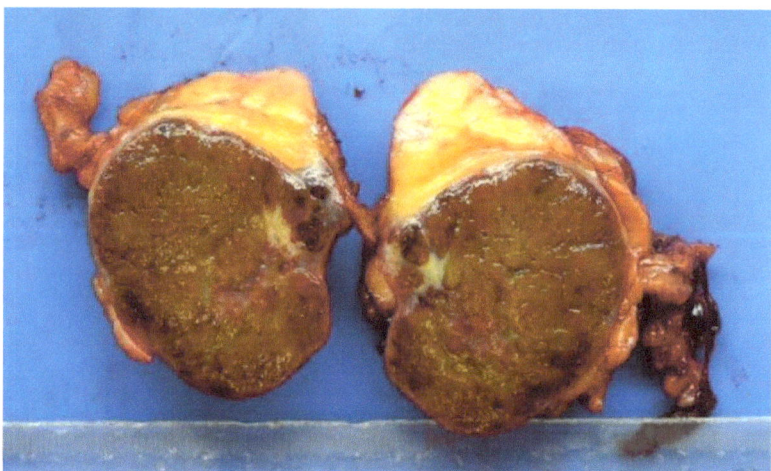

Figure 2. Oncocytoma in the right kidney of a 42-year-old man. (**A**) On the unenhanced image, the 4.8 cm lesion is isodense relative to the renal parenchyma. Enhancement is seen on the corticomedullary phase image (**B**), followed by washout on the nephrographic (**C**) and excretory (**D**) phase images. (**E**) Macroscopic view of the lesion after radical nephrectomy. Courtesy of Pr S. Ferlicot, Department of Pathology, Bicêtre.

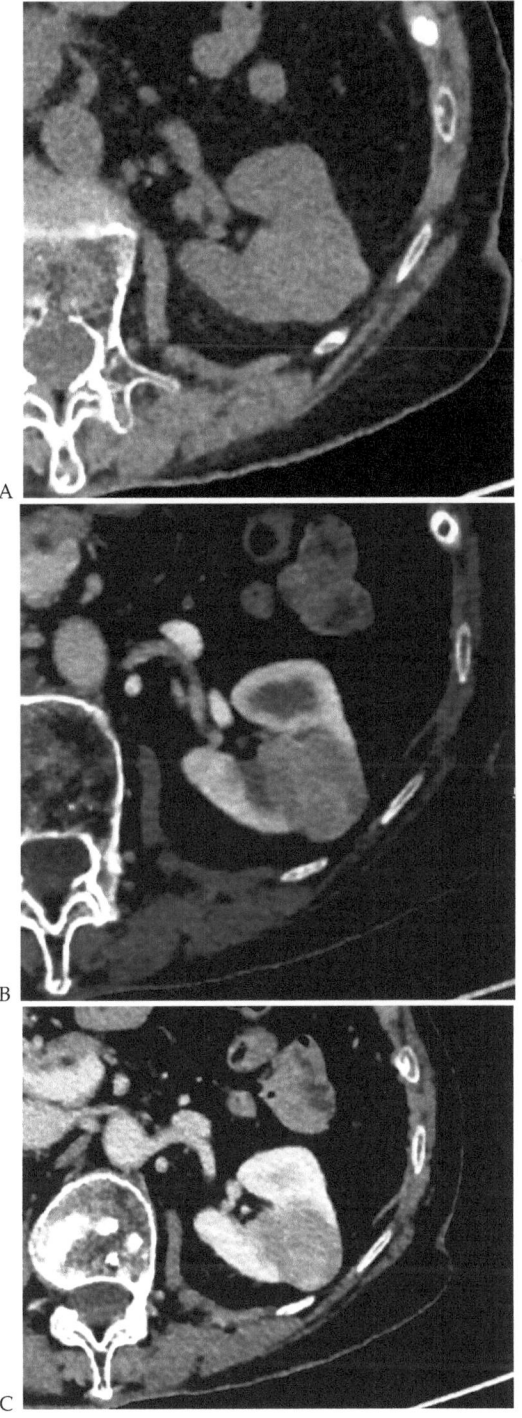

Figure 3. *Cont.*

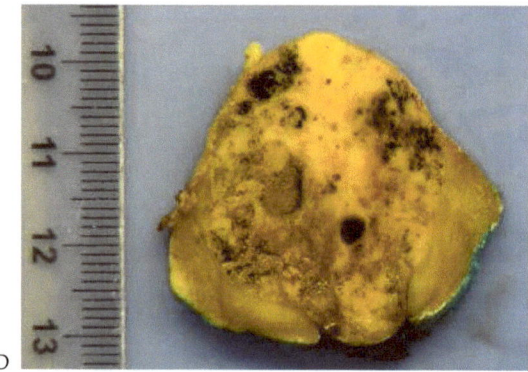

Figure 3. CT aspect of a chromophobe renal cell carcinoma in the left kidney of a 68-year-old-woman. (**A**) Unenhanced image. Presence of an isodense, homogeneous solid lesion at the medium part of the left kidney. (**B**) It appears moderately hypervascularized on the corticomedullary phase image, with hyperdense septa. (**C**) There is progressive washout on the nephrographic phase image and the lesions appears hypodense relative to the renal parenchyma (**C**). (**D**) Macroscopic view of the lesion after partial nephrectomy. Courtesy of Pr S. Ferlicot, Department of Pathology, Bicêtre Hospital.

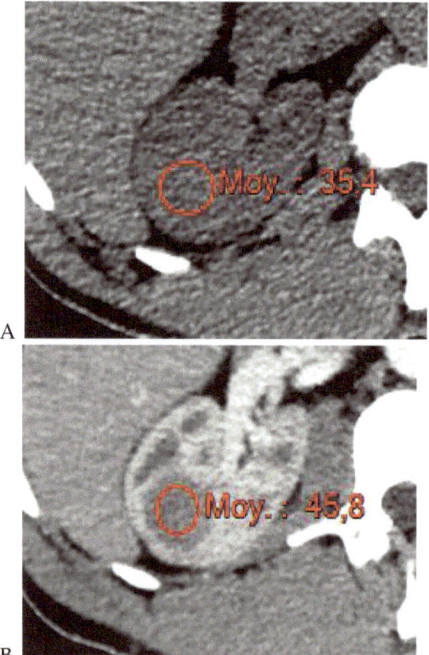

Figure 4. *Cont.*

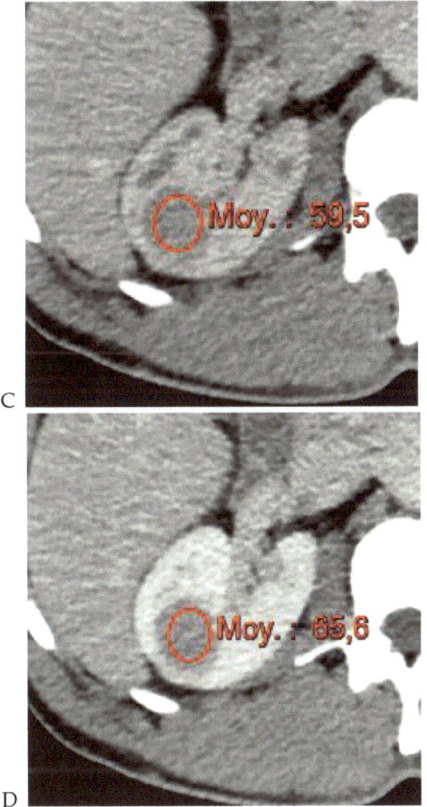

Figure 4. Multiphasic CT enhancement of a papillary renal cell carcinoma in the middle part of the right kidney of a 63-year-old woman. (**A**) Mean unenhanced attenuation was 35 HU. (**B**) Mean corticomedullary phase attenuation was 45 HU. (**C**) Mean nephrographic phase attenuation was 59 HU. (**D**) Mean excretory phase attenuation was 65 HU.

DECT offers several potential advantages over conventional CT in the evaluation of renal masses.

- It may eliminate the unwanted effects of pseudoenhancement by the improved correction of beam-hardening artifacts related to iodine [17].
- Color-coded iodine overlay images can provide advantages over conventional grayscale imaging for assessing enhancement in subcentimeter lesions, as well as for eliminating the potential errors in region of interest (ROI) positioning for renal tumors that are isodense with the renal parenchyma on the unenhanced image.
- DECT offers the possibility to obtain a direct quantification of the iodine concentration (in mg/mL) in a lesion, which represents a new option for the characterization of renal masses with equivocal enhancement, especially those with an attenuation baseline between 20 and 70 HU on unenhanced images [32,33]. They may represent either hyperdense cysts or hypovascular true enhancing tumors such as papillary RCC. In these patients, iodine quantification provides a more direct estimate of tumor blood supply and neoangiogenesis.
- A new area of research has emerged with the implementation of dual-energy maps in discriminating among RCC histologic subtypes [17,18].
- Quantification of iodine concentration is also of interest for re-evaluation after treatment. Dual-energy iodine quantification could be adopted as an imaging biomarker

of tumor viability in cases of advanced RCC treated with targeted or antiangiogenic therapies that reduce tumor perfusion with a limited effect on tumor size [17,30,34].

A meta-analysis reported that DECT had a pooled sensitivity and specificity greater than 95% for evaluation of renal masses, but the accuracy was comparable to that of conventional CT [23]. The authors concluded that larger, multi-institutional studies are needed if DECT is to replace conventional CT in the evaluation of renal masses. A recent single-center study showed a higher confidence in lesion characterization with DECT, with fewer recommendations for additional and follow-up imaging tests than dual-phase single-energy CT and similar performance to MRI [24]. Although the role of DECT to characterize renal masses is growing, the best method for the incorporation of DECT into a renal CT protocol remains to be determined [17,22,23].

2.2. Photon-Counting Detector CT

In recent years, the majority of CT instrument development has focused on photon-counting detectors for multispectral CT. Photon-counting detector CT (PCD-CT) is an emerging technology that offers new possibilities for quantification [19].

The principle of photon-counting CT (PCD-CT) is based on the use of novel energy-resolving X-ray detectors with mechanisms that differ significantly from those of conventional energy-integrating detectors (EIDs). The novel energy-resolving detectors use semiconducting materials, such as cadmium telluride or cadmium zinc telluride, which allow the direct conversion of X-ray photons into electrical signals. As a result, each photon that interacts with the detector can be individually quantified, allowing precise and individual measurement of its energy. In contrast, conventional CT scanners typically rely on EIDs, which record the total energy deposited in a pixel over a given time period, typically from a large number of photons along with electronic noise. As a result, EIDs only capture photon intensity, while PCDs also capture spectral information, allowing for a more accurate assessment of tissue attenuation properties.

The potential benefits of using a PCD instead of an EID in CT imaging include an improved signal-to-noise ratio, reduced radiation exposure to the patient, improved spatial resolution, mitigation of beam hardening artifacts, and the ability to differentiate between different contrast agents within a single image by using multiple energy bins [35,36]. Ultimately, the CT numbers obtained from conventional CT scanners are dependent on the acquisition protocol and the properties of the surrounding tissues. In contrast, photon-counting CT imparts precise physical material and/or tissue information to each pixel, allowing for more accurate tissue characterization and the visualization of subtle pathologies that may not be apparent on conventional CT images.

The first clinically approved PCD-CT system was cleared by the Food and Drug Administration (FDA) in September 2021. To date, only a few PCD-CT units (less than 30) have been installed worldwide, and clinical research is dominated by validation studies for the implementation of multispectral CT [37]. To date, no publications have specifically focused on the diagnosis of RCC using PCD-CT.

2.3. Multiparametric MR Imaging

In recent years, multiparametric MRI of the kidney has become a key imaging modality for the detection and characterization of renal masses [13,14,24,36].

The multiparametric MR imaging protocol for the evaluation of renal masses typically includes T2-weighted single-shot fast spin-echo sequences (in the axial, coronal, and/or sagittal planes), chemical shift imaging (T1-weighted two-dimensional Dixon GRE in-phase and out-of-phase images in the axial plane), axial diffusion-weighted imaging (SE EPI DWI) with multiple b-values (b = 0–50, 400–500, 800–1000 s/mm^2) with an ADC map, and dynamic 3D fat-suppressed T1-weighted sequences before and after gadolinium administration (in the axial plane) at 30 s (corticomedullary phase), 90–100 s (nephrographic phase), 180–210 s, and 5–7 min (excretory phase) [13]. Extracellular gadolinium-based contrast material is given at a dose of 0.1 mL per kilogram of body weight injected at

1–2 mL/s, followed by a 10–20 mL saline flush. Image subtraction may be performed during the contrast-enhanced phases to help detect enhancement in lesions where it is equivocal. To be considered complete, the MR protocol should include an evaluation of both kidneys and the liver.

Each radiologist should be aware of the usefulness of each sequence and its contribution to the diagnosis and ultimately cross-check the various pieces of information provided to arrive at reliable diagnostic hypotheses.

The detection of macroscopic fat in a renal mass is essential because, in the absence of calcification, it is almost always characteristic of a classic (fat-rich) angiomyolipoma, the most common solid benign renal mass. The macroscopic fat component shows a loss of signal intensity on T1-weighted fat-suppressed images. Angiomyolipomas are also characterized by the presence of an India ink artifact on opposed-phase T1-weighted images at the junction of the mass and normal renal parenchyma, indicating a fat–water interface. T1-weighted gradient-echo inversion recovery imaging allows the detection of microscopic/intracytoplasmic fat. Microscopic intracellular fat is present in clear cell RCC (Figure 5), resulting in a signal drop on opposed-phase images. A signal drop has also been described in angiomyolipomas, including fat-poor angiomyolipomas (Figure 6). Gadolinium-enhanced T1-weighted three-dimensional fat-suppressed gradient-echo imaging is useful to assess the enhancement pattern in a renal mass. It allows the differentiation of hypervascular masses from hypovascular lesions with late and slow enhancement as seen in papillary RCC (Figure 7). T2-weighted sequences are essential for differentiating cystic renal masses from solid renal masses. The T2 signal intensity of a solid renal mass is also helpful in suggesting certain histologic subtypes of RCC. Both fat-poor angiomyolipomas (Figure 6) and papillary RCCs (Figure 7) have a low signal intensity on T2-weighted images, whereas other renal masses have an intermediate or high signal intensity. Several studies have suggested the potential utility of apparent diffusion coefficient (ADC) values to further characterize a renal mass [38]. Both fatty angiomyolipomas and papillary RCCs have low ADC values.

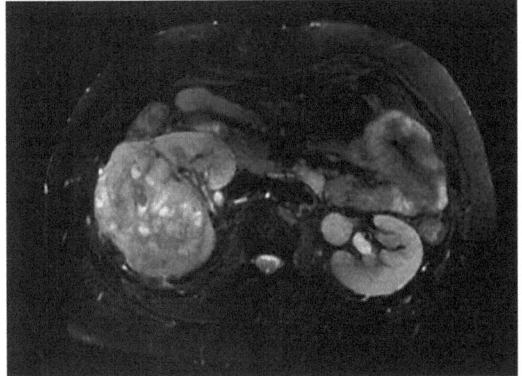 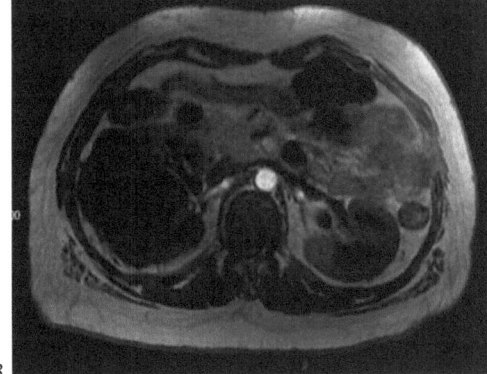

A B

Figure 5. *Cont.*

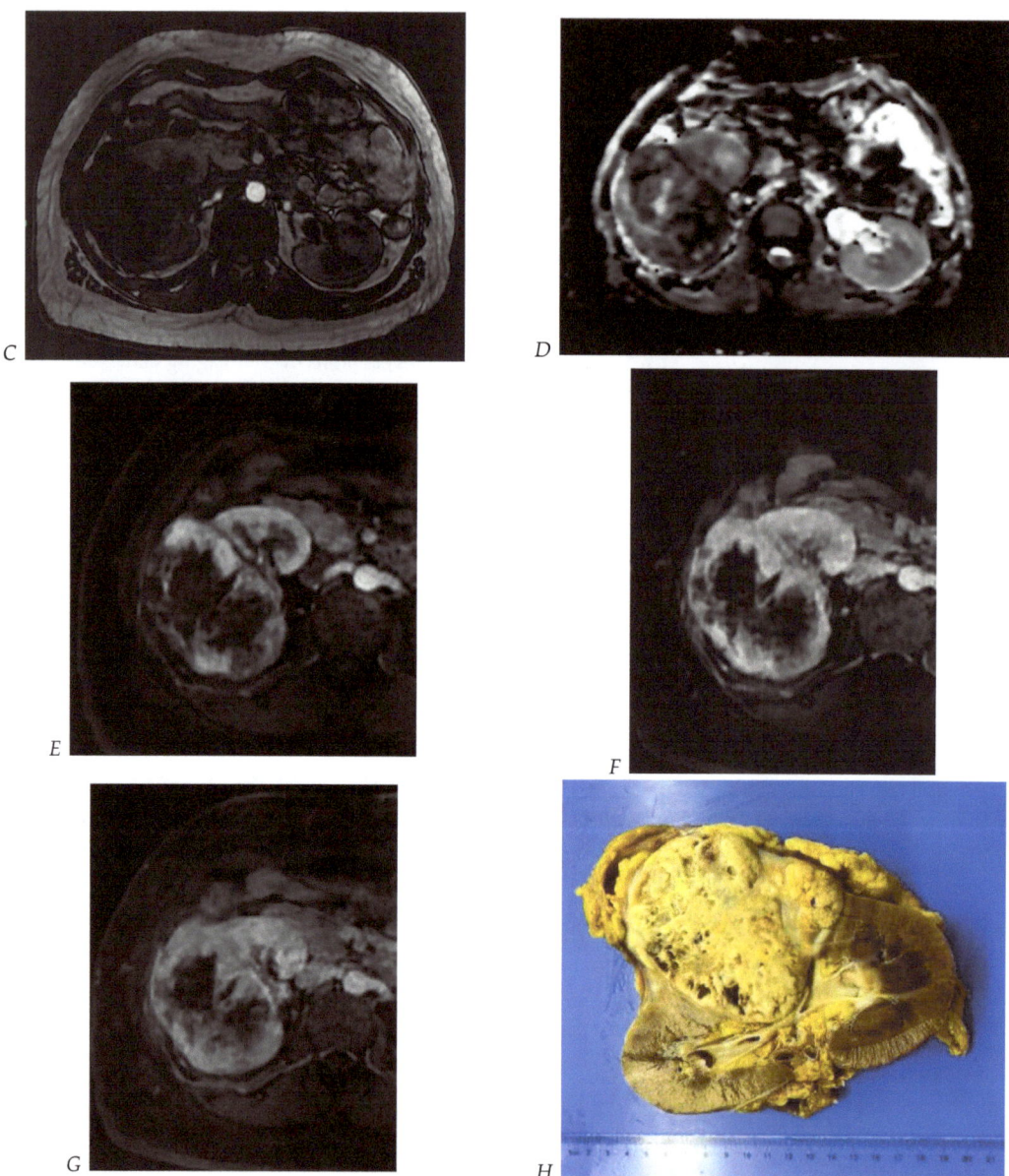

Figure 5. Clear cell renal cell carcinoma in the right kidney of a 52-year-old-man. (**A**) Coronal T2-weighted fast SE image shows a large heterogeneous mass with areas of high signal intensity compared with renal parenchyma. Transverse in-phase (**B**,**C**) opposed-phase MR images show a subtle signal loss on the opposed-phase image. (**D**) The ADC map is heterogeneous with predominant areas of restriction of tumor diffusion. Transverse gadolinium-enhanced T1-weighted gradient-echo spoiled MR images in (**E**) corticomedullary, (**F**) nephrographic, (**G**) and delayed phase images show intense and rapid peripheral enhancement during the arterial and nephrographic phases followed by a rapid washout of contrast on the delayed phase. Central necrotic areas do not enhance. (**H**) Macroscopic view of the lesion after radical nephrectomy. The lesion appears heterogeneous. Courtesy of Pr S. Ferlicot, Department of Pathology, Bicêtre Hospital.

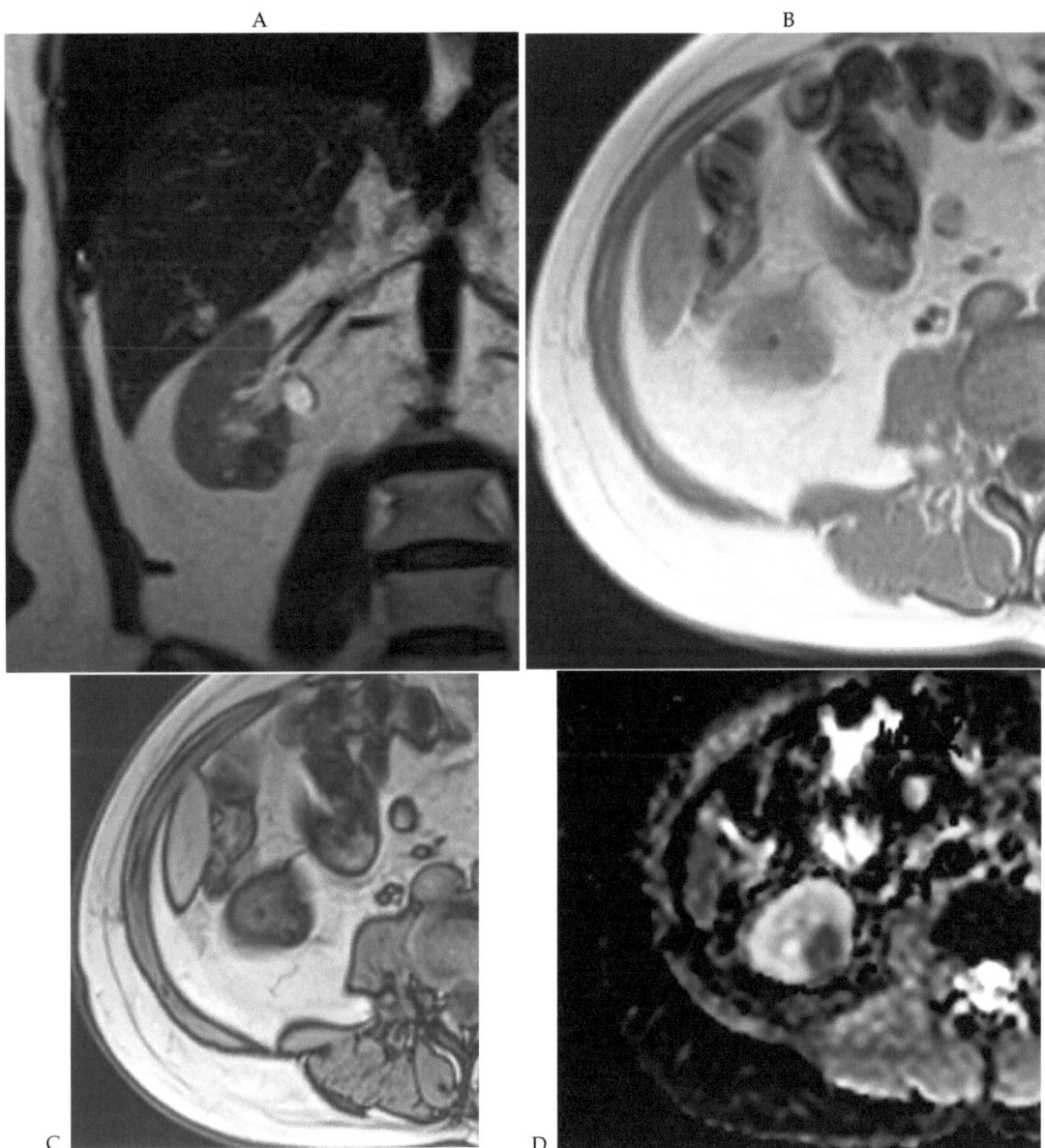

Figure 6. Cont.

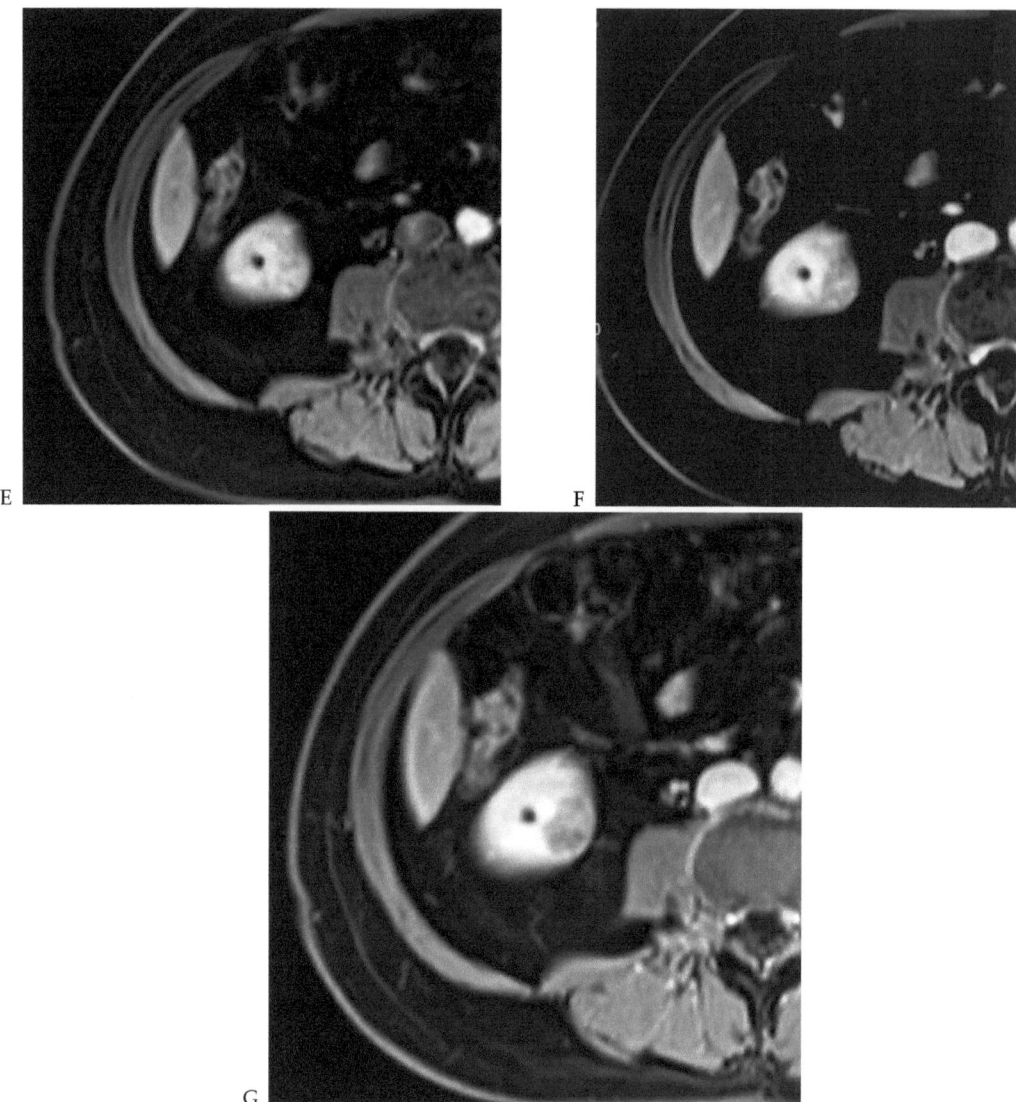

Figure 6. Fat-poor angiomyolipoma in the right kidney of a 46-year-old-man. (**A**) Coronal T2-weighted fast SE image shows the low signal intensity of the lesion compared with the renal parenchyma. Transverse in-phase (**B,C**) opposed-phase MR images show a significant loss of signal intensity on the opposed-phase image. (**D**) The ADC map shows marked restriction of tumor diffusion into the renal mass. Transverse gadolinium-enhanced T1-weighted gradient-echo spoiled MR images in (**E**) corticomedullary, (**F**) nephrographic, and (**G**) delayed phase images show early enhancement and rapid washout.

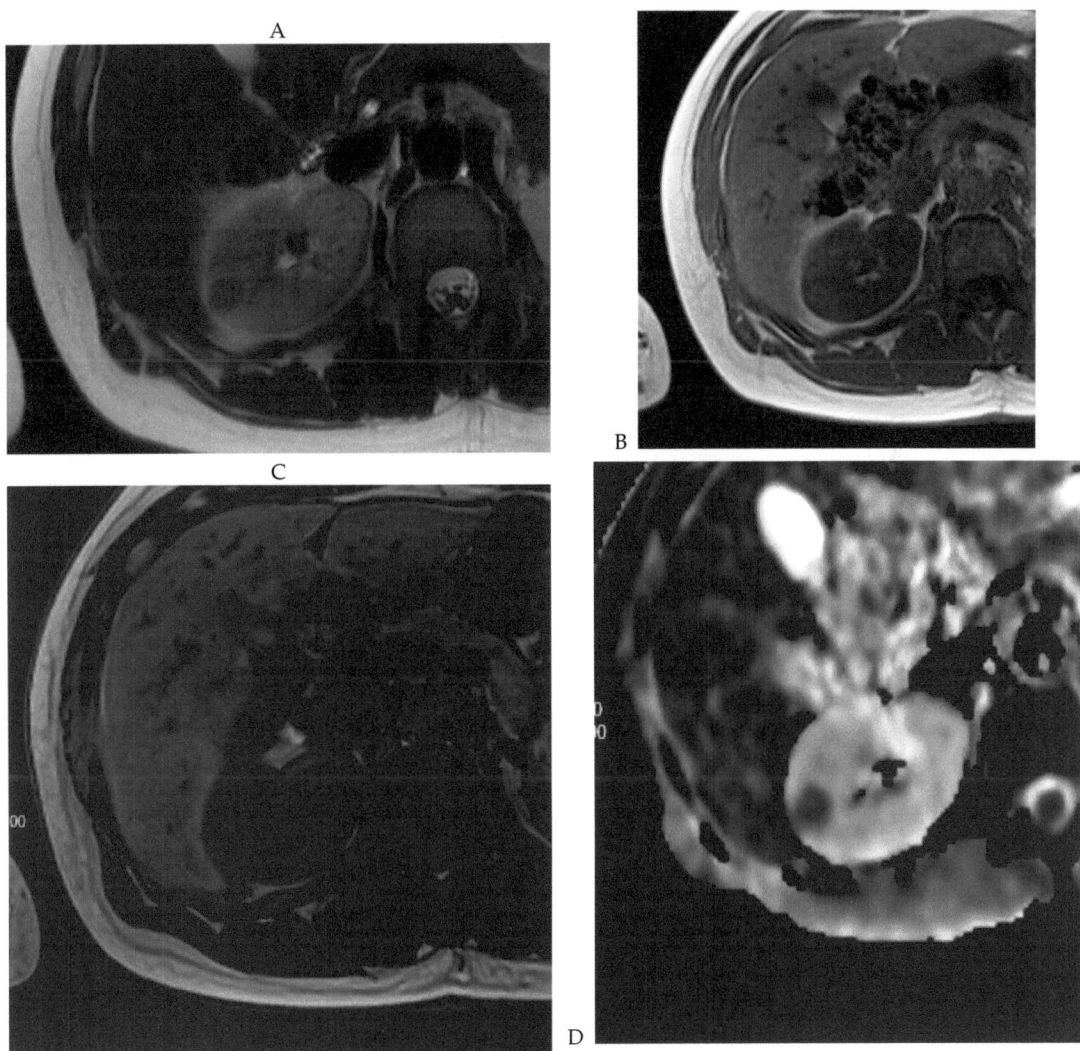

Figure 7. *Cont.*

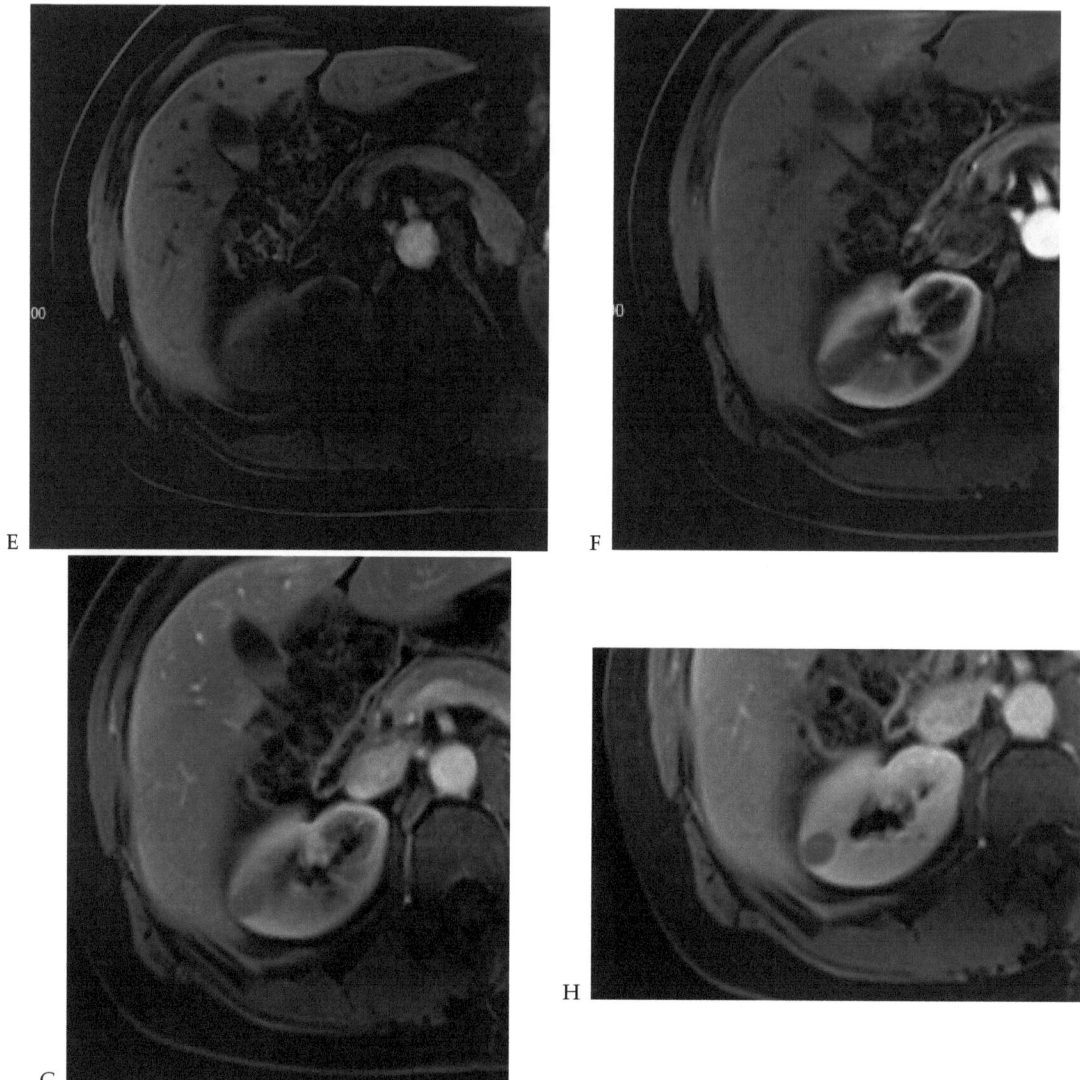

Figure 7. Papillary renal cell carcinoma in the right kidney of a 75-year-old-woman. (**A**) Axial T2-weighted fast SE image shows a homogeneous 1.8 cm mass in the posterolateral region of the right kidney, with a lower SI compared to renal parenchyma. Transverse in-phase (**B**,**C**) opposed-phase MR images do not show a significant signal loss on the opposed-phase image. (**D**) The ADC map shows restriction of tumor diffusion into the renal mass. Transverse nonenhanced (**E**) and gadolinium-enhanced T1-weighted gradient-echo spoiled MR images in (**F**) corticomedullary, (**G**) nephrographic, (**H**) and delayed phase images show progressive enhancement without washout; the mass is hypovascular compared to the renal cortex.

Cornelis et al. [12,20] proposed a stepwise reading of images organized as follows: (1) T2w images; (2) dual-shift chemical shift MR images; (3) DWI; (4) wash-in analysis of DCE images; and (5) washout analysis of DCE images. The first key feature is the predominant qualitative signal intensity of the lesion on a non-fat-suppressed T2-weighted sequence relative to the renal parenchyma. AMLs with minimal fat content and papillary

RCC have a low SI on T2-weighted images, whereas most other solid tumors appear hyperintense or heterogeneous. In addition, chromophobe RCC often appears as a heterogeneous lesion (Figure 8) with a slightly low T2 SI, which allows differentiation from clear cell RCC or renal oncocytoma [39].

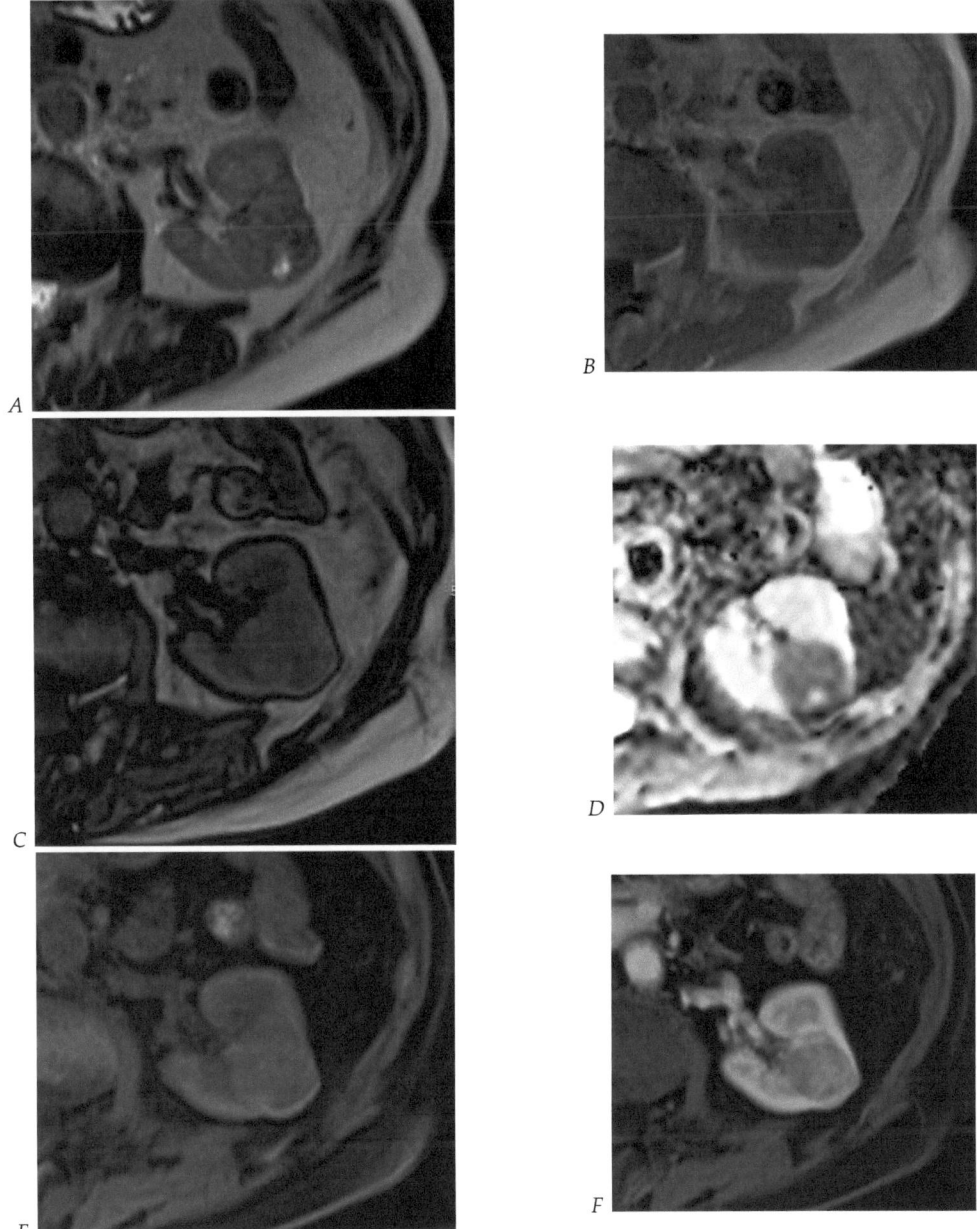

Figure 8. *Cont.*

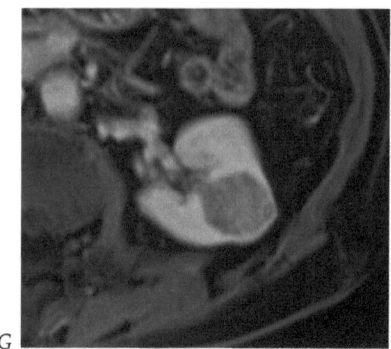
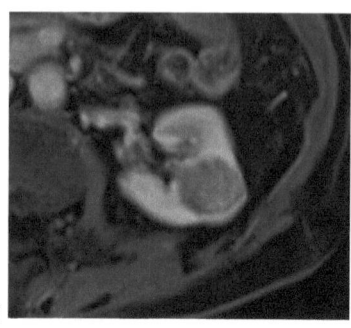

G   H

Figure 8. Same lesion as Figure 3. Chromophobe renal cell carcinoma in the left kidney of a 68-year-old-woman. (**A**) Axial T2-weighted fast SE image shows the exophytic heterogeneous isointense renal mass with a posterior hyperintense area. Transverse in-phase (**B**,**C**) opposed-phase MR images show no significant loss of signal intensity on the opposed-phase image. (**D**) The ADC map shows restriction of tumor diffusion into the renal mass. Transverse nonenhanced (**E**) and gadolinium-enhanced T1-weighted gradient-echo spoiled MR images in (**F**) corticomedullary, (**G**) nephrographic, (**H**) and delayed phase images show a mid-intense enhancement of the lesion without visible washout.

The second step is to analyze dual chemical shift MRI to look for the presence or absence of microscopic fat. Clear cell RCC (which contains intracellular microscopic fat) and fat-poor AML often show signal loss on out-of-phase sequences, whereas this has not been reported for renal oncocytoma (Figure 9). This signal loss may be seen sporadically in chromophobe or papillary RCC, but it is very rare.

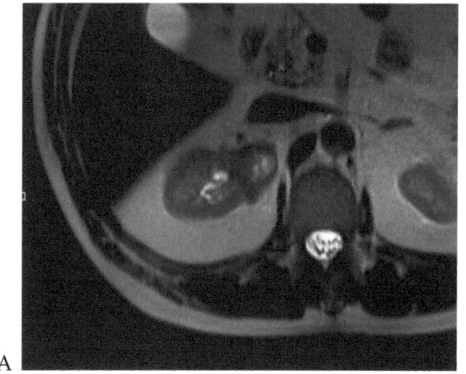
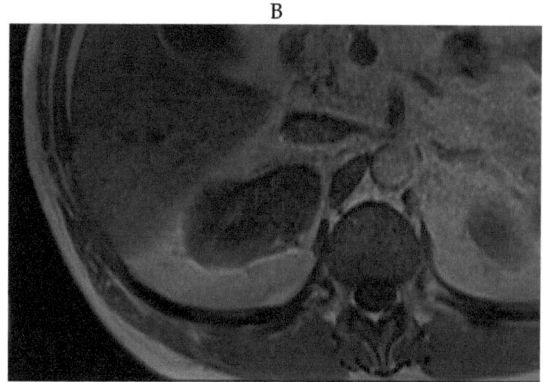

A   B

Figure 9. *Cont.*

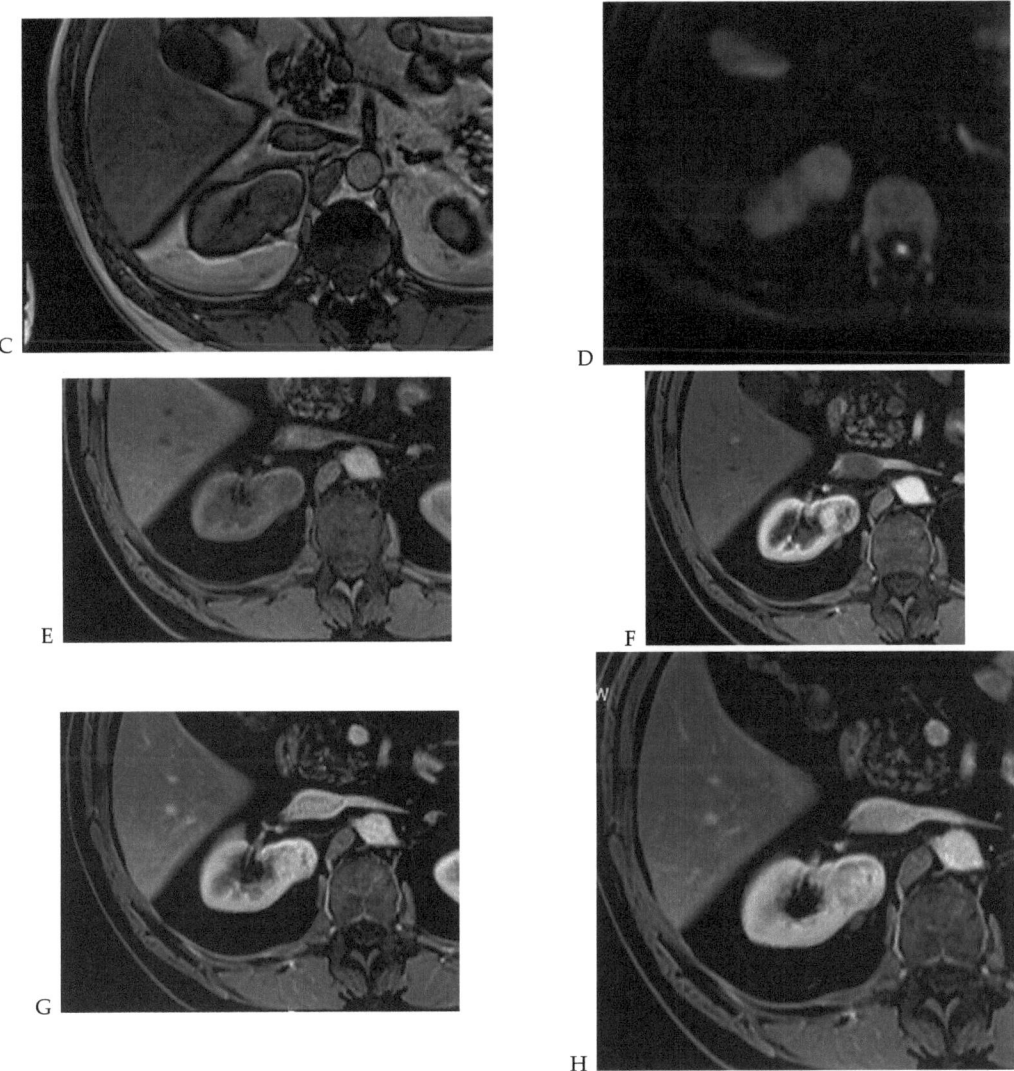

Figure 9. Same lesion as Figure 2. Oncocytoma in the right kidney of a 42-year-old man. (A) The axial T2-weighted fast SE image shows a heterogeneous lesion with a central hyperintense area. Transverse in-phase (B,C) opposed-phase MR images show no significant loss of signal intensity on the opposed-phase image. (D) The lesion is hyperintense on the diffusion-weighted image. Transverse nonenhanced (E) and gadolinium-enhanced T1-weighted gradient-echo spoiled MR images in (F) corticomedullary, (G) nephrographic, (H) and delayed phase images show early enhancement and rapid washout.

Third, the DWI sequence needs to be evaluated. Low ADC is often seen in AML and papillary RCC, while ADC remains heterogeneous but is often high in renal oncocytoma and clear cell RCC. As for T2-weighted imaging, chromophobe RCC has a slightly lower ADC compared to these last two lesions.

Finally, the analysis of DCE seems to be critical. Clear cell RCC, as well as AML, shows a rapid and intense enhancement after contrast injection in the corticomedullary phase (wash in). In oncocytoma and chromophobe RCC, the peak of enhancement is slightly delayed, but washout is observed in all of these tumor subtypes. In papillary RCC, however, enhancement is typically weak and slow, delayed, and maximal in the late phases. Therefore, washout is considered to be absent in papillary RCC. A quantitative approach was proposed by Cornelis et al. [20] to distinguish oncocytomas from chromophobe RCCs (sensitivity 25%, specificity 100%), whereas oncocytomas could be differentiated from clear cell RCC with high sensitivity (100%) and high specificity (94%). The main characteristics of solid renal tumors on multiparametric MRI are summarized in Table 1.

Table 1. Main characteristics of renal tumors on multiparametric MRI. Adapted from [12,20,39].

Tumor (Sub)Type	T2-Weighted	T1-Weighted	Fat Saturation	Dual Chemical Shift MRI	DCE T1-Weighted	DWI
Angiomyolipoma	Heterogeneous with high SI	Heterogeneous with high SI *	India ink artifact	Signal drop	Arterial enhancement	
Fat-poor angiomyolioma	Low SI			Signal drop	Arterial enhancement	Low
Oncocytoma	Heterogeneous with high SI; central scar			No	Heterogeneous moderate wash-in and washout; late segmental inversion	High
Clear cell RCC	Heterogeneous; central area (necrosis); high SI; pseudocapsule	Heterogeneous high SI of central area		Signal drop	High arterial wash-in and quick washout; heterogeneous	Heterogeneous; high
Papillary RCC	Homogeneous low signal intensity; pseudocapsule			No	Slow and low enhancement	Low
Chromophobe RCC	Heterogeneous central area (necrosis); mid SI			No	Moderate wash-in and washout	Mid

* SI: signal intensity.

Although there is growing interest in the use of multiparametric MRI for the diagnosis of renal masses, its accuracy still needs to be validated in large prospective studies.

2.4. Contrast-Enhanced Ultrasound

Kidney cancer is often discovered incidentally during an abdominal ultrasound examination. Ultrasound offers a number of advantages, including a low cost, accessibility, and the absence of ionizing radiation. It allows an initial assessment of the size of the tumor, its possible cystic nature, and its vascularization using Doppler [40,41]. However, it cannot be used to perform an exhaustive assessment of extension or to quantify tumor enhancement; moreover, its detection rate of small renal tumors is lower than that of CT, especially those smaller than 2 cm [42]. Renal contrast-enhanced ultrasound (CEUS) has been developed to enable the development of new functional applications for renal blood flow quantification [43]. Second-generation ultrasound contrast agents consist of gas microbubbles stabilized by a phospholipid shell. Measuring 3 to 7 microns, these microbubbles are small enough to pass through pulmonary capillaries and into the arterial system, yet large enough to remain strictly intravascular. There is no intra-tissue passage. Contrast agents have a short half-life (5 min), are not nephrotoxic, and are cleared via the lungs by exhalation [43]. Dynamic real-time acquisition and the use of a purely intravascular contrast agent are the two main features of CEUS that distinguish it from CT and MRI.

The purpose of renal contrast-enhanced ultrasound is to study the dynamics of contrast uptake of a lesion to aid in its characterization (Figure 10). In their recent meta-analysis of CEUS features of clear cell RCC less than 4 cm in diameter, Liu et al. [42] reported that hyperenhancement had a moderate sensitivity (67–89%) and specificity (42–75%), while fast-in contrast and heterogeneous enhancement had high diagnostic abilities (area under the curve (AUC) 0.74–0.84); however, the presence of a pseudocapsule and fast-out contrast had poor diagnostic abilities (AUC < 0.70). In 2022, Barr et al. [44] reported a pooled sensitivity of 98% and a pooled specificity of 78% of CEUS for the characterization of solid renal masses in their meta-analysis including 331 patients and 341 lesions. In addition, the high sensitivity (97%) and PPV (98.2%) of CEUS were reported for the diagnosis of RCC in small indeterminate solid renal masses on CT or MRI, excluding lipid-rich AML and cystic renal masses according to the proposed Bosniak classification 2019 [45]. In this retrospective study, CEUS also had a significantly higher sensitivity/NPV for the diagnosis of malignancy in cystic renal masses compared to CT/MRI. These results confirm the trend previously reported by Park et al. [46], who in a retrospective study of 31 cystic masses of the kidney reported diagnostic accuracies of 74% for CT and 90% for CEUS, which were not statistically different. In their series, CEUS images showed more septa in 10 (32%) lesions, more wall thickening and/or septa in 4 (13%) lesions, and more enhancement in 19 (61%) lesions. A recent meta-analysis of the diagnostic performance of CEUS in the evaluation of small renal masses reported an accuracy of 0.93 (sensitivity of 0.94, PPV of 0.95, specificity of 0.78, and NPV of 0.73) in the detection of malignant masses [47]. Although there are few high-powered randomized trials and the exact role of CEUS in the subtyping of renal cancer remains to be determined, CEUS has been included as "usually appropriate" in the American College of Radiology Appropriateness Criteria for the evaluation of indeterminate renal masses in patients with contraindications to CT/MRI contrast [48]. The use of CEUS, which varies widely from country to country, is currently increasing. Further studies are needed to clarify its role in characterizing renal cancer subtypes and stratifying the risk of malignancy of cystic lesions.

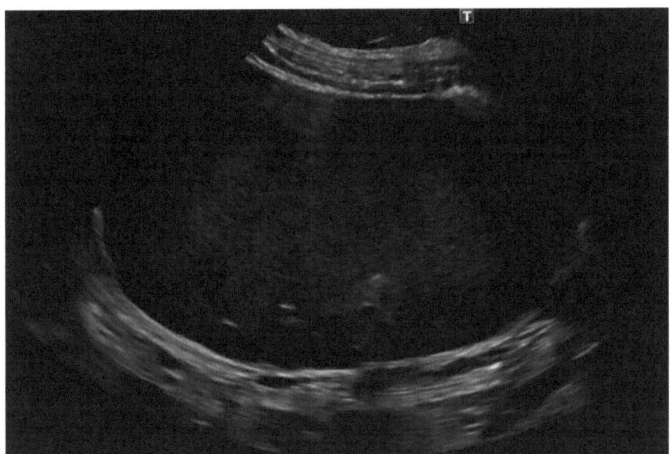

Figure 10. *Cont.*

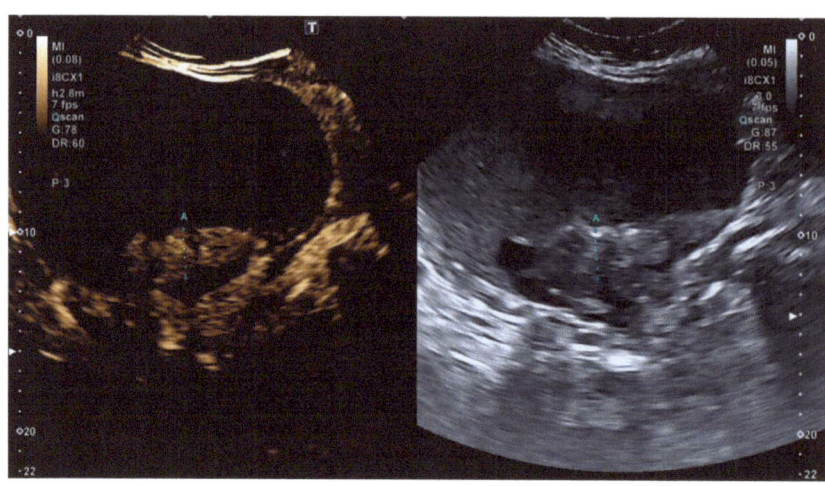

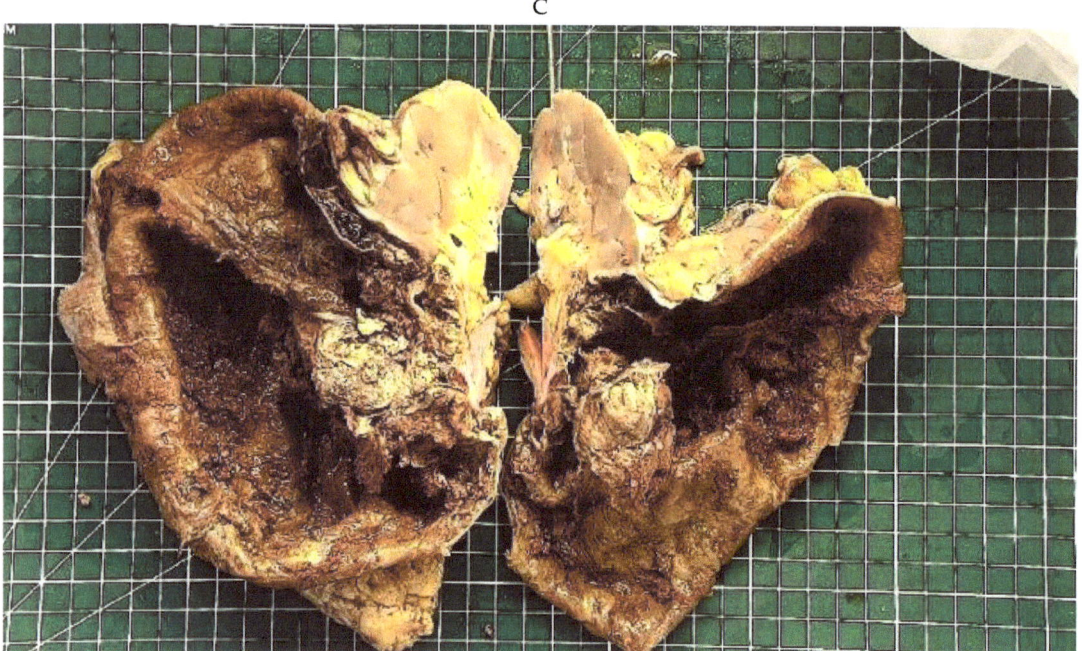

Figure 10. Papillary renal cell carcinoma in the right kidney of a 54-year-old woman. (**A**) B-mode ultrasound shows a large right cystic renal mass with heterogeneous contents and a dependent sediment. (**B**) CEUS with Sonovue® (Bracco Imaging France, Massy, France) reveals the presence of a solid enhancing component at the posterior aspect of the mass. (**C**) The mass was resected. Pathology identified a necrotic papillary renal cell carcinoma. Courtesy of Pr S. Ferlicot, Department of Pathology, Bicêtre Hospital.

2.5. Innovative Nuclear Medicine Techniques

In recent years, innovative nuclear medicine techniques have emerged as potentially valuable tools in the characterization of renal tumors. These include sestamibi SPECT/CT and PMSA PET/CT.

2.5.1. Tc-99m Sestamibi SPECT/CT

Sestamibi, a radiotracer used primarily in cardiac and parathyroid imaging, has recently received attention for its potential application in the study of renal tumors. Sestamibi SPECT/CT is a diagnostic imaging technique that combines single-photon emission computed tomography (SPECT) with computed tomography (CT) and the injection of Tc-99m sestamibi. Tc-99m sestamibi (sestamibi is short for sesta-methoxyisobutylisonitrile) is a technetium radiopharmaceutical. It is a lipophilic cationic compound that selectively accumulates in mitochondria-rich tissues, including tumors. This property is the basis for its utility in imaging solid tumors, including renal tumors. Upon administration, sestamibi undergoes cellular uptake via active transport mechanisms, resulting in its retention within tumor cells. Because oncocytic cells contain large amounts of mitochondria, oncocytomas avidly take up the Tc-99m sestamibi radiotracer. In contrast, most RCCs, especially the clear cell subtype, contain very few or no mitochondria. In addition, many RCCs express multidrug-resistant pumps that transport the radiotracer out of the cells. These two characteristics of RCCs explain why these tumors have a low radiotracer uptake [49]. In 2016, Gorin et al. [50] reported in a prospective trial that Tc-99m sestamibi could differentiate oncocytomas and hybrid oncocytic/chromophobe tumors from RCCs with a sensitivity of 87.5% (95% confidence interval [CI], 47.4–99.7%) and a specificity of 95.2% (95% CI, 83.8–99.4%). There were two falsely positive tumors in their series, and both were of the eosinophilic variant of chromophobe RCC, a rare RCC subtype. A similar diagnostic performance was reported in the meta-analysis of four articles including 117 lesions published by Wilson et al. [51] in 2020. The pooled and weighted sensitivity and specificity of Tc-99m sestamibi SPECT/CT were reported for detecting (1) renal oncocytoma versus other renal lesions at 92% (95% CI 72–98%) and 88% (95% CI 79–94%), respectively; and (2) renal oncocytoma versus chromophobe RCC at 89% and 67%, respectively. All reported studies used a tumor-to-background renal parenchyma radiotracer uptake ratio of >0.6 for positive studies. A cost-effectiveness study showed that Tc-99m sestamibi SPECT/CT followed by confirmatory biopsy could help to avoid surgery for benign small renal masses and minimize untreated malignant small renal masses, and it was cost-effective compared with existing strategies [52]. However this study had data uncertainties and included a limited number of centers from which Tc-99m sestamibi SPECT/CT performance data were collected. Tc-99m sestamibi SPECT/CT is not included in the current recommendations of the EAU guidelines [53], but it appears to be a promising imaging tool that may aid in identifying benign renal oncocytomas and hybrid oncocytic/chromophobe tumors in patients with small renal tumors.

2.5.2. PSMA PET/CT

Initially used in the management of prostate cancer, PSMA (prostate specific membrane antigen) PET/CT has a potential application in suspected RCC. PSMA is a surface receptor antigen expressed in prostate tissue and tumor-associated neovasculature. It is overexpressed in several solid tumors, including RCC. PSMA PET/CT exploits this overexpression to visualize tumor lesions with high specificity. Radiolabeled PSMA ligands, such as 68Ga-PSMA-11 and 18F-DCFPyL, bind to PSMA receptors on tumor cells, enabling the precise imaging of renal tumors. In 2018, an immunochemistry study of 227 RCC patients with a median follow-up of more than 10.0 years showed that the intensity of positive versus negative prostate-specific membrane antigen protein expression was significantly associated with overall survival [54]. There was also a clear trend toward less positive findings in papillary and chromophobe RCC cases. A large immunochemistry study [55] of n = 197 papillary RCC type 1 and n = 110 type 2 specimens showed that in papillary RCC type 1, PSMA staining was positive in only 4 of 197 (2.0%) specimens, whereas none (0/110) of the papillary RCC type 2 specimens were positive for PSMA. Clinical studies on the diagnosis of the major subtypes of RCC using PSMA PET/CT are scarce, and its diagnostic performance in this setting has not yet been established. Recent clinical studies have investigated the potential role of PSMA-PET/CT in staging RCC and detecting additional metastatic sites compared to CT or MRI [56–58]. They reported a higher sensitivity and PPV of PSMA PET/CT compared to CT, leading to a change in management in 49% of patients in Udovicich's series [59]. In the latter series, PSMA PET/CT detected additional metastases in 25% of patients compared to CT and had a significantly higher SUVmax than FDG PET/CT [59]. In Aggarwal's series [60], PSMA PET/CT performed better than CT in detecting bone metastases and worse in detecting liver lesions. Today, current EUA guidelines do not recommend PET in the management of RCC [53], but PSMA PET/CT opens new possibilities that need to be evaluated in large studies.

2.6. Radiomics

Radiomics is a rapidly evolving field of research that aims to extract quantitative metrics—so-called radiomic features—from medical images. By mathematically extracting the spatial distribution of signal intensities and pixel interrelationships, radiomics quantifies texture information using analysis methods from the field of artificial intelligence. Texture analysis provides an assessment of tumor heterogeneity by analyzing the distribution and association of pixel or voxel gray levels in the image. Radiomic features capture tissue and lesion characteristics such as heterogeneity and shape and can be used alone or in combination with demographic, histologic, genomic, or proteomic data to improve clinical decision making. It is based on the use of machine-learning algorithms that cannot be perceived by the human eye. The process of radiomics requires several steps, including image acquisition, the segmentation of a volume of interest, and the extraction of features or quantitative values, followed by final correlation with disease staging or clinical data. CT tumor texture analysis is a potentially useful emerging biomarker that has shown promise in predicting tumor histological findings, clinical outcomes [61–64], overall survival, and the response to therapy.

The current limitations of radiomics include sensitivity to variations in acquisition parameters (acquisition modes, reconstruction parameters, smoothing and segmentation thresholds) and the limited reproducibility of certain radiomic features. The mannual delineation of tumor volume is not only time-consuming, but may also be affected by inter-observer variability. Further research is needed before radiomics can become part of everyday practice.

2.7. Artificial Intelligence

Artificial intelligence (AI), including machine learning and deep learning, has ushered in a new era in the detection and characterization of renal tumors and in clinical decision making [65,66]. Regarding AI and the diagnosis of kidney cancer, several advances have been made in using artificial intelligence to aid in the detection and diagnosis of this disease, as well as in its treatment management. Here are some points to consider:

- AI can help to detect kidney cancer early by identifying subtle signs or features in medical images that may escape the human eye. This can lead to more effective treatment and improved survival [67].
- AI has been used to differentiate between benign and malignant tumors [61,68–72].
- AI has been used to determine the grade and type of malignancy and nuclear atypia of RCC [73].
- AI can be used to analyze genetic data associated with kidney cancer. By better understanding the genetic profiles of tumors, treatments can be proposed based on the specific characteristics of each patient.
- Predictive models based on AI can be developed using patient data, including clinical information, imaging data, and test results [74]. These models can help predict the risk of kidney cancer and guide treatment decisions.

3. Update of Imaging Algorithms and Guidelines Used for the Diagnosis of RCC

3.1. Bosniak Classification of Cystic Masses, Version 2019

Compared with solid masses, cystic renal masses are more likely to be benign and, if malignant, less aggressive [75,76]. Cystic renal cell carcinoma is likely to be overdiagnosed, as suggested by Schoots et al. [76]. In their meta-analysis of 3036 cystic masses, 373 (12%) were malignant and 3 (0.8%) had metastatic disease at presentation, while 49% of Bosniak III cysts were overtreated because of a benign outcome.

The Bosniak classification stratifies the risk of malignancy in cystic renal masses and divides cystic renal masses into five categories based on imaging characteristics on contrast-enhanced CT [75]. It helps to predict the risk of malignancy and suggests either follow-up or treatment. The Bosniak classification should not be used for lesions of infectious, inflammatory, or vascular etiology or in patients with hereditary cystic kidney disease. Since its introduction in 1986, it has been widely used and several refinements have been proposed. The Bosniak classification, version 2019 [75], aims to reduce interobserver variability and improve the categorization and overall accuracy of the imaging-based evaluation of cystic renal masses. The main challenges are to avoid unnecessary surgery for benign lesions and to identify cancers that require treatment. Unlike the original Bosniak classification, which did not include a precise definition of a cystic mass, the new version defines a cystic mass as one that contains less than approximately 25% enhancing tissue. It formally incorporates MRI into the classification system and includes new modality-specific criteria. It also improves the specificity of the higher-risk categories (category III and IV lesions), precisely defines wall/septa and protrusions (Table 2), and improves the clarity of radiologic reporting. It allows a greater proportion of masses to be classified in lower-risk categories. Yan et al. [77] reported improved interreader agreement, while Park et al. [78] reported increased diagnostic specificity for malignancy with the 2019 version. Soon after its release, the Bosniak classification, version 2019, was adopted worldwide, although its widespread validation is still ongoing.

Table 2. Bosniak classification for CT, version 2019. Adapted from Silvermann SG [75] and Bosniak Classification 2019 [79], https://staging.radiologyassistant.nl (accessed on 2 May 2024).

	Bosniak Classification 2019. CT
Type	Characteristics
I	Well-defined, thin ($\leq$2 mm) smooth wall. Homogeneous fluid (-9 to 20 HU). No septa or calcifications. Wall may enhance.
II	Six types, all homogeneous and well-defined with thin ($\leq$2 mm) smooth walls: - 1. Cystic masses with thin ($\leq$2 mm) and few (1–3) septa. Septa and wall may enhance. May have calcification of any type. - 2. Non-contrast CT: -9 to 20 HU. - 3. Non-contrast CT: $\geq$70 HU. - 4. Contrast CT: non-enhancing masses, 20 HU at renal mass protocol CT, may have calcification of any type. - 5. Contrast CT: masses: 21–30 HU at portal venous phase. - 6. Homogeneous low-attenuation masses that are too small to characterize.
IIF	Cystic masses with: - 1. Smooth minimally thickened (3 mm) enhancing wall. - 2. Smooth minimal thickening (3 mm) of one or more enhancing septa. - 3. Many ($\geq$4) smooth, thin ($\leq$2 mm) enhancing septa.
III	One or more enhancing thick walls or septa ($\geq$4 mm width). Enhancing irregular walls or septa (displaying $\leq$ 3 mm obtusely margined convex protrusions).
IV	One or more enhancing nodules ($\geq$4 mm convex protrusion with obtuse margins, or a convex protrusion of any size with acute margins).

3.2. Clear Cell Likelihood Score (ccLS)

The clear cell likelihood score (ccLS) is derived from multiparametric MRI with the goal of noninvasively identifying clear cell RCC, the most common subtype of renal cell carcinoma with potentially aggressive behavior. The ccLS was initially developed to address one of the limitations of imaging in renal lesion characterization, namely the lack of standardization in reporting. The first version was released in 2017 followed by a revised version in 2022 [80–82]. Automated ccLS calculators are now available online [83].

The ccLS system is a standardized framework generated using multiparametric MRI and a guiding algorithm [80,81]. It is based on a step-by-step interpretation of MR images (Table 3) and applies to small solid renal masses without macroscopic fat, less than 4 cm in diameter, with more than 25% of the lesion showing enhancement. It is based on a Likert score of the likelihood of ccRCC; the scoring options include 1 (very unlikely), 2 (unlikely), 3 (intermediate likelihood), 4 (likely), and 5 (very likely). The interpreting radiologist should follow the sequential steps shown in Table 3. They include three types of criteria: (a) eligibility criteria, to ensure that the use of the ccLS is appropriate (as typical angiomyolipomas and cystic renal masses should not be assigned a ccLS); (b) major features, which are mandatory for every renal mass; and (c) ancillary criteria, which are used in specific cases (i.e., to narrow down the differential diagnosis, if directed to do so by the flowchart). In addition, the ccLS can help stratify which patients may or may not benefit from biopsy.

Table 3. Main steps in determining ccLS (MRI clear cell likehood score).

Eligibility Criteria	
- Exclude macroscopic fat	Yes or no
- Confirm > 25% enhancement	Yes or no
Major features	
- T2-weighted imaging Signal Intensity on SSFSE sequence	Hypointense, isointense, or hyperintense
- T1-weighted corticomedullary phase enhancement	Mild, moderate, or intense
- Assess presence/absence of microscopic fat	Yes or no
Ancillary features	
- Presence of segmental enhancement inversion	Yes or no
- Restriction on DWI images	Yes or no
- Measure arterial-to-delayed enhancement ratio (akin "washout")	<1.5 or ≥1.5

In a recent cohort study of renal masses of any size, Steinberg et al. [84] reported that the PPV for clear cell RCC detection correlated with ccLS (PPV of ccLS1 was 5%, ccLS2 was 6%, ccLS3 was 35%, ccLS4 was 78%, and ccLS5 was 93%). A higher ccLS is also correlated with the faster growth of a small renal mass [85].

Integration of ccLS into clinical practice is feasible with few additional requirements beyond the typical standard multiparametric MRI acquisition protocol. It could help to guide patients to surgery, percutaneous renal biopsy, and active surveillance. ccLS use is increasing for both reporting and interdisciplinary discussion. A preliminary CT counterpart to MRI ccLS has recently been proposed [86] but is currently under evaluation.

3.3. 2017 AUA Renal Mass and Localized Renal Cancer Guidelines, Renal Mass Biopsy

The 2017 AUA guidelines focus on the evaluation and management of clinically localized sporadic renal masses suspicious for renal cell carcinoma (RCC) in adults, including solid enhancing renal tumors and Bosniak 3 and 4 complex cystic renal masses [14,49]. They focus on management considerations and follow-up of patients with RCC after intervention, but they also include general guidelines for the initial evaluation and diagnosis of RCC. They take into account patient age and comorbidities, the biological and imaging characteristics of the tumor, and renal function considerations (presence of chronic kidney disease (CKD), stage based on glomerular filtration rate (GFR), and degree of proteinuria).

An AUA guideline states that physicians should obtain high-quality multi-phase cross-sectional abdominal imaging, without specifying whether they should use CT or MRI. MRI offers the added benefits of no radiation exposure, improved characterization of lesions smaller than 2 cm and cystic lesions, and fewer allergic reactions to contrast media.

Other AUA guidelines state that the description of renal masses should include the size/complexity of the tumor, the presence or absence of macroscopic fat, and the degree of enhancement, with a threshold of 15–20 HU. They remind that "with the exception of fat-containing AML, none of the current imaging modalities can reliably distinguish between benign and malignant tumors or between indolent and aggressive tumor biology".

Regarding renal mass biopsy (RMB), the AUA guidelines state that "patients should be counseled regarding the rationale, positive and negative predictive values, potential risks, and nondiagnostic rates of RMB" and expand the usual indications for RMB. They state that clinicians should consider RMB when a mass is suspected to be hematologic, metastatic, inflammatory, or infectious, and that in the setting of a solid renal mass, "RMB should be obtained on a utility-based approach whenever it may influence management". However, RMB is not necessary in (1) young or healthy patients who are unwilling to accept the uncertainties associated with RMB; or (2) elderly or frail patients who will be managed conservatively regardless of RMB findings. They recommend performing multiple core biopsies, which are preferred over fine needle aspiration (FNA).

4. Conclusions

The diagnosis of RCC is evolving. With improved detection due to the increased use of imaging and advances in imaging technology, localized renal cancer accounts for approximately 67% of detected RCC cases. The radiologist plays a pivotal role in the detection, characterization, staging, and subsequent counseling of patients with renal cancer. The updated Bosniak classification, MRI ccLS, and updated AUA Localized Renal Cancer Panel guidelines are now available and should be considered when interpreting imaging studies and during multidisciplinary meetings. New and advanced technologies have also emerged, offering new perspectives for the future. Photon-counting detector CT, radiomics, and AI are the most promising, but further evaluation is needed to determine their exact role in daily practice and personalized medicine. With the further development and improvement of these techniques, there is no doubt that their applications in the imaging diagnosis of RCC will become increasingly widespread.

Author Contributions: M.-F.B. contributed to the design of this study, managed the literature searches, and wrote the first draft of the manuscript. C.V. managed the literature searches and wrote the first draft of the manuscript. All authors reviewed and edited the manuscript. All authors have read and agreed to the published version of the manuscript.

Funding: This research did not receive any specific grant from funding agencies in the public, commercial, or not-for-profit sectors.

Conflicts of Interest: The authors declare no conflicts of interest.

References

1. *Global Cancer Observatory: Cancer Today*; WHO International Agency for Research on Cancer: Lyon, France, 2022. Available online: https://gco.iarc.fr/today (accessed on 2 May 2024).
2. Ferlay, J.; Colombet, M.; Soerjomataram, I.; Dyba, T.; Randi, G.; Bettio, M.; Gavin, A.; Visser, O.; Bray, F. Cancer incidence and mortality patterns in Europe: Estimates for 40 countries and 25 major cancers in 2018. *Eur. J. Cancer* **2018**, *103*, 356–387. [CrossRef] [PubMed]
3. Huang, J.; Leung, D.K.; Chan, E.O.; Lok, V.; Leung, S.; Wong, I.; Lao, X.Q.; Zheng, Z.J.; Chiu, P.K.; Ng, C.F.; et al. A global trend analysis of kidney cancer incidence and mortality and their associations with smoking, alcohol consumption, and metabolic syndrome. *Eur. Urol. Focus* **2022**, *8*, 200–209. [CrossRef] [PubMed]

4. Laguna, M.P.; Algaba, F.; Cadeddu, J.; Clayman, R.; Gill, I.; Gueglio, G.; Hohenfellner, M.; Joyce, A.; Landman, J.; Lee, B.; et al. Current patterns of presentation and treatment of renal masses: A clinical research office of the endourological society prospective study. *J. Endourol.* **2014**, *28*, 861–870. [CrossRef] [PubMed]
5. Kowalewski, K.F.; Egen, L.; Fischetti, C.E.; Puliatti, S.; Juan, G.R.; Taratkin, M.; Ines, R.B.; Sidoti Abate, M.A.; Mühlbauer, J.; Wessels, F.; et al. Artificial intelligence for renal cancer: From imaging to histology and beyond. *Asian J. Urol.* **2022**, *9*, 243–252. [CrossRef] [PubMed]
6. Herts, B.R.; Silverman, S.G.; Hindman, N.M.; Uzzo, R.G.; Hartman, R.P.; Israel, G.M.; Baumgarten, D.A.; Berland, L.L.; Pandharipande, P.V. Management of the incidental renal mass on CT: A white paper of the ACR incidental findings committee. *J. Am. Coll. Radiol.* **2018**, *15*, 264–273. [CrossRef] [PubMed]
7. Corwin, M.T.; Hansra, S.S.; Loehfelm, T.W.; Lamba, R.; Fananapazir, G. Prevalence of solid tumors in incidentally detected homogeneous renal masses measuring > 20 HU on portal venous phase CT. *AJR Am. J. Roentgenol.* **2018**, *211*, W173–W177. [CrossRef] [PubMed]
8. Lane, B.R.; Babineau, D.; Kattan, M.W.; Novick, A.C.; Gill, I.S.; Zhou, M.; Weight, C.J.; Campbell, S.C. A preoperative prognostic nomogram for solid enhancing renal tumors 7 cm or less amenable to partial nephrectomy. *J. Urol.* **2007**, *178*, 429–434. [CrossRef] [PubMed]
9. Young, J.R.; Margolis, D.; Sauk, S.; Pantuck, A.J.; Sayre, J.; Raman, S.S. Clear cell renal cell carcinoma: Discrimination from other renal cell carcinoma subtypes and oncocytoma at multiphasic multidetector CT. *Radiology* **2013**, *267*, 444–453. [CrossRef] [PubMed]
10. Cheville, J.C.; Lohse, C.M.; Zincke, H.; Weaver, A.L.; Blute, M.L. Comparisons of outcome and prognostic features among histologic subtypes of renal cell carcinoma. *Am. J. Surg. Pathol.* **2003**, *27*, 612–624. [CrossRef]
11. Abou Elkassem, A.M.; Lo, S.S.; Gunn, A.J.; Shuch, B.M.; Dewitt-Foy, M.E.; Abouassaly, R.; Vaidya, S.S.; Clark, J.I.; Louie, A.V.; Siva, S.; et al. Role of imaging in renal cell carcinoma: A multidisciplinary perspective. *Radiographics* **2021**, *41*, 1387–1407. [CrossRef]
12. Cornelis, F.; Tricaud, E.; Lasserre, A.S.; Petitpierre, F.; Bernhard, J.C.; Le Bras, Y.; Yacoub, M.; Bouzgarrou, M.; Ravaud, A.; Grenier, N. Routinely performed multiparametric magnetic resonance imaging helps to differentiate common subtypes of renal tumours. *Eur. Radiol.* **2014**, *24*, 1068–1080. [CrossRef] [PubMed]
13. Lopes Vendrami, C.; Parada Villavicencio, C.; DeJulio, T.J.; Chatterjee, A.; Casalino, D.D.; Horowitz, J.M.; Oberlin, D.T.; Yang, G.Y.; Nikolaidis, P.; Miller, F.H. Differentiation of solid renal tumors with multiparametric MR Imaging. *Radiographics* **2017**, *37*, 2026–2042. [CrossRef] [PubMed]
14. Ward, R.D.; Tanaka, H.; Campbell, S.C.; Remer, E.M. 2017 AUA Renal mass and localized renal cancer guidelines: Imaging implications. *Radiographics* **2018**, *38*, 2021–2033. [CrossRef] [PubMed]
15. Campbell, S.; Uzzo, R.G.; Allaf, M.E.; Bass, E.B.; Cadeddu, J.A.; Chang, A.; Clark, P.E.; Davis, B.J.; Derweesh, I.H.; Giambarresi, L.; et al. Renal mass and localized renal cancer: AUA guideline. *J. Urol.* **2017**, *198*, 520–529. [CrossRef] [PubMed]
16. Schawkat, K.; Krajewski, K.M. Insights into renal cell carcinoma with novel imaging approaches. *Hematol. Oncol. Clin. N. Am.* **2023**, *37*, 863–875. [CrossRef] [PubMed]
17. Mileto, A.; Nelson, R.C.; Samei, E.; Jaffe, T.A.; Paulson, E.K.; Barina, A.; Choudhury, K.R.; Wilson, J.M.; Marin, D. Impact of dual-energy multi-detector row CT with virtual monochromatic imaging on renal cyst pseudoenhancement: In vitro and in vivo study. *Radiology* **2014**, *272*, 767–776. [CrossRef] [PubMed]
18. Dai, C.; Cao, Y.; Jia, Y.; Ding, Y.; Sheng, R.; Zeng, M.; Zhou, J. Differentiation of renal cell carcinoma subtypes with different iodine quantification methods using single-phase contrast-enhanced dual-energy CT: Areal vs. volumetric analyses. *Abdom. Radiol. (NY)* **2018**, *43*, 672–678. [CrossRef] [PubMed]
19. Decker, J.A.; Bette, S.; Lubina, N.; Rippel, K.; Braun, F.; Risch, F.; Woźnicki, P.; Wollny, C.; Scheurig-Muenkler, C.; Kroencke, T.J.; et al. Low-dose CT of the abdomen: Initial experience on a novel photon-counting detector CT and comparison with energy-integrating detector CT. *Eur. J. Radiol.* **2022**, *148*, 110181. [CrossRef] [PubMed]
20. Cornelis, F.; Grenier, N. Multiparametric magnetic resonance imaging of solid renal tumors: A practical algorithm. *Semin Ultrasound CT MR* **2017**, *38*, 47–58. [CrossRef]
21. Suarez-Ibarrola, R.; Hein, S.; Reis, G.; Gratzke, C.; Miernik, A. Current and future applications of machine and deep learning in urology: A review of the literature on urolithiasis, renal cell carcinoma, and bladder and prostate cancer. *World J. Urol.* **2020**, *38*, 2329–2347. [CrossRef]
22. Bellini, D.; Panvini, N.; Laghi, A.; Marin, D.; Patel, B.V.; Wang, C.L.; Carbone, I.; Mileto, A. Systematic review and meta-analysis investigating the diagnostic yield of dual-energy CT for renal mass assessment. *AJR Am. J. Roentgenol.* **2019**, *212*, 1044–1053. [CrossRef] [PubMed]
23. Salameh, J.P.; McInnes, M.D.F.; McGrath, T.A.; Salameh, G.; Schieda, N. Diagnostic accuracy of dual-energy ct for evaluation of renal masses: Systematic review and meta-analysis. *AJR Am. J. Roentgenol.* **2019**, *212*, W100–W105. [CrossRef] [PubMed]
24. Pourvaziri, A.; Mojtahed, A.; Hahn, P.F.; Gee, M.S.; Kambadakone, A.; Sahani, D.V. Renal lesion characterization: Clinical utility of single-phase dual-energy CT compared to MRI and dual-phase single-energy CT. *Eur. Radiol.* **2023**, *33*, 1318–1328. [CrossRef] [PubMed]
25. Xiao, J.M.; Hippe, D.S.; Zecevic, M.; Zamora, D.A.; Cai, L.M.; Toia, G.V.; Chandler, A.G.; Dighe, M.K.; O'Malley, R.B.; Shuman, W.P.; et al. Virtual unenhanced dual-energy CT images obtained with a multimaterial decomposition algorithm: Diagnostic value for renal mass and urinary stone evaluation. *Radiology* **2021**, *298*, 611–619. [CrossRef] [PubMed]

26. Bucolo, G.M.; Ascenti, V.; Barbera, S.; Fontana, F.; Aricò, F.M.; Piacentino, F.; Coppola, A.; Cicero, G.; Marino, M.A.; Booz, C.; et al. Virtual non-contrast spectral CT in renal masses: Is it time to discard conventional unenhanced phase? *Clin. Med.* **2023**, *12*, 4718. [CrossRef]
27. Graser, A.; Becker, C.R.; Staehler, M.; Clevert, D.A.; Macari, M.; Arndt, N.; Nikolaou, K.; Sommer, W.; Stief, C.; Reiser, M.F.; et al. Single-phase dual-energy CT allows for characterization of renal masses as benign or malignant. *Investig. Radiol.* **2010**, *45*, 399–405. [CrossRef] [PubMed]
28. Graser, A.; Johnson, T.R.; Hecht, E.M.; Becker, C.R.; Leidecker, C.; Staehler, M.; Stief, C.G.; Hildebrandt, H.; Godoy, M.C.; Finn, M.E.; et al. Dual-energy CT in patients suspected of having renal masses: Can virtual nonenhanced images replace true nonenhanced images? *Radiology* **2009**, *252*, 433–440. [CrossRef] [PubMed]
29. Lennartz, S.; Pisuchpen, N.; Parakh, A.; Cao, J.; Baliyan, V.; Sahani, D.; Hahn, P.F.; Kambadakone, A. Virtual unenhanced images: Qualitative and quantitative comparison between different dual-energy CT scanners in a patient and phantom study. *Investig. Radiol.* **2022**, *57*, 52–61. [CrossRef]
30. Chandarana, H.; Megibow, A.J.; Cohen, B.A.; Srinivasan, R.; Kim, D.; Leidecker, C.; Macari, M. Iodine quantification with dual-energy CT: Phantom study and preliminary experience with renal masses. *AJR Am. J. Roentgenol.* **2011**, *196*, W693–W700. [CrossRef]
31. Shen, L.; Yoon, L.; Mullane, P.C.; Liang, T.; Tse, J.R. World Health Organization (WHO) 2022 classification update: Radiologic and pathologic features of papillary renal cell carcinomas. *Acad. Radiol.* **2024**, S1076-6332(24)00056-4. [CrossRef]
32. Ascenti, G.; Krauss, B.; Mazziotti, S.; Mileto, A.; Settineri, N.; Vinci, S.; Donato, R.; Gaeta, M. Dual-energy computed tomography (DECT) in renal masses: Nonlinear versus linear blending. *Acad. Radiol.* **2012**, *19*, 1186–1193. [CrossRef]
33. Mileto, A.; Sofue, K.; Marin, D. Imaging the renal lesion with dual-energy multidetector CT and multi-energy applications in clinical practice: What can it truly do for you? *Eur. Radiol.* **2016**, *26*, 3677–3690. [CrossRef]
34. Brufau, B.P.; Cerqueda, C.S.; Villalba, L.B.; Izquierdo, R.S.; González, B.M.; Molina, C.N. Metastatic renal cell carcinoma: Radiologic findings and assessment of response to targeted antiangiogenic therapy by using multidetector CT. *Radiographics* **2013**, *33*, 1691–13716. [CrossRef]
35. Schade, K.A.; Mergen, V.; Sartoretti, T.; Alkadhi, H.; Euler, A. Pseudoenhancement in cystic renal lesions–impact of virtual monoenergetic images of photon-counting detector CT on lesion classification. *Acad. Radiol.* **2023**, *30* (Suppl. S1), S305–S313. [CrossRef] [PubMed]
36. Ramamurthy, N.K.; Moosavi, B.; McInnes, M.D.; Flood, T.A.; Schieda, N. Multiparametric MRI of solid renal masses: Pearls and pitfalls. *Clin. Radiol.* **2015**, *70*, 304–316. [CrossRef] [PubMed]
37. Douek, P.C.; Bocalini, S.; Oei, E.H.G.; Cormode, D.P.; Pourmorteza, A.; Boussel, L.; Si-Mohamed, S.A.; Budde, R.P.J. Clinical applications of photon-counting CT: A review of pioneer studies and a glimpse into the future. *Radiology* **2023**, *309*, e:222432. [CrossRef] [PubMed]
38. Rosenkrantz, A.B.; Niver, B.E.; Fitzgerald, E.F.; Babb, J.S.; Chandarana, H.; Melamed, J. Utility of the apparent diffusion coefficient for distinguishing clear cell renal cell carcinoma of low and high nuclear grade. *AJR Am. J. Roentgenol.* **2010**, *195*, W344–W351. [CrossRef]
39. Rosenkrantz, A.B.; Hindman, N.; Fitzgerald, E.F.; Niver, B.E.; Melamed, J.; Babb, J.S. MRI features of renal oncocytoma and chromophobe renal cell carcinoma. *AJR Am. J. Roentgenol.* **2010**, *195*, W421–W427. [CrossRef]
40. Hélénon, O.; Correas, J.M.; Balleyguier, C.; Ghouadni, M.; Cornud, F. Ultrasound of renal tumors. *Eur. Radiol.* **2001**, *11*, 1890–1901. [CrossRef]
41. King, K.G. Use of contrast ultrasound for renal mass evaluation. *Radiol. Clin. N. Am.* **2020**, *58*, 935–949. [CrossRef]
42. Liu, Y.; Kan, Y.; Zhang, J.; Li, N.; Wang, Y. Characteristics of contrast-enhanced ultrasound for diagnosis of solid clear cell renal cell carcinomas 4 cm: A meta-analysis. *Cancer Med.* **2021**, *10*, 8288–8299. [CrossRef] [PubMed]
43. Barr, R.G.; Wilson, S.R.; Lyshchik, A.; McCarville, B.; Darge, K.; Grant, E.; Robbin, M.; Wilmann, J.K.; Chong, W.K.; Fleischer, A.; et al. Contrast-enhanced Ultrasound-State of the Art in North America: Society of Radiologists in Ultrasound White Paper. *Ultrasound Q.* **2020**, *36* (4S Suppl. S1), S1–S39. [CrossRef] [PubMed]
44. Barr, R.G. Use of lumason/sonovue in contrast-enhanced ultrasound of the kidney for characterization of renal masses-a meta-analysis. *Abdom. Radiol. (NY)* **2022**, *47*, 272–287. [CrossRef] [PubMed]
45. Elbanna, K.Y.; Jang, H.J.; Kim, T.K.; Khalili, K.; Guimarães, L.S.; Atri, M. The added value of contrast-enhanced ultrasound in evaluation of indeterminate small solid renal masses and risk stratification of cystic renal lesions. *Eur. Radiol.* **2021**, *31*, 8468–8477. [CrossRef] [PubMed]
46. Park, B.K.; Kim, B.; Kim, S.H.; Ko, K.; Lee, H.M.; Choi, H.Y. Assessment of cystic renal masses based on Bosniak classification: Comparison of CT and contrast-enhanced US. *Eur. J. Radiol.* **2007**, *61*, 310–314. [CrossRef] [PubMed]
47. Tufano, A.; Antonelli, L.; Di Pierro, G.B.; Flammia, R.S.; Minelli, R.; Anceschi, U.; Leonardo, C.; Franco, G.; Drudi, F.M.; Cantisani, V. Diagnostic performance of contrast-enhanced ultrasound in the evaluation of small Rrenal masses: A systematic review and meta-analysis. *Diagnostics* **2022**, *12*, 2310. [CrossRef] [PubMed]
48. Expert Panel on Urologic Imaging; Wang, Z.J.; Nikolaidis, P.; Khatri, G.; Dogra, V.S.; Ganeshan, D.; Goldfarb, S.; Gore, J.L.; Gupta, R.T.; Hartman, R.P.; et al. ACR Appropriateness Criteria(R) Indeterminate Renal Mass. *J. Am. Coll. Radiol.* **2020**, *17* (11S), S415–S428. [CrossRef] [PubMed]

49. Campbell, S.P.; Tzortzakakis, A.; Javadi, M.S.; Karlsson, M.; Solnes, L.B.; Axelsson, R.; Allaf, M.E.; Gorin, M.A.; Rowe, S.P. ^{99m}Tc-sestamibi SPECT/CT for the characterization of renal masses: A pictorial guide. *Br. J. Radiol.* **2018**, *91*, 20170526. [CrossRef] [PubMed]
50. Gorin, M.A.; Rowe, S.P.; Baras, A.S.; Solnes, L.B.; Ball, M.W.; Pierorazio, P.M.; Pavlovich, C.P.; Epstein, J.I.; Javadi, M.S.; Allaf, M.E. Prospective evaluation of (99m)Tc-sestamibi SPECT/CT for the diagnosis of renal oncocytomas and hybrid oncocytic/chromophobe tumors. *Eur. Urol.* **2016**, *69*, 413–416. [CrossRef]
51. Wilson, M.P.; Katlariwala, P.; Murad, M.H.; Abele, J.; McInnes, M.D.F.; Low, G. Diagnostic accuracy of 99mTc-sestamibi SPECT/CT for detecting renal oncocytomas and other benign renal lesions: A systematic review and meta-analysis. *Abdom. Radiol. (NY)* **2020**, *45*, 2532–2541. [CrossRef]
52. Su, Z.T.; Patel, H.D.; Huang, M.M.; Meyer, A.R.; Pavlovich, C.P.; Pierorazio, P.M.; Javadi, M.S.; Allaf, M.E.; Rowe, S.P.; Gorin, M.A. Cost-effectiveness analysis of ^{99m}Tc-sestamibi SPECT/CT to guide management of small renal masses. *Eur. Urol. Focus* **2021**, *7*, 827–834. [CrossRef] [PubMed]
53. Ljungberg, B.; Albiges, L.; Abu-Ghanem, Y.; Bedke, J.; Capitanio, U.; Dabestani, S.; Fernández-Pello, S.; Giles, R.H.; Hofmann, F.; Hora, M.; et al. European Association of Urology guidelines on renal cell carcinoma: The 2022 update. *Eur. Urol.* **2022**, *82*, 399–410. [CrossRef] [PubMed]
54. Spatz, S.; Tolkach, Y.; Jung, K.; Stephan, C.; Busch, J.; Ralla, B.; Rabien, A.; Feldmann, G.; Brossart, P.; Bundschuh, R.A.; et al. Comprehensive evaluation of Prostate Specific Membrane Antigen expression in the vasculature of renal tumors: Implications for imaging studies and prognostic role. *J. Urol.* **2018**, *199*, 370–377. [CrossRef] [PubMed]
55. Zschäbitz, S.; Erlmeier, F.; Stöhr, M.; Herrmann, E.; Polifka, I.; Agaimy, A.; Trojan, L.; Ströbel, P.; Becker, F.; Wülfing, C.; et al. Expression of Prostate-specific Membrane Antigen (PSMA) in papillary renal cell carcinoma–Overview and Report on a Large Multicenter Cohort. *J. Cancer* **2022**, *13*, 706–1712. [CrossRef]
56. Rhee, H.; Blazak, J.; Tham, C.M.; Ng, K.L.; Shepherd, B.; Lawson, M.; Preston, J.; Vela, I.; Thomas, P.; Wood, S. Pilot study: Use of gallium-68 PSMA PET for detection of metastatic lesions in patients with renal tumour. *EJNMMI Res.* **2016**, *6*, 76. [CrossRef]
57. Rhee, H.; Ng, K.L.; Tse, B.W.; Yeh, M.C.; Russell, P.J.; Nelson, C.; Thomas, P.; Samaratunga, H.; Vela, I.; Gobe, G.; et al. Using prostate specific membrane antigen (PSMA) expression in clear cell renal cell carcinoma for imaging advanced disease. *Pathology* **2016**, *48*, 613–616. [CrossRef]
58. Meyer, A.R.; Carducci, M.A.; Denmeade, S.R.; Markowski, M.C.; Pomper, M.G.; Pierorazio, P.M.; Allaf, M.E.; Rowe, S.P.; Gorin, M.A. Improved identification of patients with oligometastatic clear cell renal cell carcinoma with PSMA-targeted (18)F-DCFPyL PET/CT. *Ann. Nucl. Med.* **2019**, *33*, 617–623. [CrossRef] [PubMed]
59. Udovicich, C.; Callahan, J.; Bressel, M.; Ong, W.L.; Perera, M.; Tran, B.; Azad, A.; Haran, S.; Moon, D.; Chander, S.; et al. Impact of Prostate-specific Membrane Antigen Positron Emission Tomography/Computed Tomography in the management of oligometastatic renal cell carcinoma. *Eur. Urol. Open Sci.* **2022**, *44*, 60–68. [CrossRef]
60. Aggarwal, P.; Singh, H.; Das, C.K.; Mavuduru, R.S.; Kakkar, N.; Lal, A.; Gorsi, U.; Kumar, R.; Mittal, B.R. Potential role of 68Ga-PSMA PET/CT in metastatic renal cell cancer: A prospective study. *Eur. J. Radiol.* **2024**, *17*, 111218. [CrossRef]
61. Uhlig, J.; Biggemann, L.; Nietert, M.M.; Beißbarth, T.; Lotz, J.; Kim, H.S.; Trojan, L.; Uhlig, A. Discriminating malignant and benign clinical T1 renal masses on computed tomography: A pragmatic radiomics and machine learning approach. *Medicine* **2020**, *99*, e19725. [CrossRef]
62. Uhlig, J.; Leha, A.; Delonge, L.M.; Haack, A.M.; Shuch, B.; Kim, H.S.; Bremmer, F.; Trojan, L.; Lotz, J.; Uhlig, A. Radiomic features and Machine Learning for the discrimination of renal tumor histological subtypes: A pragmatic study using clinical-routine Computed Tomography. *Cancers* **2020**, *12*, 3010. [CrossRef] [PubMed]
63. Lubner, M.G.; Stabo, N.; Abel, E.J.; Del Rio, A.M.; Pickhardt, P.J. CT textural analysis of large primary renal cell carcinomas: Pretreatment tumor heterogeneity correlates with histologic findings and clinical outcomes. *AJR Am. J. Roentgenol.* **2016**, *207*, 96–105. [CrossRef] [PubMed]
64. Ursprung, S.; Beer, L.; Bruining, A.; Woitek, R.; Stewart, G.D.; Gallagher, F.A.; Sala, E. Radiomics of computed tomography and magnetic resonance imaging in renal cell carcinoma-a systematic review and meta-analysis. *Eur. Radiol.* **2020**, *30*, 3558–3566. [CrossRef] [PubMed]
65. Zhou, T.; Guan, J.; Feng, B.; Xue, H.; Cui, J.; Kuang, Q.; Chen, Y.; Xu, K.; Lin, F.; Cui, E.; et al. Distinguishing common renal cell carcinomas from benign renal tumors based on machine learning: Comparing various CT imaging phases, slices, tumor sizes, and ROI segmentation strategies. *Eur. Radiol.* **2023**, *33*, 4323–4332. [CrossRef] [PubMed]
66. Raman, A.G.; Fisher, D.; Yap, F.; Oberai, A.; Duddalwar, V.A. Radiomics and artificial intelligence: Renal cell carcinoma. *Urol. Clin. N. Am.* **2024**, *51*, 35–45. [CrossRef] [PubMed]
67. Sassa, N.; Kameya, Y.; Takahashi, T.; Matsukawa, Y.; Majima, T.; Tsuruta, K.; Kobayashi, I.; Kajikawa, K.; Kawanishi, H.; Kurosu, H.; et al. Creation of synthetic contrast-enhanced computed tomography images using deep neural networks to screen for renal cell carcinoma. *Nagoya J. Med. Sci.* **2023**, *85*, 713–724. [PubMed]
68. Oberai, A.; Varghese, B.; Cen, S.; Angelini, T.; Hwang, D.; Gill, I.; Aron, M.; Lau, C.; Duddalwar, V. Deep learning based classification of solid lipid-poor contrast enhancing renal masses using contrast enhanced CT. *Br. J. Radiol.* **2020**, *93*, 20200002. [CrossRef] [PubMed]

69. Baghdadi, A.; Aldhaam, N.A.; Elsayed, A.S.; Hussein, A.A.; Cavuoto, L.A.; Kauffman, E.; Guru, K.A. Automated differentiation of benign renal oncocytoma and chromophobe renal cell carcinoma on computed tomography using deep learning. *BJU Int.* **2020**, *125*, 553–560. [CrossRef]
70. Kocak, B.; Kaya, O.K.; Erdim, C.; Kus, E.A.; Kilickesmez, O. Artificial intelligence in renal mass characterization: A systematic review of methodologic items related to modeling, performance evaluation, clinical utility, and transparency. *AJR Am. J. Roentgenol.* **2020**, *215*, 1113–1122. [CrossRef]
71. Han, S.; Hwang, S.I.; Lee, H.J. The classification of renal cancer in 3-phase CT images using a deep learning method. *J. Digit Imaging* **2019**, *32*, 638–643. [CrossRef]
72. Uhlig, J.; Uhlig, A.; Bachanek, S.; Onur, M.R.; Kinner, S.; Geisel, D.; Köhler, M.; Preibsch, H.; Puesken, M.; Schramm, D.; et al. Primary renal sarcomas: Imaging features and discrimination from non-sarcoma renal tumors. *Eur. Radiol.* **2022**, *32*, 981–989. [CrossRef] [PubMed]
73. Sim, K.C.; Han, N.Y.; Cho, Y.; Sung, D.J.; Park, B.J.; Kim, M.J.; Han, Y.E. Machine learning-based magnetic resonance radiomics analysis for predicting low- and high-grade clear cell renal cell carcinoma. *J. Comput. Assist. Tomogr.* **2023**, *47*, 873–881. [CrossRef] [PubMed]
74. Nie, P.; Liu, S.; Zhou, R.; Li, X.; Zhi, K.; Wang, Y.; Dai, Z.; Zhao, L.; Wang, N.; Zhao, X.; et al. A preoperative CT-based deep learning radiomics model in predicting the stage, size, grade and necrosis score and outcome in localized clear cell renal cell carcinoma: A multicenter study. *Eur. J. Radiol.* **2023**, *166*, 111018. [CrossRef] [PubMed]
75. Silverman, S.G.; Pedrosa, I.; Ellis, J.H.; Hindman, N.M.; Schieda, N.; Smith, A.D.; Remer, E.M.; Shinagare, A.B.; Curci, N.E.; Raman, S.S.; et al. Bosniak classification of cystic renal masses, version 2019: An update proposal and needs assessment. *Radiology* **2019**, *292*, 475–488. [CrossRef]
76. Schoots, I.G.; Zaccai, K.; Hunink, M.G.; Verhagen, P.C.M.S. Bosniak classification for complex renal cysts reevaluated: A systematic review. *J. Urol.* **2017**, *198*, 12–21. [CrossRef]
77. Yan, J.H.; Chan, J.; Osman, H.; Munir, J.; Alrasheed, S.; Flood, T.A.; Schieda, N. Bosniak Classification version 2019: Validation and comparison to original classification in pathologically confirmed cystic masses. *Eur. Radiol.* **2021**, *31*, 9579–9587. [CrossRef]
78. Park, M.Y.; Park, K.J.; Kim, M.H.; Kim, J.K. Bosniak classification of cystic renal masses version 2019: Comparison with version 2005 for class distribution, diagnostic performance, and interreader agreement using CT and MRI. *AJR Am. J. Roentgenol.* **2021**, *217*, 1367–1376. [CrossRef] [PubMed]
79. Bosniak Classification 2019. Available online: https://staging.radiologyassistant.nl (accessed on 2 May 2024).
80. Shetty, A.S.; Fraum, T.J.; Ballard, D.H.; Hoegger, M.J.; Itani, M.; Rajput, M.Z.; Lanier, M.H.; Cusworth, B.M.; Mehrsheikh, A.L.; Cabrera-Lebron, J.A.; et al. Renal mass imaging with MRI clear cell likelihood score: A user's guide. *Radiographics* **2023**, *43*, e220209. [CrossRef]
81. Canvasser, N.E.; Kay, F.U.; Xi, Y.; Pinho, D.F.; Costa, D.; de Leon, A.D.; Khatri, G.; Leyendecker, J.R.; Yokoo, T.; Lay, A.; et al. Diagnostic accuracy of multiparametric magnetic resonance imaging to identify clear cell renal cell carcinoma in cT1a renal masses. *J. Urol.* **2017**, *198*, 780–786. [CrossRef]
82. Pedrosa, I.; Cadeddu, J.A. How We Do It: Managing the indeterminate renal mass with the MRI clear cell likelihood score. *Radiology* **2022**, *302*, 256–269. [CrossRef]
83. ccLS Calculator. Available online: https://cclsrads.com/ (accessed on 3 May 2024).
84. Steinberg, R.L.; Rasmussen, R.G.; Johnson, B.A.; Ghandour, R.; De Leon, A.D.; Xi, Y.; Yokoo, T.; Kim, S.; Kapur, P.; Cadeddu, J.A.; et al. Prospective performance of clear cell likelihood scores (ccLS) in renal masses evaluated with multiparametric magnetic resonance imaging. *Eur. Radiol.* **2021**, *31*, 314–324. [CrossRef] [PubMed]
85. Rasmussen, R.G.; Xi, Y.; Sibley, R.C., 3rd; Lee, C.J.; Cadeddu, J.A.; Pedrosa, I. Association of clear cell likelihood score on MRI and growth kinetics of small solid renal masses on active surveillance. *AJR Am. J. Roentgenol.* **2022**, *218*, 101–110. [CrossRef] [PubMed]
86. Al Nasibi, K.; Pickovsky, J.S.; Eldehimi, F.; Flood, T.A.; Lavallee, L.T.; Tsampalieros, A.K.; Schieda, N. Development of a multiparametric renal CT algorithm for diagnosis of clear cell renal cell carcinoma among small ($\leq$4 cm) solid renal masses. *AJR Am. J. Roentgenol.* **2022**, *219*, 814–823. [CrossRef] [PubMed]

Disclaimer/Publisher's Note: The statements, opinions and data contained in all publications are solely those of the individual author(s) and contributor(s) and not of MDPI and/or the editor(s). MDPI and/or the editor(s) disclaim responsibility for any injury to people or property resulting from any ideas, methods, instructions or products referred to in the content.

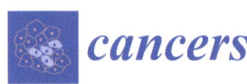

Article

Multiparametric Ultrasound for Focal Testicular Pathology: A Ten-Year Retrospective Review

Dean Y. Huang [1,2,*], Majed Alsadiq [3], Gibran T. Yusuf [1,2], Annamaria Deganello [1,2], Maria E. Sellars [1] and Paul S. Sidhu [1,2]

1. Department of Clinical Radiology, King's College Hospital, London SE5 9RS, UK
2. Department of Imaging Sciences, School of Biomedical Engineering and Imaging Sciences, Faculty of Life Sciences and Medicine, King's College London, London SE1 7EH, UK
3. Department of Imaging, The Royal London Hospital, London E1 1FR, UK
* Correspondence: dean.huang@nhs.net; Tel.: +44-(0)203-299-(4599/4164)

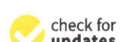

Simple Summary: In our retrospective study at a tertiary centre, we reviewed the use of contrast-enhanced ultrasound (CEUS) and strain elastography (SE) as adjuncts to conventional greyscale and colour Doppler US (CDUS) for evaluating focal testicular abnormalities over a decade. This study highlights the potential of advanced ultrasound techniques to provide deeper insights into the characteristics of testicular abnormalities. In particular, we observed that contrast-enhanced ultrasound could detect vascular enhancement in all malignant cases, even those not identified by conventional CDUS, and more conclusively confirm benignity. While SE alone offered no distinctive advantage, incorporating a combination of CEUS and SE into the evaluation of focal testicular abnormalities improved diagnostic performance metrics over conventional CDUS. Our research underscores the enhanced performance achieved by utilising these advanced ultrasound techniques. The comprehensive diagnostic assessment provided by these techniques could facilitate a shift towards more conservative management of testicular lesions, supporting the preference for organ-preserving methods over more radical surgeries.

Citation: Huang, D.Y.; Alsadiq, M.; Yusuf, G.T.; Deganello, A.; Sellars, M.E.; Sidhu, P.S. Multiparametric Ultrasound for Focal Testicular Pathology: A Ten-Year Retrospective Review. *Cancers* **2024**, *16*, 2309. https://doi.org/10.3390/cancers16132309

Academic Editors: Fumitaka Koga and Michael J. Spinella

Received: 21 March 2024
Revised: 21 June 2024
Accepted: 22 June 2024
Published: 24 June 2024

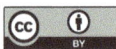

Copyright: © 2024 by the authors. Licensee MDPI, Basel, Switzerland. This article is an open access article distributed under the terms and conditions of the Creative Commons Attribution (CC BY) license (https://creativecommons.org/licenses/by/4.0/).

Abstract: Conventional ultrasonography (US), including greyscale imaging and colour Doppler US (CDUS), is pivotal for diagnosing scrotal pathologies, but it has limited specificity. Historically, solid focal testicular abnormalities often led to radical orchidectomy. This retrospective study evaluated the utilisation of contrast-enhanced ultrasound (CEUS) and strain elastography (SE) in investigating intratesticular focal abnormalities. A total of 124 cases were analysed. This study underscored the superior diagnostic capabilities of CEUS in detecting vascular enhancement in all malignant cases, even those with undetectable vascularity by CDUS. It also highlighted the potential of CEUS in identifying distinctive vascular patterns in benign vascular tumours. Definitive confirmation of benignity could be obtained when the absence of enhancement was demonstrated on CEUS. While SE alone offered no distinctive advantage in differentiating between benign and malignant pathologies, we demonstrated that incorporating a combination of CEUS and SE into the evaluation of focal testicular abnormalities could improve diagnostic performance metrics over conventional CDUS. Our findings underscore the role of advanced ultrasound techniques in enhancing the evaluation of focal testicular abnormalities in clinical practice and could aid a shift towards testis-sparing management strategies.

Keywords: multiparametric; ultrasound; testicular cancer; testis-sparing surgery; orchiectomy

1. Introduction

Conventional ultrasonography (US), including greyscale imaging and colour Doppler US (CDUS), stands as the cornerstone for evaluating scrotal pathologies due to its high resolution, availability, cost-effectiveness, and absence of ionizing radiation [1–4]. Despite its widespread use, the specificity of greyscale ultrasound in characterising scrotal masses remains limited, often leaving the nature of such lesions ambiguous [5–7]. Traditionally, solid testicular lesions, especially those presenting as palpable lumps, have led to radical orchidectomy [8,9]. However, the landscape of scrotal ultrasonography has evolved significantly with advancements in technology and technique, including high frequency, tissue harmonic, and compound imaging. This evolution, alongside a broader spectrum of clinical applications, has increased the detection of small, incidental focal testicular lesions, many of which are benign. Indeed, recent literature suggests a predominance of benignity in these cases, with Leydig cell tumours with low malignant potential (LCT-LMP) constituting a significant fraction among small, impalpable, incidentally discovered testicular nodules [10,11].

This shift in the diagnostic landscape necessitates a reconsideration of radical orchiectomy for focal testicular abnormalities, pivoting towards more organ-sparing approaches when there is a high likelihood of benignity [12]. Yet, despite improved imaging modalities and diagnostic aids, including tumour markers and second-line MRI as recommended by the European Society of Urogenital Radiology (ESUR) [13], significant diagnostic ambiguity persists. This uncertainty complicates the selection of benign lesions for testis-sparing management, underlining a gap in the current diagnostic toolkit.

Contrast-enhanced ultrasound (CEUS) and ultrasound strain elastography (SE) have emerged as valuable adjuncts to traditional ultrasonography, offering insights into vascularisation and tissue elasticity not available through conventional US alone [14,15]. These modalities have shown promise in distinguishing malignant from benign lesions [16,17], guiding management decisions towards more conservative, organ-preserving strategies [18–21]. Since their adoption in 2008, CEUS and SE have become integral to the multidisciplinary evaluation of testicular abnormalities in our institution [22–34], marking a significant advance in our approach to scrotal pathology.

The main aim of our retrospective review was to share our decade-long clinical experience with utilising a combination of advanced ultrasound techniques, an approach termed multiparametric ultrasound (MPUS) [18,35], including CEUS and SE, in assessing focal testicular abnormalities. We seek to elucidate how CEUS and SE features correlate with clinical outcomes across a broad spectrum of clinical presentations.

2. Materials and Methods

2.1. Study Design and Ethical Considerations

This retrospective study assessed the diagnostic accuracy of MPUS in characterising intratesticular focal abnormalities over a ten-year period (2009–2019) at King's College Hospital, London, United Kingdom. Between 2009 and 2019, 12,981 testicular ultrasound examinations were performed in our department for the following indications: evaluation and location of palpable scrotal masses, detection of primary tumours, follow-up of patients with testicular microlithiasis, follow-up of patients with previous lymphoma, acute scrotum, scrotal trauma, localisation of the undescended testis, detection of varicoceles in infertile men, and evaluation of testicular ischaemia. From an initial dataset of all scrotal ultrasound examinations, 124 consecutive cases of focal testicular abnormalities investigated by MPUS were selected for analysis. Institutional Review Board approval was obtained, with all procedures performed in accordance with ethical standards and patient confidentiality guidelines.

2.2. Patient Cohort and Data Acquisition

Eligible cases were identified from the departmental ultrasound database based on the inclusion criteria of having undergone MPUS, comprising greyscale US, CDUS, CEUS, and SE. Comprehensive clinical data, including the patients' ages, clinical presentations, tumour markers, histopathological reports, and follow-up outcomes, were extracted from electronic patient records. Imaging data were retrieved from the institution's Picture Archiving and Communication System.

2.3. Ultrasound Examination Techniques

The ultrasound examinations were conducted by a team of three radiologists, each with extensive expertise in scrotal ultrasonography and a significant range of experience in MPUS (5–15 years). Prior to the sonographic evaluation, informed verbal consent was obtained from all participants as part of routine clinical practice in our hospital. All scrotal ultrasound studies were conducted utilizing either an Acuson Sequoia (Siemens Mountain View, CA, USA) with a 15L8w transducer or an S2000 system (Siemens Medical Solutions, Mountain View, CA, USA) equipped with either a 14L5 or a 9L4 linear array transducer. Strain elastography examinations were carried out on an HV900 system (Hi-RTE™, Hitachi Medical Corporation, Tokyo, Japan) employing a 14–6 MHz linear transducer and Hitachi real-time tissue elastography.

Scrotal ultrasound was performed with the patient in the supine position, holding the penis lifted onto the abdomen and covered. Standardised greyscale US pre-sets were used with abnormalities imaged in both axial and longitudinal planes in accordance with established protocol [2]. The operators varied the pulse repetition frequency, focal zone, gain, and wall filter as necessary to obtain optimal sonograms in each case. Colour Doppler ultrasound was performed with the highest signal gain setting possible without the appearance of background noise and low pulse-repetition frequencies (0.2–0.4) to maximise sensitivity to slow flow velocities. CEUS and SE assessments were undertaken following the identification of a focal intratesticular abnormality via initial greyscale and CDUS evaluations as part of our clinical practice. CEUS examinations employed bolus injection of ultrasound contrast agents for contrast administration. Harmonic imaging with a low-mechanical index technique (Cadence contrast pulse sequencing (CPS™); Siemens Medical Solutions, Mountain View, CA, USA) was utilised, setting the mechanical index at or below 0.10, typically implemented at 10–20 frames per second during the enhancement phase. A bolus injection of 4.8 mL of SonoVue™ (Bracco SpA, Milan, Italy), a sulphur hexafluoride microbubble contrast agent, was administered, followed by a 10 mL normal saline flush via a 20-gauge cannula inserted in the antecubital vein. During CEUS examinations, one examiner maintained the transducer over the area of interest while a second radiologist administered the ultrasound contrast agent. Continuous observation was performed from the time of arrival of the microbubbles for at least 90 s after injection of ultrasound contrast agent in the majority of cases. All utilised ultrasound systems featured dual-screen display capabilities, enabling the simultaneous presentation of the underlying modified greyscale image alongside the CEUS image, allowing the operator to retain the interrogated abnormality within the field of view throughout the entire examination. Ultrasound SE examinations were conducted in real time using a freehand technique. Each abnormality was assessed by applying gentle pressure, which was adjusted according to the on-screen quality indicator scale for compression strain. The stiffness of the abnormality was compared to the surrounding tissue and visually represented through colour coding, with the stiffest areas depicted in blue, the softest tissues in red, and areas of intermediate elasticity in green to yellow on the display. All static images and cine loops were preserved within our picture archiving and communication system (PACS, Centricity, GE Healthcare, Germany) or in our institution's upgraded picture archiving and communication system (SECTRA, Linköping, Sweden) (Figures 1–4).

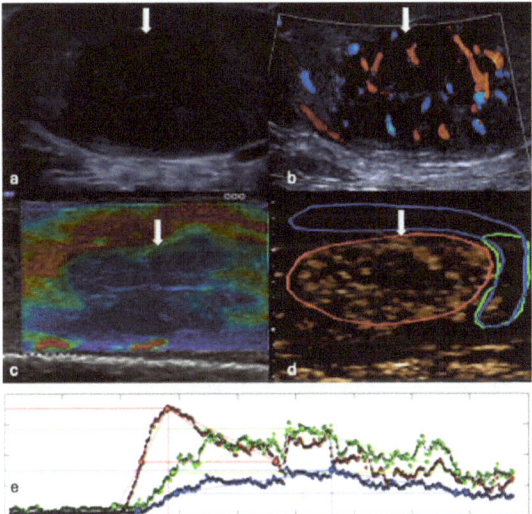

Figure 1. MPUS of a testicular seminoma. (**a**) Greyscale US reveals a large, multiloculated hypoechoic mass (white arrow). (**b**) CDUS demonstrates that the lesion (white arrow) is vascularised. (**c**) On SE, the lesion (white arrow) exhibits uniformly hard tissue stiffness, appearing blue. (**d**) On CEUS the lesion (white arrow) shows enhancement, with late-phase washout evident on the CEUS time–intensity curve (x-axis: time; y-axis: signal intensity) (**e**). Red region of interest (ROI) = lesion; blue and green ROIs = surrounding parenchyma.

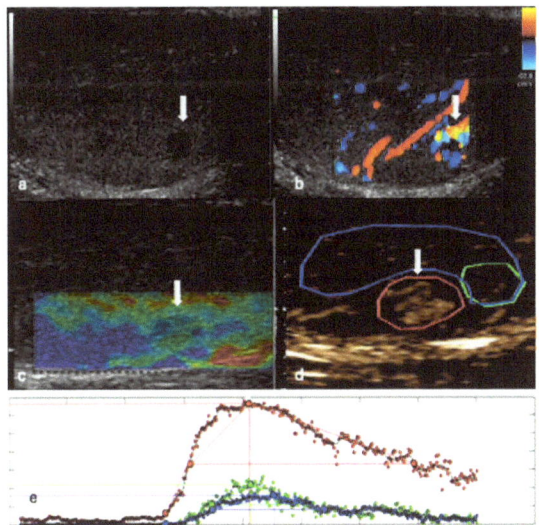

Figure 2. MPUS of a leydig cell tumour. (**a**) Greyscale US shows small, well-defined lesions (white arrow) with homogeneous low reflectivity. (**b**) CDUS indicates that the lesion (white arrow) is highly vascularised. (**c**) SE identifies the lesion (white arrow) as mildly hard, depicted in shades of green and blue. (**d**) CEUS demonstrates a hyper-enhancing lesion (white arrow), with prolonged hyper-enhancement relative to the surrounding parenchyma in the late phase on the CEUS time–intensity curve (x-axis: time; y-axis: intensity) (**e**). Red region of interest (ROI) = lesion; blue and green ROIs = surrounding parenchyma.

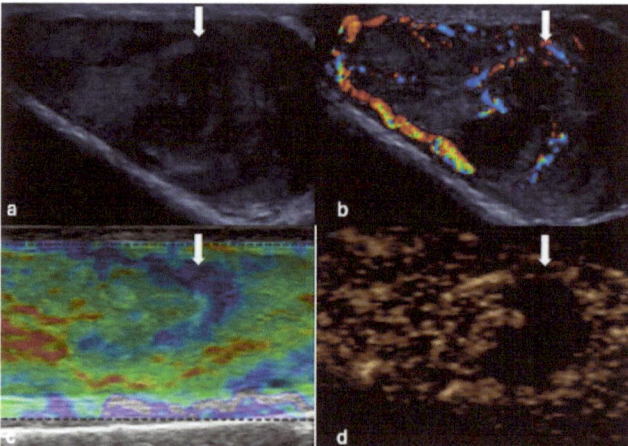

Figure 3. MPUS of a segmental infarction. (**a**) Greyscale US shows a lesion (white arrow) with a low echogenic centre and surrounding high echogenicity. (**b**) CDUS indicates that no colour Doppler signal is present within the lesion (white arrow). (**c**) On SE, this lesion (white arrow) demonstrates a predominantly green signal consistent with a "soft" lesion. (**d**) CEUS conclusively demonstrates the absence of enhancement within the central aspects of the lesion (white arrow).

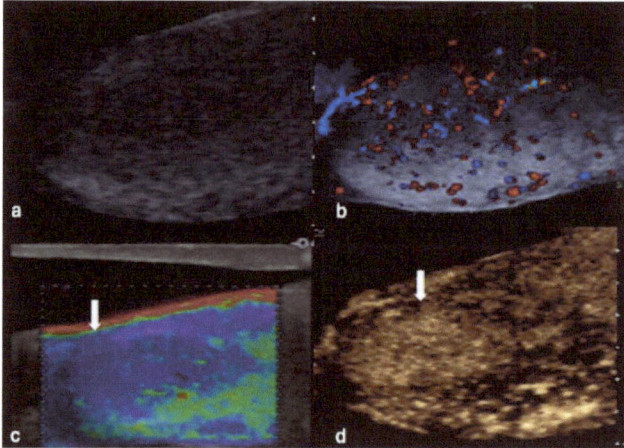

Figure 4. MPUS of a testicular lymphoma. (**a**) Greyscale ultrasound shows diffuse enlargement of the testis with ill-defined, extensive decreased echogenicity in the majority of the testis. (**b**) CDUS indicates that hypervascularity is present within the testis. (**c**) SE demonstrates a hard lesion (white arrow), which is not clearly depicted on greyscale US. (**d**) CEUS demonstrates hyper-enhancement of the lesion (white arrow).

2.4. Clinical Decision Making and Intervention

Management decisions for identified focal intratesticular abnormalities were formulated by a multidisciplinary team comprising urologists, oncologists, radiologists, and histopathologists. Criteria for radical orchiectomy included definitive malignant ultrasound features, elevated tumour markers, and evidence of metastasis. Conversely, lesions considered likely benign were managed with either surveillance or testis-sparing surgery (TSS). Criteria for TSS selection encompassed abnormality size under 2 cm, a safe distance between the mass and rete testis, negative tumour markers in patients, and the absence of metastatic disease ascertained by computed tomography staging evaluation.

The standard surgical technique for managing intratesticular abnormalities is the inguinal approach. In the context of TSS, the procedure involves exteriorisation of the testis followed by incision of the tunica vaginalis to facilitate direct examination. Localisation of the tumour is achieved either through manual palpation or via intraoperative ultrasound guidance. Additionally, intraoperative frozen section examinations are employed at the discretion of the surgical team to aid in immediate histopathological evaluation.

2.5. Data Analysis

Two experienced reviewers, each with over five years of expertise in scrotal ultrasonography and blinded to the other's evaluations, independently recorded the ultrasound features of each lesion. To ensure the objectivity and integrity of our data analysis, both reviewers were completely blinded to all clinical information, including the presence or absence of raised tumour markers and distant metastasis. The reviewers' assessments were based solely on the imaging data presented to them, devoid of any preconceived notions about the patients' clinical status. Discrepancies were resolved through joint discussions between the reviewers to reach a consensus. The assessment focused on documenting essential sonographic characteristics, such as size, echogenicity, vascular patterns, contrast enhancement properties, and strain elastography findings. Strain elastography results were analysed using a colour-coded scheme to delineate varying degrees of tissue stiffness in accordance with established criteria for testicular strain elastography [26,36].

Quantitative CEUS of time–intensity curves (TICs) was performed to evaluate perfusion parameters, facilitating a comparative study between histologically verified benign and malignant lesions, including specific analysis within the two largest homogeneous groups of malignant seminomas and benign Leydig cell tumours with low malignant potential. Exclusions from the TIC analysis were made in instances of compromised image loop storage, alterations in imaging planes, or adjustments in receiver gain settings. Pixel intensity data, expressed in grey levels, were converted to echo-power units (arbitrary units, au) using MATLAB (version R2015a), facilitating a more precise analysis of the echo intensity within the region of interest (ROI). This conversion was followed by the application of a gamma variate curve fitting to the raw data, from which various perfusion parameters were calculated based on the fitted model (Figure 5).

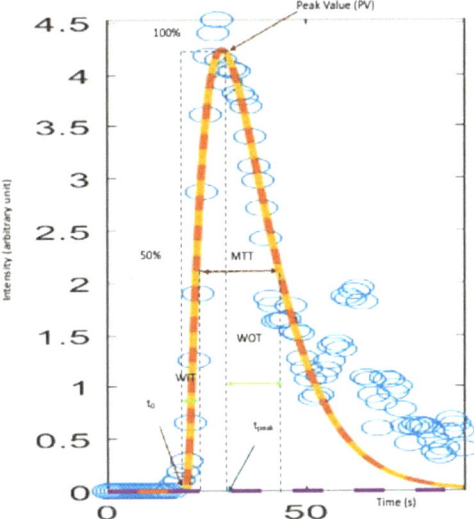

Figure 5. Quantitative CEUS analysis of an intratesticular abnormality. Perfusion parameters derived from the time–intensity curve (blue circles: intensity data entries) with curve-fitting (orange curve)

include the following: tmax (time to peak, TTP): time needed from contrast injection to maximum intensity (s); peak value (PV): the maximum intensity on the TIC curve (arbitrary units, arb); wash-in time (WIT) (raise time): time from 5% intensity to 50% intensity (s); wash-out time (WOT): time from the peak of the TIC curve to the 50% PV value (s); inflow rate (5 s): calculated as the rate of rise in the first 5 s from t0 (arb/s); inflow rate: calculated as the rate of rise over tpeak-t0 (arb/s); outflow rate (5 s): calculated as the rate of outflow in the first 5 s from PV (arb/s); outflow rate: calculated as peak enhancement divided by WOT for the descending slope to reach a contrast signal intensity of zero or the end of the curve (arb/s); MTT (mean transit time, full width at half maximum, FWHM): The time between the half-amplitude values on each side of the maximum (s).

2.6. Reference Standards and Diagnostic Criteria

Final diagnoses were confirmed either through histopathological examination of specimens obtained via surgical intervention or through a minimum follow-up period of twelve months for non-surgical cases. Lesions were identified as malignant based on the presence of malignant histological features in the analysed specimens, including instances of burnt-out tumours. Conversely, lesions were classified as benign following histopathological analysis of excised material or orchiectomy specimens that confirmed benign histological characteristics, including Leydig cell tumours with low malignant potential, as delineated by specific histological criteria [37–39]. Furthermore, lesions demonstrating no change, stability, or reduction in size during follow-up were also classified as benign.

2.7. Statistical Analyses

Quantitative data were presented as either mean ± standard deviation for normally distributed variables or median and interquartile range for variables not following a normal distribution. For participants presenting with multiple testicular lesions, the largest abnormality was selected for inclusion in the statistical comparison of ultrasound features between benign and malignant categories. The Mann–Whitney U test was applied to evaluate significant differences in continuous variables across the two groups. Interobserver reliability was quantified using Cohen's kappa coefficient for the two independent reviewers. Variations in categorical data between benign and malignant lesions were assessed using Pearson's Chi-squared test and Fisher's exact test as appropriate. The McNemar test was used to compare sensitivity, specificity, and accuracy, and bootstrapping was used to quantify appropriate confidence intervals and obtain the significance of the difference for positive predictive values (PPVs) and negative predictive values (NPVs) between groups. The DeLong test was used to compare the area under the curve (AUC) for the receiver operating characteristic (ROC) curves between ultrasound techniques. Logistic regression analysis was conducted to examine the influence of specific sonographic features on the probability of a lesion being malignant, utilising Nagelkerke R^2 and the Hosmer and Lemeshow test as measures of goodness-of-fit. The Wilcoxon signed-rank test was used for comparing perfusion parameters between each lesion and its adjacent normal testicular tissue. All statistical analyses were performed using SPSS software (version 29, IBM), with a significance threshold set at $p < 0.05$.

3. Results

A total of 124 MPUS examinations conducted to evaluate intratesticular focal abnormalities were included. This cohort comprised 78 benign and 46 malignant diagnoses. The demographic analysis (Table 1) demonstrated no significant age difference between patients with benign and those with malignant testicular abnormalities ($p = 0.27$). A significant difference ($p = 0.005$) was observed in the palpability of the focal abnormalities, with a greater prevalence in malignant cases compared to benign cases. Elevated tumour markers were noted only in 9 out of 46 patients with malignant lesions and none in patients with a benign diagnosis.

Histopathological analysis was available for 76 cases (Table 2), identifying 46 as malignant and 30 as benign. Among these, 16 patients underwent testis-sparing surgery, with all abnormalities in this subset confirmed as benign. For the remaining 48 cases not undergoing surgery, benignity was determined based on observed stability or regression during the follow-up period.

Table 1. Summary of clinical features.

	Malignant	Benign	p-Value Benign vs. Malignant
Number of patients	46	78	
Age (mean ± standard deviation)	37.13 ± 10.29	39.55 ± 23.51	$p = 0.27$
Site (number (%))			
Right	28 (60.87%)	33 (42.31%)	$p = 0.05$
Left	17 (36.70%)	39 (50.00%)	$p = 0.16$
Bilateral	1 (2.17%)	6 (7.69%)	$p = 0.20$
Clinical Presentation (number (%))			
Palpable lump	29 (63.04%)	29 (37.18%)	$p = 0.005$
Pain	7 (15.22%)	24 (30.77%)	$p = 0.05$
Trauma	0	6 (7.69%)	$p = 0.05$
Inflammatory	2 (4.34%)	3 (3.85%)	$p = 0.89$
Infertility	0	3 (3.85%)	$p = 0.18$
Post-surgery	0	2 (2.56%)	$p = 0.27$
Asymptomatic	8 (17.39%)	11 (14.10%)	$p = 0.62$
Positive Tumour Markers (number (%))	9 (19.57%)	0	$p < 0.001$
Clinical Management (number, (%))	Orchiectomy: 46 (100%)	Orchiectomy: 14 (17.94%) Testis-sparing surgery: 16 (20.51%) Follow-up: 48 (61.54%)	

Table 2. Histopathological analysis of 76 surgical cases.

Variables	Orchiectomy	Testis-Sparing Surgery
Number of patients	60	16
Histological diagnosis: Malignant		
Seminoma	29	0
Mixed germ cell tumours	12	0
Lymphoma	2	0
Burnt-out tumour	1	0
Metastasis (prostate primary)	1	0
Sarcoma	1	0
Total	46	0
Histological Diagnosis: Benign		
Leydig cell tumour with low malignant potential	7	9
Sertoli cell tumour	0	1
Global testicular infarct	6	0
Abscess	2	0
Adenomatoid tumour (intratesticular)	1	1
Epidermoid cyst	1	1
Fibrotic change	1	1
Calcified haematoma	0	1
Lipomatous hamartoma	1	0
Inflammatory reaction	1	0
Lobular capillary haemangioma	1	0
Sarcoidosis	0	1
TB	1	0
Mature teratoma	1	1
Total	14	16

MPUS Characteristics

The sonographic features observed are summarised in Table 3. High interrater reliability was demonstrated, with a Cohen's kappa coefficient of 0.96 for greyscale ultrasound, 0.94 for CDUS, 0.96 for CEUS, and 0.93 for strain elastography. The average dimension of the focal abnormalities was 15.26 ± 13.20 mm. A significant difference ($p < 0.001$) in size was observed, with benign abnormalities measuring 10.02 ± 6.80 mm and malignant abnormalities 21.12 ± 12.19 mm. Among the 124 evaluated abnormalities, 93 (75.0%) presented as predominantly hypoechoic on greyscale ultrasound, with three abnormalities being isoechoic and two hyperechoic. Additionally, 26 abnormalities (21.0%) demonstrated mixed echogenicity. No significant differences were detected between benign and malignant categories concerning the hypoechoic appearance, the presence of macro-calcification, or irregular margins. Similarly, the incidence of testicular microlithiasis (TML) did not significantly differ between the groups.

Table 3. Summary of comparative MPUS features between the benign and malignant groups.

MP-US Features	Benign (All Lesions, n = 78)	Malignant (All Lesions, n = 46)	p-Value (All Lesions, Benign vs. Malignant)	Benign (<10 mm, n = 46)	Malignant (<10 mm, n = 7)	p-Value (<10 mm, Benign vs. Malignant)
Maximal dimension (mm)	10.02 ± 6.80	21.12 ± 12.19	$p < 0.001$	5.25 +/− 2.25	5.59 +/− 2.55	$p = 0.72$
Echogenicity			$p = 0.83$			$p = 0.31$
Not hypoechoic	20	11		6	0	
Hypoechoic	58	35		40	7	
Margin			$p = 0.65$			$p = 0.92$
Well-circumscribed	49	27		32	5	
Poorly circumscribed	29	19		14	2	
Testicular Microlithiasis			$p = 0.89$			$p = 0.79$
Not present	71	37		41	6	
Present	7	9		5	1	
CDUS vascularity			$p < 0.001$			$p = 0.67$
Not present	37	5		17	2	
Present	41	41		29	5	
CEUS enhancement			$p < 0.001$			$p = 0.17$
Not present	29	0		10	0	
Present	49	46		36	7	
CEUS homogeneous enhancement			$p = 0.08$			$p = 0.52$
Heterogenous enhancement	7	14		2	0	
Homogeneous enhancement	42	32		34	7	
CEUS early hyperenhancement			$p = 0.72$			$p = 0.83$
Not present	22	19		14	4	
Present	27	27		22	3	
CEUS late hyperenhancement			$p = 0.002$			$p = 0.44$
Not present	29	40		20	5	
Present	20	6		16	2	
Strain elastography			$p = 0.07$			$p = 0.52$
Soft	28	6		19	2	
Hard	50	40		27	5	

Vascularisation, as detected by CDUS, was observed in 89.10% (41/46) of malignant abnormalities and 52.56% (41/78) of benign abnormalities, yielding a statistically significant difference ($p < 0.001$). Nonetheless, CDUS did not detect vascularisation in 10.87% (5/46) of malignant abnormalities, including three seminomas, one mixed germ cell tumour, and one burnt-out tumour. During contrast-enhanced ultrasound (CEUS) examination, enhancement was observed in all malignant abnormalities (46/46, 100%) but also in 37.18% (49 out of 78) of benign abnormalities. Notably, CEUS detected enhancement in all 5 malignant abnormalities, which were initially characterised as 'avascular' by CDUS, while all 29 abnormalities lacking enhancement on CEUS were benign. Within the subset of 95 abnormalities demonstrating enhancement on CEUS, there were no statistically significant differences between benign and malignant groups regarding homogeneous enhancement or early (within 40 s of contrast injection) hyperenhancement. However, a significant distinction was observed in late (40–90 s post-contrast injection) hyperenhancement on CEUS.

Additionally, in comparing the two largest histologically verified homogeneous groups of vascular tumours—malignant seminomas and LCT-LMP—significant differences ($p = 0.04$) in late hyperenhancement between the two groups were observed, with seminomas (5/29, 17.24%) and LCT-LMP (8/17, 47.06%) demonstrating late hyperenhancement. Strain elastography revealed no significant differences in increased tissue stiffness between benign and malignant abnormalities. Likewise, comparisons of stiffness between seminomas and LCT-LMP showed no significant differences, with increased stiffness observed in 13 out of 17 LCT cases and 27 out of 29 seminomas during strain elastography analysis ($p = 0.174$). A subset of 53 lesions smaller than 10 mm, comprising 7 malignant and 46 benign lesions, was also analysed (Table 3). No statistically significant differences were noted between the benign and malignant groups in terms of margin, presence of microlithiasis, CDUS vascularity, CEUS enhancement, the presence of prolonged hyperenhancement on CEUS, or stiffness on SE. However, it is worth noting that two out of the seven malignant lesions displayed no vascularity on CDUS. Both of these malignant lesions showed enhancement on CEUS, and all lesions < 10 mm that demonstrated no enhancement were benign.

The comparative analysis of imaging modalities, including conventional CDUS, CEUS, SE, and their combined application (CEUS+SE), is summarised in Table 4. CEUS achieved the highest sensitivity but had a low specificity of 37.18% (95% CI: 26.50 to 48.87). In terms of specificity, the combination of CEUS and SE showed the best performance at 60.26% (95% CI: 48.54 to 71.17), which was significantly higher than conventional CDUS ($p = 0.04$). Although it did not reach statistical significance when compared to CDUS ($p = 0.12$), the accuracy rate of the combined CEUS and SE approach (70.16%, 95% CI: 61.29 to 78.04%) suggests an improvement compared to CDUS (62.90%, 95% CI: 53.77 to 71.40%), CEUS (60.48%, 95% CI: 51.31 to 69.14%), or SE (54.84%, 95% CI: 45.65 to 63.79%). Other diagnostic performance metrics did not show significant differences among these diagnostic tests.

Table 4. Performance metrics of CDUS, CEUS, and SE.

	CDUS	CEUS	p-Value CDUS vs. CEUS	SE	p-Value CDUS vs. SE	CEUS + SE	p-Value CDUS vs. CEUS + SE
TP	41	46		40		40	
FP	41	49		50		31	
TN	37	29		28		47	
FN	5	0		6		6	
Sensitivity (%)	89.13 (76.43–96.38)	100.00 (92.29–100.00)	$p = 0.004$	86.96 (73.74–95.06)	$p = 0.28$	86.96 (73.74–95.06)	$p = 0.05$
Specificity (%)	47.44 (36.01–59.07)	37.18 (26.50–48.87)	$p = 0.06$	35.90 (25.34–47.56)	$p = 0.18$	60.26 (48.54–71.17)	$p = 0.04$
PPV (%)	50.00 (39.20–61.10)	48.42 (38.20–58.60)	$p = 0.33$	44.44 (34.70–54.70)	$p = 0.10$	56.34 (45.20–67.50)	$p = 0.09$
NPV (%)	88.10 (78.80–96.30)	100 (100.00–100.00)	$p = 0.12$	82.35 (69.00–94.10)	$p = 0.27$	88.68 (78.80–96.30)	$p = 0.49$
Accuracy (%)	62.90 (53.77–71.40)	60.48 (51.31–69.14)	$p = 0.79$	54.84 (45.65–63.79)	$p = 0.25$	70.16 (61.29–78.04)	$p = 0.12$
AUC	0.68 (0.61–0.76)	0.69 (0.63–0.74)	$p = 0.93$	0.61 (0.54–0.69)	$p = 0.15$	0.74 (0.66–0.81)	$p = 0.19$

This table summarises the performance metrics (values and respective 95% confidence interval) of CDUS, CEUS, SE, and CEUS + SE. For CDUS, the presence of hypervascularity indicates malignancy. For CEUS, the presence of enhancement indicates malignancy. For SE, hardness indicates malignancy. For CEUS + SE, the presence of both enhancement and hardness indicates malignancy. TP = true positive, FP = false positive, TN = true negative, and FN = false negative. LR = likelihood ratio. PPV = positive predictive value. NPV = negative predictive value. AUC = area under the ROC curve.

A multivariable logistic regression analysis (Table 5) was conducted to evaluate the contribution of various sonographic features identified as independent predictors of malignancy in abnormalities enhanced on CEUS. Investigated factors encompassed lesion size larger than 10 mm, homogeneous enhancement, early hyperenhancement, absence of late hyperenhancement, and increased tissue stiffness as determined by SE. The model demonstrated significant predictive capability (Nagelkerke $R^2 = 0.49$), fitting the data well ($\chi^2(6) = 5.31$, $p = 0.50$), correctly classifying 75.50% of benign cases and 84.80% of malignant cases, with an overall accuracy of 80.00%. Within this model, two features had a statistically significant effect on the outcome: lesion size larger than 10 mm and absence of late hyperenhancement. The findings of a lesion size larger than 10 mm had a highly significant effect on the outcome ($p < 0.001$), with an odds ratio (OR) of 9.72 (95% CI: 2.97 to 31.86), indicating that for an enhancing lesion, having a size larger than 10 mm increases the odds of malignancy by nearly ten times. The absence of late hyperenhancement on CEUS was also significant ($p = 0.01$) with an OR of 5.81 (95% CI: 1.43 to 23.65), suggesting that for an enhancing abnormality, the absence of late hyperenhancement increases the odds of malignancy by approximately six times.

Table 5. Multivariable logistic regression analysis to evaluate the contribution of various features identified via CEUS and SE as independent predictors of malignancy.

Sonographic Features	ß Coefficient	Standard Errors	p-Value	OR	95% Confidence Intervals for OR	
					Lower	Upper
Lesion size > 10 mm	2.27	0.61	$p < 0.001$	9.72	2.97	31.86
Homogeneous enhancement	0.12	0.69	$p = 0.86$	1.13	0.29	4.33
Early hyperenhancement	0.84	0.62	$p = 0.18$	2.32	0.68	7.90
Absence of late hyperenhancement on CEUS	1.76	0.72	$p = 0.01$	5.81	1.43	23.65
Increased tissue stiffness on SE	1.03	0.69	$p = 0.13$	2.81	0.73	10.79

In the comparative quantitative analysis of perfusion parameters derived from time–intensity curves during CEUS evaluations, normalisation of data relative to the surrounding parenchyma (lesion-to-parenchyma ratios) revealed no statistically significant differences in all parameters between benign and malignant groups (Table 6). Nonetheless, a notable distinction was identified in the perfusion parameters between histologically confirmed seminomas and LCT-LMP: seminomas exhibited a significantly shorter washout time compared to the adjacent parenchyma (35.30 ± 6.61 s vs. 44.88 ± 15.23 s; $p = 0.03$), in contrast to LCT-LMP, which did not show a statistically significant difference in washout time to the surrounding parenchyma (25.13 ± 12.20 s vs. 34.12 ± 16.90 s, $p = 0.25$).

Table 6. Summary of comparative perfusion parameters for the benign and malignant groups.

DCE-US Parameters	Diagnosis	Lesion/Parenchyma Ratio			p-Value (Benign vs. Malignant)
		Mean	Std. Deviation	Std. Error Mean	
TTP	Benign	0.85	0.18	0.05	$p = 0.41$
	Malignant	0.89	0.21	0.04	
PV	Benign	11.77	18.73	5.70	$p = 0.73$
	Malignant	10.08	22.09	3.68	
WIT	Benign	2.13	2.69	0.72	$p = 0.25$
	Malignant	2.06	4.88	0.81	
WOT	Benign	1.02	0.72	0.19	$p = 0.98$
	Malignant	1.64	4.27	0.71	
Inflow Rate	Benign	13.38	27.92	7.46	$p = 0.49$
	Malignant	22.44	73.66	12.28	
Inflow Rate (5 s)	Benign	10.86	18.41	4.92	$p = 0.56$
	Malignant	12.95	20.00	3.50	
Outflow Rate	Benign	18.84	37.84	10.11	$p = 0.13$
	Malignant	18.50	40.83	7.31	
Outflow Rate (5 s)	Benign	17.51	21.91	5.86	$p = 0.12$
	Malignant	18.87	23.37	8.57	
MTT	Benign	1.07	0.80	0.21	$p = 0.52$
	Malignant	1.10	0.68	0.11	

4. Discussion

In this study from a tertiary centre, we describe our decade-long experience with multiparametric ultrasound, including CEUS and SE, in evaluating focal testicular abnormalities. To our knowledge, this series represents the largest cohort published to date [18,40–42]. We evaluated the contribution these techniques bring to clinical practice. All malignant lesions demonstrated enhancement on CEUS, including 10.8% of malignant tumours that were deemed 'avascular' on CDUS in our cohort. Conversely, lesions without CEUS enhancement were uniformly benign. Our cohort also revealed that late hyperenhancement on CEUS in benign enhancing tumours, such as in Leydig cell tumours with low malignant potential, offers a potential feature for distinguishing these from malignant tumours, such as seminomas. This study also showed that by integrating CEUS and the combination of CEUS and SE, the diagnostic performance of ultrasound imaging in differentiating benign and malignant focal testicular abnormalities was improved. Specifically, CEUS showed a higher sensitivity when compared to CDUS, and CEUS+SE showed higher specificity when compared to CDUS. Notably, during our decade-long clinical experience, all patients who opted for testis-sparing surgery instead of radical orchiectomy following MPUS assessments were confirmed to have benign conditions.

In our study, a statistically significant difference was observed in the association of lesion size and final diagnosis between the benign and the malignant groups in our cohort of patients. In a study by Eifler et al. [43] based on 49 lesions in 145 men referred for azoospermia who underwent ultrasonographic analysis, the investigators proposed an algorithm based on tumour markers and the size and vascularity of the lesions. They suggested that a lesion < 5 mm, characterised by an absence of vascularity and negative tumour markers, could be followed by serial US monitoring. A further study by Scandura et al. [44] reported the majority of testicular lesions < 10 mm identified by radiology were benign. In our study, it was shown that for an enhancing lesion, having a size larger than 10 mm increases the odds of malignancy by nearly ten times. However, we found that greyscale ultrasound did not demonstrate statistically significant differences in features such as margin, hypoechoic nature, or the presence of microlithiasis between benign and malignant testicular lesions. The lack of significant differences in these observed greyscale sonographic features suggests that these parameters alone are insufficient for reliable differentiation, underscoring the limitation of greyscale US.

The descriptive statistical analysis of various ultrasound modalities, including CDUS, CEUS, and SE, demonstrated high sensitivity across these techniques, aligning with findings reported in existing literature [16,18,45,46]. However, all examined modalities exhibited low specificity in our study, with SE identified as the least specific technique. Existing research on the diagnostic accuracy of SE for evaluating testicular lesions presents divergent outcomes [46–49]. For instance, Grasso et al. [50] compared B-mode plus colour Doppler ultrasound to real-time elastography (RTE) in 41 patients and noted the inability to differentiate malignant from benign lesions based solely on elastography. Goddi et al. [48] reported an SE sensitivity of 87.5% with a specificity of 98.2% in a large series of 144 testicular lesions but comprising a clear majority of benign lesions (112 of 144, 77%). Aigner et al. [47] reported similar sensitivity (100%) and specificity (81%) in 62 patients. Conversely, Marsaud et al. [51] subsequently reported a sensitivity for strain elastography to be 96% in 34 patients (26 malignant), but specificity proved to be as low as 37.5%. Schrodeer et al. [46] reported a specificity of 25%, with only one-quarter of non-neoplastic lesions being correctly identified by SE in their study. Our findings support the notion that SE, when used alone, is not definitive in distinguishing between malignant and benign abnormalities. This observation aligns with current guidelines regarding the use of elastography in evaluating testicular focal abnormalities [15]. However, our data indicate that SE could still provide added value in diagnosing focal testicular abnormalities. In our cohort, combining SE with CEUS significantly improves specificity compared to using conventional CDUS alone.

In our study, CEUS exhibited high sensitivity for intratesticular malignant tumours (100%). Notably, CEUS identified enhancement in all malignant lesions across our cohort, including instances where CDUS could not ascertain tissue vascularisation, such as malignant lesions < 10 mm. This reinforces the notion that CEUS offers superior capabilities in depicting vascular flow [14]. Although CDUS is widely used in the evaluation of most intratesticular tumours, the technique is not without limitations. Ma et al. [52] showed that a substantial proportion (36.5%) of hypoechoic testicular lesions that were avascular on CDUS were malignant in their cohort. Our findings, therefore, underscore the distinctive clinical advantages of CEUS over CDUS. The adjunctive application of CEUS facilitates the timely identification of testicular malignancies, which may otherwise not exhibit a vascular signal on CDUS, thereby mitigating the risk of diagnostic delays. The importance of not missing any tumour is crucial not only for immediate treatment outcomes but also for long-term prognosis and survival, particularly in the context of malignancies where early detection can significantly influence the treatment approach and outcome [53].

Our study determined that lesions exhibiting no enhancement on CEUS were invariably benign, lending credence to the interpretation that the absence of vascularity on CEUS is a robust indicator of benignity, as supported by the low incidence of false negatives in related research with CEUS [16,20]. Our finding substantiates the view that lack of vascularity on CEUS can be interpreted as a strong indicator of benignity. The confirmation of the absence of vascularisation with CEUS excludes ('rule out') a malignant diagnosis more reliably than CDUS. Examples of such cases include epidermoid cysts and hard infarctions, which can be conclusively considered to be benign when no internal enhancement is demonstrated on CEUS. In practical terms, this finding indicates that adjunct CEUS allows increased diagnostic confidence when a focal intratesticular lesion is encountered in routine urological practice, allowing accurate triaging of patients for conservative management, such as watchful waiting or testis-sparing surgery, versus the alternative of an unnecessary orchiectomy, in a clinically appropriate setting.

A significant portion of our cohort featured vascular benign abnormalities, such as LCT-LMP. This prevalence of vascular benign lesions contributed to misclassifications by both CDUS and CEUS when the detection of increased perfusion in lesions is solely relied on as a binary marker for malignancy. However, our findings indicate that for an enhancing abnormality, the absence of late hyperenhancement raises the likelihood of malignancy by approximately six times, highlighting the unique benefits of CEUS. While the investigation of tissue vascularisation is not the prerogative of CEUS alone, in our investigation, CEUS exhibited the capability to identify a distinct vascular pattern of prolonged enhancement, potentially aiding in the differential diagnosis of benign vascular testicular lesions, such as LCT-LMP, a finding corroborated by other groups [16,54]. These observations in our study hold significant clinical implications, as small incidental Leydig cell tumours are more likely to have a benign course [55,56], and distinct vascular patterns for LCT-LMP on CEUS may inform decisions to forego orchiectomy in favour of more conservative organ-sparing approaches for vascular focal lesions presumed to be LCT-LMP [57,58], contingent upon clinical judgment (e.g., negative tumour markers, normal staging computed tomography, and patient suitability).

All patients who underwent testis-sparing surgery in our cohort had benign diagnoses. In clinical settings, imaging findings, along with clinical risk and biochemical assessment, allow increased confidence for the most appropriate clinical management pathway to be instituted by the multi-disciplinary team caring for patients. If a testicular lesion can be shown to be of a high probability to be benign pre-operatively, the organ-sparing approach to small testicular lesion represents a valid treatment, as testis-sparing surgery can provide accurate histological diagnosis and optimal oncological efficacy yet preclude the risk of removal of a testicle bearing a benign lesion. Muller et al. [59] reported their experience in testis-sparing surgery for incidentally detected testicular lesions < 5 mm. All patients who opted for testis-sparing surgery instead of radical orchiectomy following MPUS assessments were confirmed to have benign conditions during our decade-long clinical experience. Our experience showed the utility of advanced ultrasound techniques in preoperative characterisation could aid in facilitating the formulation of optimal clinical management strategies.

This study is subject to some limitations. Primarily, it was structured as a retrospective analysis, which may impact the prospective applicability of the findings. Our study encompasses a wide range of cases encountered in routine clinical practice at our tertiary care centre over a ten-year period. Our dataset includes clinically impalpable lesions incidentally discovered in adult men presenting with symptoms such as scrotal pain or subfertility. Including both palpable and impalpable lesions allows us to assess the effectiveness of ultrasound in a realistic clinical setting and reflect the heterogeneity observed in routine practice. However, this broad inclusion complicates the extraction of precise guidance for populations with specific clinical presentations. The series size was modest, covering a wide spectrum of testicular pathologies but with limited cases per specific condition, such as malignant lesions < 10 mm. This suggests a need for future studies on a larger scale to validate these results with greater statistical power. Additionally, this study focused on a select group of patients with focal testicular abnormalities identified through greyscale ultrasound, risking selection bias. The operator-dependent nature of ultrasound also presents a challenge in ensuring consistent and reproducible results across different examiners. Lastly, non-surgical cases managed as benign were not confirmed histologically, leaving room for diagnostic uncertainty.

5. Conclusions

Our decade-long experience indicates that integrating advanced ultrasound technologies, such as contrast-enhanced ultrasound and strain elastography, could refine the diagnosis of focal intratesticular abnormalities. Future research should continue to explore and validate the clinical benefits of these technologies, aiming to establish clear protocols that optimise their use in everyday medical practice.

Author Contributions: Conceptualization, P.S.S. and D.Y.H.; methodology, D.Y.H.; formal analysis, D.Y.H. and M.A.; investigation, D.Y.H., G.T.Y., A.D., M.E.S. and P.S.S.; data curation, D.Y.H. and M.A.; writing—original draft preparation, D.Y.H.; writing—review and editing, D.Y.H. and P.S.S.; supervision, P.S.S.; project administration, D.Y.H.; funding acquisition, not applicable. All authors have read and agreed to the published version of the manuscript.

Funding: This research received no external funding.

Institutional Review Board Statement: This study was conducted in accordance with the Declaration of Helsinki, and the protocol was approved by the Ethics Committee of the Institutional Review Board of King's College Hospital NHS Foundation Trust (project identification code: KCH14-102 (IRAS 148856). Date of approval: 12 October 2018).

Informed Consent Statement: Waived due to the retrospective nature of this study.

Data Availability Statement: The datasets presented in this article are unavailable due to privacy restrictions.

Conflicts of Interest: The authors declare no conflicts of interest.

References

1. Tsili, A.C.; Bougia, C.K.; Pappa, O.; Argyropoulou, M.I. Ultrasonography of the scrotum: Revisiting a classic technique. *Eur. J. Radiol.* **2021**, *145*, 110000. [CrossRef] [PubMed]
2. Dogra, V.S.; Gottlieb, R.H.; Oka, M.; Rubens, D.J. Sonography of the Scrotum. *Radiology* **2003**, *227*, 18–36. [CrossRef] [PubMed]
3. Bhatt, S.; Jafri, S.Z.H.; Wasserman, N.; Dogra, V.S. Non neoplastic intratesticular masses. *Diagn. Interv. Radiol.* **2009**, *17*, 52–63. [CrossRef] [PubMed]
4. Bhatt, S.; Dogra, V.S. Role of US in Testicular and Scrotal Trauma. *RadioGraphics* **2008**, *28*, 1617–1629. [CrossRef] [PubMed]
5. Woodward, P.J.; Sohaey, R.; O'donoghue, M.J.; Green, D.E. From the Archives of the AFIP. *RadioGraphics* **2002**, *22*, 189–216. [CrossRef] [PubMed]
6. McDonald, M.W.; Reed, A.B.; Tran, P.T.; Evans, L.A. Testicular Tumor Ultrasound Characteristics and Association with Histopathology. *Urol. Int.* **2011**, *89*, 196–202. [CrossRef] [PubMed]

7. Mirochnik, B.; Bhargava, P.; Dighe, M.K.; Kanth, N. Ultrasound Evaluation of Scrotal Pathology. *Radiol. Clin. North Am.* **2012**, *50*, 317–332. [CrossRef] [PubMed]
8. Altaffer, L.F.; Steele, S.M. Scrotal Explorations Negative for Malignancy. *J. Urol.* **1980**, *124*, 617–619. [CrossRef] [PubMed]
9. Toren, P.J.; Roberts, M.; Lecker, I.; Grober, E.D.; Jarvi, K.; Lo, K.C. Small Incidentally Discovered Testicular Masses in Infertile Men—Is Active Surveillance the New Standard of Care? *J. Urol.* **2010**, *183*, 1373–1377. [CrossRef]
10. Carmignani, L.; Gadda, F.; Mancini, M.; Gazzano, G.; Nerva, F.; Rocco, F.; Colpi, G.M. DETECTION OF TESTICULAR ULTRASONOGRAPHIC LESIONS IN SEVERE MALE INFERTILITY. *J. Urol.* **2004**, *172*, 1045–1047. [CrossRef]
11. Carmignani, L.; Gadda, F.; Gazzano, G.; Nerva, F.; Mancini, M.; Ferruti, M.; Bulfamante, G.; Bosari, S.; Coggi, G.; Rocco, F.; et al. High Incidence of Benign Testicular Neoplasms Diagnosed by Ultrasound. *J. Urol.* **2003**, *170*, 1783–1786. [CrossRef] [PubMed]
12. Zuniga, A.; Lawrentschuk, N.; Jewett, M.A.S. Organ-sparing approaches for testicular masses. *Nat. Rev. Urol.* **2010**, *7*, 454–464. [CrossRef] [PubMed]
13. Tsili, A.C.; Bertolotto, M.; Turgut, A.T.; Dogra, V.; Freeman, S.; Rocher, L.; Belfield, J.; Studniarek, M.; Ntorkou, A.; Derchi, L.E.; et al. MRI of the scrotum: Recommendations of the ESUR Scrotal and Penile Imaging Working Group. *Eur. Radiol.* **2017**, *28*, 31–43. [CrossRef] [PubMed]
14. Sidhu, P.S.; Cantisani, V.; Dietrich, C.F.; Gilja, O.H.; Saftoiu, A.; Bartels, E.; Bertolotto, M.; Calliada, F.; Clevert, D.-A.; Cosgrove, D.; et al. The EFSUMB Guidelines and Recommendations for the Clinical Practice of Contrast-Enhanced Ultrasound (CEUS) in Non-Hepatic Applications: Update 2017 (Long Version). *Ultraschall Med.-Eur. J. Ultrasound* **2018**, *39*, e2–e44. [CrossRef] [PubMed]
15. Săftoiu, A.; Gilja, O.H.; Sidhu, P.S.; Dietrich, C.F.; Cantisani, V.; Amy, D.; Bachmann-Nielsen, M.; Bob, F.; Bojunga, J.; Brock, M.; et al. The EFSUMB Guidelines and Recommendations for the Clinical Practice of Elastography in Non-Hepatic Applications: Update 2018. *Ultraschall Med.* **2019**, *40*, 425–453. [CrossRef] [PubMed]
16. Isidori, A.M.; Pozza, C.; Gianfrilli, D.; Giannetta, E.; Lemma, A.; Pofi, R.; Barbagallo, F.; Manganaro, L.; Martino, G.; Lombardo, F.; et al. Differential Diagnosis of Nonpalpable Testicular Lesions: Qualitative and Quantitative Contrast-enhanced US of Benign and Malignant Testicular Tumors. *Radiology* **2014**, *273*, 606–618. [CrossRef] [PubMed]
17. Fang, C.; Huang, D.Y.; Sidhu, P.S. Elastography of focal testicular lesions: Current concepts and utility. *Ultrasonography* **2019**, *38*, 302–310. [CrossRef] [PubMed]
18. Auer, T.; De Zordo, T.; Dejaco, C.; Gruber, L.; Pichler, R.; Jaschke, W.; Dogra, V.S.; Aigner, F. Value of Multiparametric US in the Assessment of Intratesticular Lesions. *Radiology* **2017**, *285*, 640–649. [CrossRef] [PubMed]
19. Bertolotto, M.; Muça, M.; Currò, F.; Bucci, S.; Rocher, L.; Cova, M.A. Multiparametric US for scrotal diseases. *Abdom. Imaging* **2018**, *43*, 899–917. [CrossRef]
20. Pinto, S.P.; Huang, D.Y.; Dinesh, A.A.; Sidhu, P.S.; Ahmed, K. A Systematic Review on the Use of Qualitative and Quantitative Contrast-enhanced Ultrasound in Diagnosing Testicular Abnormalities. *Urology* **2021**, *154*, 16–23. [CrossRef]
21. Ager, M.; Donegan, S.; Boeri, L.; de Castro, J.M.; Donaldson, J.F.; Omar, M.I.; Dimitropoulos, K.; Tharakan, T.; Janisch, F.; Muilwijk, T.; et al. Radiological features characterising indeterminate testes masses: A systematic review and meta-analysis. *BJU Int.* **2022**, *131*, 288–300. [CrossRef] [PubMed]
22. Patel, K.; Sellars, M.E.; Clarke, J.L.; Sidhu, P.S.; Frcr, K.P.; Mbbs, F.M.E.S.; Msc, J.L.C.; Bsc, M.P.S.S. Features of Testicular Epidermoid Cysts on Contrast-Enhanced Sonography and Real-time Tissue Elastography. *J. Ultrasound Med.* **2012**, *31*, 115–122. [CrossRef] [PubMed]
23. Lung, P.F.C.; Jaffer, O.S.; Sellars, M.E.; Sriprasad, S.; Kooiman, G.G.; Sidhu, P.S. Contrast-Enhanced Ultrasound in the Evaluation of Focal Testicular Complications Secondary to Epididymitis. *Am. J. Roentgenol.* **2012**, *199*, W345–W354. [CrossRef] [PubMed]
24. Hedayati, V.; E Sellars, M.; Sharma, D.M.; Sidhu, P.S. Contrast-enhanced ultrasound in testicular trauma: Role in directing exploration, debridement and organ salvage. *Br. J. Radiol.* **2012**, *85*, e65–e68. [CrossRef] [PubMed]
25. Yusuf, G.; Konstantatou, E.; Sellars, M.E.; Huang, D.Y.; Sidhu, P.S. Multiparametric Sonography of Testicular Hematomas. *J. Ultrasound Med.* **2015**, *34*, 1319–1328. [CrossRef] [PubMed]
26. Konstantatou, E.; Fang, C.; Romanos, O.; Derchi, L.E.; Bertolotto, M.; Valentino, M.; Kalogeropoulou, C.; Sidhu, P.S. Evaluation of Intratesticular Lesions With Strain Elastography Using Strain Ratio and Color Map Visual Grading: Differentiation of Neoplastic and Nonneoplastic Lesions. *J. Ultrasound Med.* **2018**, *38*, 223–232. [CrossRef] [PubMed]
27. Yusuf, G.; Sellars, M.E.; Kooiman, G.G.; Diaz-Cano, S.; Sidhu, P.S. Global Testicular Infarction in the Presence of Epididymitis. *J. Ultrasound Med.* **2013**, *32*, 175–180. [CrossRef] [PubMed]
28. Rafailidis, V.; Robbie, H.; Konstantatou, E.; Huang, D.Y.; Deganello, A.; E Sellars, M.; Cantisani, V.; Isidori, A.M.; Sidhu, P.S. Sonographic imaging of extra-testicular focal lesions: Comparison of grey-scale, colour Doppler and contrast-enhanced ultrasound. *Ultrasound* **2016**, *24*, 23–33. [CrossRef] [PubMed]
29. Patel, K.V.; Huang, D.Y.; Sidhu, P.S. Metachronous bilateral segmental testicular infarction: Multi-parametric ultrasound imaging with grey-scale ultrasound, Doppler ultrasound, contrast-enhanced ultrasound (CEUS) and real-time tissue elastography (RTE). *J. Ultrasound* **2014**, *17*, 233–238. [CrossRef]
30. Zebari, S.; Huang, D.Y.; Wilkins, C.J.; Sidhu, P.S. Acute Testicular Segmental Infarct Following Endovascular Repair of a Juxta-renal Abdominal Aortic Aneurysm: Case Report and Literature Review. *Urology* **2019**, *126*, 5–9. [CrossRef]

31. Kachramanoglou, C.; Rafailidis, V.; Philippidou, M.; Bertolotto, M.; Huang, D.Y.; Deganello, A.; Sellars, M.E.; Sidhu, P.S. Multiparametric Sonography of Hematologic Malignancies of the Testis: Grayscale, Color Doppler, and Contrast-Enhanced Ultrasound and Strain Elastographic Appearances With Histologic Correlation. *J. Ultrasound Med.* **2016**, *36*, 409–420. [CrossRef] [PubMed]
32. Huang, D.Y.; Sidhu, P.S. Focal testicular lesions: Colour Doppler ultrasound, contrast-enhanced ultrasound and tissue elastography as adjuvants to the diagnosis. *Br. J. Radiol.* **2012**, *85*, S41–S53. [CrossRef] [PubMed]
33. Huang, D.Y.; Pesapane, F.; Rafailidis, V.; Deganello, A.; Sellars, M.E.; Sidhu, P.S. The role of multiparametric ultrasound in the diagnosis of paediatric scrotal pathology. *Br. J. Radiol.* **2020**, *93*, 20200063. [CrossRef] [PubMed]
34. Mansoor, N.M.; Huang, D.Y.; Sidhu, P.S. Multiparametric ultrasound imaging characteristics of multiple testicular adrenal rest tumours in congenital adrenal hyperplasia. *Ultrasound* **2022**, *30*, 80–84. [CrossRef] [PubMed]
35. Sidhu, P.S. Multiparametric Ultrasound (MPUS) Imaging: Terminology Describing the Many Aspects of Ultrasonography. *Ultraschall Med.* **2015**, *36*, 315–317. [CrossRef]
36. Itoh, A.; Ueno, E.; Tohno, E.; Kamma, H.; Takahashi, H.; Shiina, T.; Yamakawa, M.; Matsumura, T. Breast Disease: Clinical Application of US Elastography for Diagnosis. *Radiology* **2006**, *239*, 341–350. [CrossRef]
37. Kim, I.; Young, R.H.; Scully, R.E. Leydig cell tumors of the testis. *Am. J. Surg. Pathol.* **1985**, *9*, 177–192. [CrossRef]
38. Farkas, L.M.; Székely, J.G.; Pusztai, C.; Baki, M. High Frequency of Metastatic Leydig Cell Testicular Tumours. *Oncology* **2000**, *59*, 118–121. [CrossRef]
39. Di Tonno, F.; Tavolini, I.M.; Belmonte, P.; Bertoldin, R.; Cossaro, E.; Curti, P.; D'incà, G.; Fandella, A.; Guaitoli, P.; Guazzieri, S.; et al. Lessons from 52 Patients with Leydig Cell Tumor of the Testis: The GUONE (North-Eastern Uro-Oncological Group, Italy) Experience. *Urol. Int.* **2009**, *82*, 152–157. [CrossRef] [PubMed]
40. Sun, L.-P.; Xu, H.-X.; Liu, H.; Dong, L.; Xiang, L.-H.; Xu, G.; Wan, J.; Fang, Y.; Ding, S.-S.; Jin, Y. Multiparametric ultrasound for the assessment of testicular lesions with negative tumoral markers. *Asian J. Androl.* **2023**, *25*, 50–57. [CrossRef]
41. Reginelli, A.; D'andrea, A.; Clemente, A.; Izzo, A.; Urraro, F.; Scala, F.; Nardone, V.; Guida, C.; Scialpi, M.; Cappabianca, S. Does multiparametric US improve diagnostic accuracy in the characterization of small testicular masses? *Gland. Surg.* **2019**, *8*, S136–S141. [CrossRef] [PubMed]
42. Schwarze, V.; Marschner, C.; Sabel, B.; de Figueiredo, G.N.; Marcon, J.; Ingrisch, M.; Knösel, T.; Rübenthaler, J.; Clevert, D.-A. Multiparametric ultrasonographic analysis of testicular tumors: A single-center experience in a collective of 49 patients. *Scand. J. Urol.* **2020**, *54*, 241–247. [CrossRef] [PubMed]
43. Eifler, J.B., Jr.; King, P.; Schlegel, P.N. Incidental Testicular Lesions Found During Infertility Evaluation are Usually Benign and May be Managed Conservatively. *J. Urol.* **2008**, *180*, 261–265. [CrossRef] [PubMed]
44. Scandura, G.; Verrill, C.; Protheroe, A.; Joseph, J.; Ansell, W.; Sakhdev, A.; Shamash, J.; Berney, D.M. Incidentally detected testicular lesions <10 mm in diameter: Can orchidectomy be avoided? *BJU Int.* **2017**, *121*, 575–582. [CrossRef] [PubMed]
45. Luzurier, A.; Maxwell, F.; Correas, J.; Benoit, G.; Izard, V.; Ferlicot, S.; Teglas, J.; Bellin, M.; Rocher, L. Qualitative and quantitative contrast-enhanced ultrasonography for the characterisation of non-palpable testicular tumours. *Clin. Radiol.* **2018**, *73*, 322.e1–322.e9. [CrossRef] [PubMed]
46. Schröder, C.; Lock, G.; Schmidt, C.; Löning, T.; Dieckmann, K.-P. Real-Time Elastography and Contrast-Enhanced Ultrasonography in the Evaluation of Testicular Masses: A Comparative Prospective Study. *Ultrasound Med. Biol.* **2016**, *42*, 1807–1815. [CrossRef] [PubMed]
47. Aigner, F.; De Zordo, T.; Pallwein-Prettner, L.; Junker, D.; Schäfer, G.; Pichler, R.; Leonhartsberger, N.; Pinggera, G.; Dogra, V.S.; Frauscher, F. Real-time Sonoelastography for the Evaluation of Testicular Lesions. *Radiology* **2012**, *263*, 584–589. [CrossRef] [PubMed]
48. Goddi, A.; Sacchi, A.; Magistretti, G.; Almolla, J.; Salvadore, M. Real-time tissue elastography for testicular lesion assessment. *Eur. Radiol.* **2011**, *22*, 721–730. [CrossRef] [PubMed]
49. Pozza, C.; Gianfrilli, D.; Fattorini, G.; Giannetta, E.; Barbagallo, F.; Nicolai, E.; Cristini, C.; Di Pierro, G.B.; Franco, G.; Lenzi, A.; et al. Diagnostic value of qualitative and strain ratio elastography in the differential diagnosis of non-palpable testicular lesions. *Andrology* **2016**, *4*, 1193–1203. [CrossRef] [PubMed]
50. Grasso, M.; Blanco, S.; Raber, M.; Nespoli, L. Elasto-sonography of the testis: Preliminary experience. *Arch. Ital. Urol. Androl.* **2010**, *82*, 160–163.
51. Marsaud, A.; Durand, M.; Raffaelli, C.; Carpentier, X.; Rouscoff, Y.; Tibi, B.; Floc'h, A.; De Villeneuve, M.; Haider, R.; Ambrosetti, D.; et al. Apport de l'élastographie en temps réel pour la caractérisation des masses testiculaires. *Progres En Urol.* **2015**, *25*, 75–82. [CrossRef]
52. Ma, W.; Sarasohn, D.; Zheng, J.; Vargas, H.A.; Bach, A. Causes of Avascular Hypoechoic Testicular Lesions Detected at Scrotal Ultrasound: Can They Be Considered Benign? *Am. J. Roentgenol.* **2017**, *209*, 110–115. [CrossRef] [PubMed]
53. Patrikidou, A.; Cazzaniga, W.; Berney, D.; Boormans, J.; de Angst, I.; Di Nardo, D.; Fankhauser, C.; Fischer, S.; Gravina, C.; Gremmels, H.; et al. European Association of Urology Guidelines on Testicular Cancer: 2023 Update. *Eur. Urol.* **2023**, *84*, 289–301. [CrossRef] [PubMed]
54. Maxwell, F.; Savignac, A.; Bekdache, O.; Calvez, S.; Lebacle, C.; Arama, E.; Garrouche, N.; Rocher, L. Leydig Cell Tumors of the Testis: An Update of the Imaging Characteristics of a Not So Rare Lesion. *Cancers* **2022**, *14*, 3652. [CrossRef]

55. Nicolai, N.; Necchi, A.; Raggi, D.; Biasoni, D.; Catanzaro, M.; Piva, L.; Stagni, S.; Maffezzini, M.; Torelli, T.; Faré, E.; et al. Clinical Outcome in Testicular Sex Cord Stromal Tumors: Testis Sparing vs Radical Orchiectomy and Management of Advanced Disease. *Urology* **2015**, *85*, 402–406. [CrossRef] [PubMed]
56. Westlander, G.; Ekerhovd, E.; Granberg, S.; Hanson, L.; Hanson, C.; Bergh, C. Testicular ultrasonography and extended chromosome analysis in men with nonmosaic Klinefelter syndrome: A prospective study of possible predictive factors for successful sperm recovery. *Fertil. Steril.* **2001**, *75*, 1102–1105. [CrossRef] [PubMed]
57. Bozzini, G.; Ratti, D.; Carmignani, L. Treatment of Leydig cell tumors of the testis: Can testis-sparing surgery replace radical orchidectomy? Results of a systematic review. *Actas Urol Esp* **2017**, *41*, 146–154. [CrossRef] [PubMed]
58. Laclergerie, F.; Mouillet, G.; Frontczak, A.; Balssa, L.; Eschwege, P.; Saussine, C.; Larré, S.; Cormier, L.; Vuillemin, A.T.; Kleinclauss, F. Testicle-sparing surgery versus radical orchiectomy in the management of Leydig cell tumors: Results from a multicenter study. *World J. Urol.* **2017**, *36*, 427–433. [CrossRef] [PubMed]
59. Müller, T.; Gozzi, C.; Akkad, T.; Pallwein, L.; Bartsch, G.; Steiner, H. Management of incidental impalpable intratesticular masses of $\leq$ 5 mm in diameter. *BJU Int.* **2006**, *98*, 1001–1004. [CrossRef]

Disclaimer/Publisher's Note: The statements, opinions and data contained in all publications are solely those of the individual author(s) and contributor(s) and not of MDPI and/or the editor(s). MDPI and/or the editor(s) disclaim responsibility for any injury to people or property resulting from any ideas, methods, instructions or products referred to in the content.

MDPI AG
Grosspeteranlage 5
4052 Basel
Switzerland
Tel.: +41 61 683 77 34

Cancers Editorial Office
E-mail: cancers@mdpi.com
www.mdpi.com/journal/cancers

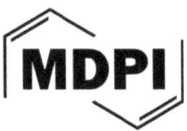

Disclaimer/Publisher's Note: The title and front matter of this reprint are at the discretion of the Guest Editor. The publisher is not responsible for their content or any associated concerns. The statements, opinions and data contained in all individual articles are solely those of the individual Editor and contributors and not of MDPI. MDPI disclaims responsibility for any injury to people or property resulting from any ideas, methods, instructions or products referred to in the content.

www.ingramcontent.com/pod-product-compliance
Lightning Source LLC
LaVergne TN
LVHW072329090526
838202LV00019B/2382